The Treatment of Knotty Diseases

—— with Chinese Acupuncture and Chinese Herbal Medicine

Compiled by   Shao Nian-fang
Translated by   Xiao Gong (MD, TCM Professor)
                   Zuo Lian-jun
Examined and
    Revised by   Xiao Gong

Shandong Science and Technology Press

First Edition 1990

Published by
  Shandong Science and Technology Press
    34 Yuhan Lu, Jinan, China
Printed by
  Weifang Xinhua Printing House
    99 Gongnong Lu, Weifang, China
Distributed by
  China International Book Trading Corporation
    21 Chegongzhuang Xilu, Beijing 100044, China
      P. O. Box 399, Beijing, China

Printed in the People's Republic of China

Forward

Through more than twenty years medical practice, the author has experienced a number of difficult diseases or syndromes which were already treated in many ways and in not a few modern hospitals of high rank without much effect, or even resisted to treatment thus forming really difficult and knotty problems. To those cases, according to the theory of traditional Chinese medicine (TCM) and its application, the principle of syndrome differentiation and treatment, a coordinated combination of herbal medicine, acupuncture and other treatment has been the adopted scheme, among them many has obtained prominent therapeutic effects, and not a few even reached the state of clinical cure. These clinical material has been included and sorted out in this book.

In this book, 58 kinds of diseases or syndromes included, and to each kind discussion goes on under four main headings, namely the brief introduction, the TCM syndrome differentiation and treatment, the case report and the personal experience. The brief introduction denotes the general conception in western medicine including a few words about its etiological and therapeutic progress, and it corresponds to the category of the syndromes in TCM. The syndrome differentiation and treatment part is the central core of each paragraph, under this the pathogenesis in brief is for the disease or syndrome as a whole and followed by division into types and to each type the key points of pathogenesis is for the special type of a disease or syndrome and then followed in order by chief manifestations, therapeutic principle, prescriptions and drugs, acupoints, with emphasis on the practical application to each disease. In case report one or two successful cases included for example, and the inferences can be drawn for other cases. The personal experience is an expression of author's special understanding, clinical experience, and the prevailing effective recipes and drugs, clinical therapy is the focal point of this book, as to theoretical consideration only dealt with simply and briefly by cutting out the superfluous meaning or words.

The distinguishing characteristics of this book are:

1. This is a writing about commonly met difficult and knotty diseases or syndromes in the general clinic.

2. With emphasis on TCM syndrome differentiation and treatment as a special feature.

3. The integration of various therapeutic methods of TCM such as ready made medicines, including the traditional *Gao* (soft extracts for oral intake, and adhesive plasters for external use), *Dan* (refined powders or granules), *Wan* (the large bolus and the small pills), *San* (powder, including decoction powder), and the up to date tablets, infusion granules, and injections. The decoction

recipes and modifications, acupuncture therapy and other therapeutic measures such as digital pressing and massage and others included.

4. The close correlation of theoretical consideration and practice, with special preference to clinical practice.

Besides, for the convenience of the reader, the nominations of diseases are in term of the western medicine.

Shao Nian-fang

CONTENTS

Knotty fever 1
Lupus erythematosis 17
Alopecia areata 24
Myasthenia gravis 28
Recurrent aphtha 34
Cerebral vascular accident 38
Coma 50
Brain atrophy 62
Dementia senilis 68
Rhythmic palatopharyngo laryngeal muscular
    clonus 74
Meniere's syndrome 80
Trigeminal neuralgia 85
Facial neuritis 91
Acute infectious polyneuritis 97
Epilepsy 106
Schizophrenia 111
Nervous tinnitus and deafness 121
Hydrocephalus after intracranial operation 127
Coronary atherosclerotic heart disease 133
Variant angina pectoris 145
Acute myocardial infarction 151
Shock 158
Congestive myocarditis 167
Gall bladder-heart syndrome 171

Viral myocarditis	175
Sick sinus syndrome	181
Cardiac arrhythmia	189
Migraine	201
Hyperlipoidemia	206
Respiratory and cardiac failure of pulmonary encephalopathy	212
Heart failure of chronic pulmonary heart disease	218
Lung abscess	225
Tuberculous pleuritis with effusion	231
Carcinoma of lung	240
Esophageal carcinoma and gastric carcinoma	247
Atrophic gastritis	259
Chronic nonspecific ulcerative colitis	264
Senile constipation	269
Cirrhosis of liver with ascites	273
Cholelithiasis	282
Nephrolithiasis	287
Hypertrophy of prostate gland	292
Nephrosis syndrome	299
Primary thrombocytopenic purpura	308
Leukopenia of unknown origin	314
Aplastic anemia	319
Epidemic hemorrhagic fever	326
Cervical spondylopathy	335
Brachial plexus neuritis	341
Chronic recurrent urticaria	346

Functional metrorrhagia ·····351
Habitual abortion ·····357
Myoma of uterus ·····363
Dysmenorrhea·····368
Impotence·····373
Climacteric syndrome ·····378
Senile hyperthyroidism ·····382
Postconcussional syndrome of the brain·····388
Index of Prescriptions ·····394

Knotty fever

Fever is a common symptom of many diseases. There are numerous causes and the pathological changes are rather complicated. The mental status, constitutional varieties of patients, their reactions to medicine, and the influences of environment all together alter the fundamental principles of fever and make its diagnosis a knotty problem. Thus in modern medicine innomination, a title of 'fever of unknown origin', 'fever its cause to be determined' usually given. In some cases with ascertained diagnosis, the treatment still remains unsettled, with the use of a lot of antibiotics, antipyretics, and other physical measures to keep down the temperature without evident effect. This kind of fever remains a knotty problem, so we called it 'knotty fever'. It is not unusual to find out in accordance with the principles of syndrome differentiation and treatment of TCM the satisfactory therapeutic effects.

I. TCM syndrome differentiation and treatment

Fever may be classified into exterior syndrome, exterior-interior syndrome, and interior syndrome.

Pathogenesis in brief: Exuberance of *yang* will be *shi* (sthenia), fever in that case is usually acute in onset. *Yin* deficiency will be *xu* (asthenia), fever in that case is usually of low-grade. The fever due to obstruction and stagnation of phlegm and blood will usually be lingering and resistant to treatment.

(I) Exterior syndrome

Key points of pathogenesis: The invasion of the *wei* superficial (*wei* is for protection) induces the disharmony of *ying* (inside the vessel) and *wei* (outside the vessel), it's due to cold or heat, syndrome differentiation will make out clear distinction.

1. Exterior cold syndrome

Chief manifestations: Severe aversion to cold, slight fever, anhidrosis, colla pain and stiffness, general aching, tongue coat thin and white, pulse floating and tense.

Therapeutic principle: To relieve exterior syndrome with pungent and warm diaphoretic drugs.

(1) Patent drug: *Jing Fang Bai Du San* 10g, take its infusion with boiling water, t.i.d.

(2) Decoction recipe: *Jing Fang Jie Du Tang* with modifications:

Schizonepeta 12g, Ledebouriella root 12g, Pueraria root 18g, Dahurian angelica root 10g, Notopterygium root 10g, Chinese green onion 30mm Fresh zingiberis 3 slices, Glycyrrhiza root 3g, for oral administration after being decocted in water, one dose a day.

Plus-minus (Addition or diminution of ingredients): With manifestations of dampness such as heaviness of limbs, epigastric oppressions and anorexia, agastache, eupatorium, atractylodes rhizome, poria should be added; with prominent general aching and anhidrosis, ephedra may be necessary.

(3) Acupoints: *Fengfu, Fengchi, Waiguan, Fengmen, Hegu, Taiyang, Yingxiang, Taiyuan* (all reducing in manipulation).

2. Exterior heat syndrome

Chief manifestations: Fever severe, chillness mild, headache, snuffy nose, cough, slight thirst, throat dry and sore, redness of tongue margins and tip, tongue coat thin, white or yellow, pulse floating and rapid.

Therapeutic principle: To relieve exterior syndrome with pungent and cold diaphoretic drugs.

(1) Patent drug:

①*Yin Qiao Jie Du Wan* one pill t.i.d.

②*Xi Ling Jie Du Pian* 12 tablets t.i.d.

③*Qiang Li Yin Qiao Pian* 8 tablets t.i.d.

(2) Decoction recipe: *Yin Qiao San* with modifications: Honeysuckle flower 30g, Forsythiae fruit 12g, Platycodon root 10g, Peppermint 10g, Bitter apricot seed(stir-fried) 10g, Schizonepeta 10g, Lophatherum 10g, Scutellaria root 12g, Licorice root 3g, for oral administration after being decocted in water, one dose a day.

Plus-minus: For high fever and sore throat add isatis root, subprostrate sophora root, gypsum, anemarrhena rhizome; for severe haedache add mulberry leaf, chrysanthemum flower; for severe cough, add loquat leaf, peucedanum root, thunberg fritillariae bulb, mulberry bark; in case complicated with summer heat and dampness with manifestations of epigastric fullness, nausea, dark urine, tongue coat slimmy, with addition of Elscholtzia, hyacinth bean flower, agastache, *Liu Yi San*; complicated with dryness, with the appearance of thirst, dry cough without sputum, add glehnia and ophiopogon root thunberg fritillariae bulb, trichosanthes root, peach rind; no remission of high fever, add *Zi Xue San*; in weak patient, add American ginseng.

(3) Acupoints: *Quchi, Waiguan, Hegu, Quze*(reducing method of manipulation). Exuberance of evil heat, add *Dazhui, Xiangu*(reducing method of manipulation); sorethroat, hoarseness of voice, add *Yuji, Shaoshang* (reducing method of manipulation).

(II) Exterior-interior syndrome

Key points of pathogenesis: Invasion of pathogenic evils into *Shaoyang*, location at half way exterior and half way interior, a reflection of struggle between the *zhen qi* (the genuine energen) and the pathogenic evils.

Chief manifestations: Alternations of seizures of chill and fever. Painful fullness of chest and hypochondrium, vexation, nausea, anorexia, bitter taste in mouth and dryness of pharynx, dizziness and blurred vision, tongue coat white and wet, pulse taut.

Therapeutic principle: To mediate the exterior and the interior.

1. Patent drug: *Xiao Yao Wan* 5g t.i.d. and *Long Dan Xie Gan Wan* 5g t.i.d.

2. Decoction recipe: *Xiao Chai Hu Tang*:

Bupleurum root 24g, Scutellaria root 15g, Pinellia tuber 10g, Ginseng 10g, Fresh ginger 3 slices, Ziziphi jujuba fruit 3 pieces, Licorice 3g, for oral administration after being decocted in water, one dose a day.

Plus-minus: In case of coldness in exterior and heat in interior, ginseng should be withdrawn and ephedra, gypsum, apricot kernel, houttuynia, mulberry bark added; for heat in exterior and interior, ginseng should be withdrawn and honeysuckle flower, forsythia fruit, capejasmine fruit, rhubarb may be added.

3. Acupoints: *Dazhui, Taodao, Jianshi, Houxi, Xiangu, Hegu* (all with reducing method of manipulation).

(III) Interior syndrome

〖Excess Syndrome〗

Key Points of pathogenesis: Invasion of pathogen evils into the interior at *qi, yin* or blood system or stage, exuberance of pathogens, and syndrome of excess, the disease state critical in most cases.

1. Exuberance of heat in *qi* system

Chief manifestations: High fever, thirst, sweating, painful swelling of gum, with erosion or bleeding, tongue proper red with yellow and dry coat, pulse full and large.

Therapeutic principle: To clear off the evil heat and promote saliva secretion.

(1) Patent drug: *Zi Xue San* 5g t.i.d. to be taken with boiled water.

(2) Decoction recipe: *Bai Hu Tang* with modifications:

5

Gypsum 60~120g, Anemarrhena rhizome 30g, Trichosanthes root 20g, Pseudostellaria root 30g, Bupleurum root 30g, Isatis root 45g, Honeysuckle flower 30g, Paris rhizome 20g, Licorice 6g, for oral administration after being decocted in water, one dose a day.

Plus-minus: Coma and delirium, constipation, rhubarb and mirabilite and grass-leaved sweetflag rhizome to be added; high fever and purpura, rhinoceros horn powder, scrophularia root, moutan bark; painful swelling of gum, coptis root and capejasmine fruit; pulmonary stasis with poisonous heat, cough and dyspnea with plenty sputum, reed rhizome, houttuynia, mulberry bark, and scutellaria root added.

(3)Acupoints: *Dazhi, Hegu Xiangu* (reducing technique). For Coma, add *Renzhong, Shixuan* (reducing technique).

2. Noxious heat invasion in *yin* system

Chief manifestations: High fever at night, dysphoria, insomnia, thirst without much drink. In severe cases, coma, delirium, skin rash vague in appearance, tongue proper red and dry. Pulse thin and rapid.

Therapeutic principle: To clean off the noxious heat in the *yin* system.

(1)Patent drug: *Zhi Bao Dan*, one bolus t.i.d. or *Zi Xue San*, dosage as mentioned before. These can be given by nasal tube or through rectum infusion.

(2)Decoction recipe: *Qing ying Tang* with modifications:

Rhinoceros horn powder 3g (to be swallowed with

boiled water) or Water buffalo horn 30g (to be decocted before hand), Rehmannia root 30g, Scrophularia root 30g, Ophiopogon root 30g, Coptis root 10g, Honey suckle flower 45g, Forsythia fruit 20g, Lophatherum 10g, Moutan bark 15g, for oral administration after being decocted in water, one dose a day.

Plus-minus: In case with high fever, grass-leaved sweetflag rhizome, curcuma root, and *Niu Huang Qing Xin Wan* given through nasal tube; with profuse secretion of salva and sputum, with further addition of bamboo juice, artificial bezoar powder.

(3)Acupoints: *Shixuan*(with bleeding),*Baihui*, *Dazhui*, *Quchi*, *Hegu* (All reducing technique). Phlegm stagnation with cloudiness of mind, *Laogong*, *Fenglong*, *Yanglingquan* (all reducing technique).

3. Noxious heat invasion of heart

Chief manifestations: High fever, coma, irritability and delirium, tongue proper deep red, tongue coat yellow and dry, pulse thin and rapid.

Therapeutic principle: To clean off cardiac heat and restore consciousness.

(1) Patent drug:

①*Qing Kai Ling* injection or *Xing Nao Jing* injection 15~30ml added to 5% glucose in distill water 500ml intravenous drippling, 1~2 times daily.

②*An Gong Niu Huang Wan* or *Zhi Bao Dan*, one bolus, two or three times a day, or by route of nasal feeding.

(2) Decoction recipe: *Qing Gong Tang* with modifica-

tions:

Rhinoceros horn powder 5g (to be swallowed with boiled water) or Buffalo horn 30g (to be decocted beforehand), Scrophularia root 30g, Ophiopogon root 30g, Lotus plumule 10g, Forsythia seed 10g, Lophatherum leaflet 10g, Grassleaved sweetflag rhizome 12g, Curcuma root 10g, Calcite 30g, to be decocted in water, for oral admimstration or by mean of nasal tube.

Plus-minus: In cases of mental confusion due to phlegm with development of coma, *Hou Zao San* 0.1g nasal spray; wind produced due to extreme heat with the development of convulsion, antelope's horn powder 5g to be given with drink water and uncaria stem with hooks; in cases with skin eruptions, hemoptysis, hematemesis, epistaxis due to blood heat, gypsum, anemarrhena rhizome, capejasmine fruit, moutan bark may be added.

(3)Acupoints: *Shixuan, Shierjing* (puncture to bleed), *Baihui, Yintang, Dazhui, Quchi, Hegu* (all reducing tech nigue). Mental confusion due to phlegm, *Laogong, Fenglong, Yanglingquan* (all reducing technique); for convulsion *Xingjian, Siguan, Yanglingquan* (all reducing technique); excess of blood, toxic heat, *Quze, Weizhong* (puncture to bleed).

4. Damp heat of liver and biliary tract

Chief manifestations: Fever, thirst, bitter taste of mouth, hypochondriac pain, epigastric fullness and abdominal distention, nausea, vomiting, scanty dark urine.

Tongue proper red, yellow and slimmy tongue coat, pulse taut, slippery and rapid.

Therapeutic principle: To clean off the damp heat of liver and biliary tract.

(1) Patent drug: *Long Dan Xie Gan Wan* 10g t.i.d.

(2) Decoction recipe: *Hao Qin Qing Dan Tang* with modifications:

Sweet wormwood 24g, Scutellaria root 15g, Tangerine peel 10g, Bamboo shavings 6g, Pinellia tuber 12g, Curcuma root 12g, Red poria 15g; Bitter orange 10g, Coptis root 6g, *Bi Yu San* 10g, for oral administration after being decocted in water, one dose a day.

Plus-minus: Exuberance of damp heat with jaundice, add oriental wormwood and capejasmine fruit; with dark urine and constipation rhubarb should be used.

(3) Acupoints: *Taichong, Qimeng, Riyue, Danshu, Yanglingquan, Jianli, Ganshu* (all reducing technique).

5. Damp heat of urinary bladder

Chief manifestations: Fever, frequent urination, dysuria with difficult and painful passage such as drippling and urgency, lumbar pain, tongue proper red, tongue coat yellow and slimmy, pulse slippery and rapid.

Therapeutic principle: To clear off the damp heat in the lower burner.

(1) Patent drug: *Long Dan Xie Gan Wan* 10g t.i.d. to be taken with congongrass rhizome 30g decocted infusion.

(2) Decoction recipe: *Ba Zheng San* With modificatcons:

9

Common knotgrass 15g, Chinese pink herb 20g, Plantain herb 30g, *Mutong* (Sichuang clematis stem or Manshurian aristolochia stem) 10g, Capejasmine fruit 10g, Talc 24g, Motherwort 30g, Honey-suckle flower 30g, Rush pith 3g, Rhubarb 6g, Licorice 6g, for oral administration after being decocted in water, one dose a day.

Plus-minus: For dark urine, plus small thistle, cogongrass rhizome; for turbid urination, plus yam and pyrrosia leaf.

(3) Acupoints: *Shenshu, Pangguangshu, Zhongji, Yinlingquan, Shuifen* (all reducing technique).

【Deficiency syndrome】

Key points of pathogenesis: The decline of the pathogenic evil, the deficiency of both *qi* and *yin*, the disharmony of *zang* and *fu*, low grade fever.

1. Fever with *qi* deficiency

Chief manifestations: Fever higher after fatigue, accompanied with dizziness, malaise, shortness of breath, aversion to talk, spontaneous sweating, easy to catch cold, anorexia and loose stool. Tongue proper light in color, tongue coat thin and white. Pulse thin and weak.

Therapeutic principle: To strengthen the spleen and to replenish the *qi*, to allay the fever with drugs of sweet and warm in nature.

(1) Patent drug: *Bu Zhong Yi Qi Wan*, one bolus t.i.d.

(2) Decoction recipe: *Bu Zhong Yi Qi Tang* with

modifications:

Astragalus root 15g, Dangshen 15g, White atractylodes rhizome 12g, Chinese angelica root 12g, Tangerine peel 12g, Cimicifuga rhizome 10g, Bupleurum root 15g, Immature bitter orange (stir-fried) 10g, Licorice 3g, for oral administration after being decocted in water, one dose a day.

Plus-minus: To arrest much spontaneous sweating, oyster shell powder, floating wheat added, chillness and fever, sweating with aversion to wind, cinnamon twig, white peony root should be added; fever, chillness with cold limbs, pallor of face, pulse deep fine and weak, pertains to *yang* deficiency, *Jin Gui Shen Qi Wan*, one bolus, t.i.d.

(3)Acupoints: *Feishu, Pishu, Zusanli, Guanyuan, Qihai* (moxibustion in all cases).

2. Fever due to *yin* deficiency

Chief manifestations: Fever in the afternoon or at night, hotness over palms and soles, hectic or tidal fever, vexation, insomnia, flush of cheeks, night sweat, dryness of mouth and pharynx, dark urine and constipation. Tongue proper red with scanty coat, pulse thin and rapid.

Therapeutic principle: To nourish the *yin* and to clear the evil heat.

(1) Patent drug: *Zhi Bai Di Huang Wan*, one bolus t.i.d.

(2) Decoction recipe: *Qing Gu San* with modifications: Stellaria root 18g, Wolfberry bark 15g, Picrorhiza rhizome 12g, Anemarrhena 12g, Sweet wormwood 12g, Large-leaf gentian root 12g, Turtle shell 24g, Wild jujuba seed 24g, Licorice 3g for oral administration after being decocted in water, one dose a day.

Plus-minus: Severe *yin* deficiency, rehmannia root scrophularia root, prepared fleeceflower root; accompanied with *qi* deficiency, malaise, pseudostellaria root, glehnia root, ophiopogon root added; with flare up of wind, wriggling (squirming) of hands and feet, turtle shell, white poeny, oyster shell, rehmannia to be added.

(3) Acupoints: *Shenshu, Taixi, Ganshu, Xinshu* (all reinforcing technique), *Xingjian, Daling* (all reducing technique).

II. Case reports

Case 1: Ms. Sun, 54 years old, cadre, first visit on January 25, 1988. In the past she had rheumatoid arthritis, postsequale of wind-stroke, pulmonary heart disease, she was confined to bed for three years. Recently she caught cold and thus had fever, cough with sputum, dyspnea. A diagnosis of chronic bronchitis complicated with acute infection was made and penicillin, streptomycin, gentamicin, erythromycin, already used for more than ten days with some drop of temperature. Now she still had fever (body temperature 39.4°C), cough with scanty sticky sputum, some dyspnea, malaise, anorexia, mouth dry, vexation and listlessness. Tongue proper deep red, without coat. pulse thin rapid without strength. Blood WBC 16,500, neutrophil 85% lymphocyte 15%. Fluorescopy of chest, chronic bronchitis complicated with acute infection.

TCM syndrome differentiation and treatment: Prostrated fever with damage of *qi* and *yin*. The therapeutic principle is to replenish the *qi* and *yin*, to clear off the heat and to resolve the phlegm.

Recipe: American ginseng 12g, Glehnia root 30g, Ophiopogon root 24g, Stellaria root 24g, Wolfberry bark 24g, Mulberry bark 15g, Thunberg fritillaria bulb 12g, Sweet wormwood 18g, Peel of mongolian snakegourd 15g, Honeysuckle flower 30g, Houttuynia 24g, Licorice 3g, to be decocted with water oral intake, with simultaneous take of *An Gong Niu Huang Wan* 1 bolus each time.

Therapeutic effect: After three days medication of above prescription, fever subsided and mind clear. Body temperature 36.5°C, still had some cough, blood WBC 8,500, continuous use of the above prescription with some modification for a few days to strengthen the therapeutic results.

Case 2: Liu, male, 6 months old, brought to our clinic first on August 3, 1972. The infant had a fever of 38.2°C on the third day after birth, sneezing, vomiting and diarrhea, restlessness, and cry. On the 13th day with the appearance of drowsiness and easily frightened, a diagnosis of septicaemia made in a hospital, and he was admitted to the hospital on March 15,1972. During hospitalization, kanamycin, erythromycin, penicillin, hydrocortisone and other drugs were given. He was discharged on March 31,1972 after three days' normal temperature. But he had to be readmitted on April 16 on account of high fever up to 39°C. With further addition of tetracycline, chloromycin, pentamicin, and transfusion of whole blood and plasma several times, the temperature remained high, blood culture showed staphylococcus albus, and he was discharged on his family's request. On the second day he was brought to our hospital, the child was restless and cry with sweating all over the body, vomiting of milk, diarrhea, flush of face, finger venules dark purple. Tongue tip red, tongue coat white and slimmy.

TCM syndrome differentiation and treatment: His mother had three abortions previous to his birth, and had frequent attacks of fever during this pregnancy. The infant was rather thin after delivery. This accounted for congenital deficiency, the toxic heat invaded the channels and collaterals, and the prolonged course made further depletion of essence, thus *yin* deficiency and exuberance of toxic heat and knotty fever resulted. The therapeutic principle should be to replenish the essence, to clear off the toxic heat and activate the channels.

Recipe: Glehnia root 5g, Ophiopogon root 6g, Sweet wormwood 6g, Wolfberry bark 5g, Swallowort root 5g, Lotus seed 10g, Bamboo shaving 6g, Lotus leaf half sheet, Luffa 6g, Honeysuckle flower 6g, Cereal sprout 10g, to be decocted with water, one dose a day.

The second visit on August 9: Sneezing stopped, fever lower, no vomiting after medication, night sleep not sound. In the afternoon, spiritless, much urination. Tongue and finger venule the same as last visit.

Recipe: Rehmannia 6g, Glehnia root 5g, Sweet wormwood 5g, Lotus seed 6g, Cereal sprout 10g, Catechu 2g, Wolfberry bark 6g, Hyacinth bean pod 12g, Luffy 5g, Bamboo shaving 5g, Lotus leaf half sheet, Arctium fruit 1g, to be decocted with water, one dose daily.

The third visit on August 22: After medication no fever at day time, after midnight, still feverish, fever subsided in the morning, mild cough, some red rash over skin, spirit better. Tongue coat thin and white, Finger venules light red in colour.

Recipe: Glehnia root 6g, Lotus seed 10g, Bamboo shaving 10g, Wolfberry bark 3g, Sweet wormwood 5g, Honeysuckle flower 10g, Thunberg fritillarian bulb 5g, Arctium fruit 1g, *Tianzhuhuang* 3g, Swallowwort root 5g, to be decocted with water, one dose a day.

The fourth visit on August 27: After medication, no fever, spirit and feeding recovered. The sleep still not sound. Milk curds in stool, urine appears normal. Tongue coat and finger venules same as last visit.

Recipe: The same prescription as last visit with further addition of cereal sprout 10g, one prescription dose a day.

The fifth visit on November 16: The petechiae all

over the body become itching, restlessness, loose stool. Tongue coat white, finger venule light red in color.

Recipe: Glehnia root 6g, Lotus seed 10g, Phaseolus seed 10g, Arctium fruit 1g, Bamboo shaving 10g, Rice sprout 12g, Cicada slough 3g, Honeysuckle vine 6g, Hyacinth bean flower 6g, Forsythia fruit 5g, to be decocted with water, one prescription dose a day.

The sixth visit on January 5, 1973: After medication all symptoms disappeared. Spirit and appetite good, stool slight loose. Tongue coat white, index finger venules light red.

Recipe: Glehnia root 3g, Lotus seed 5g, Cicada slough 3g, Arctium fruit 3g, Honeysuckle vine 6g, to be decocted with water, one prescription dose every other day, continuous medication for one month to fortify the therapeutic effects.

Follow up visit 6 months later, infant appeared healthy.

II. Personal experience

The pathogenesis of fever varies and is complicated especially after the use of numerous antibiotics. In such cases, we have to grasp firmly the principles of TCM syndrome differential diagnosis and treatment, in cases of *qi* deficiency to replenish the vital energy; to replenish the *yin*, while the essence is deficient, and to warm up the *yang* in cases of *yang* asthenia, while encountering cases of high fever with leucocytosis, not to think only of clearing away heat and detoxification.

Many patent Chinese herb drugs in treating fever are in the form of bolus or tablets, it's better to crash and melt it before use, or to make infusion with boiled water. In order to obtain satisfactory result large dosages have to be given, in some cases as much as 5 times the usual dosage, given in the remarks of patent drugs.

As to knotted fever, we have to differentiate the various etiological factors, external affections or internal damage, the nature of fever, the types of fever, the pathogenesis of fever, etc. In all, with more complete understanding of these mentioned above and fully conscious of the treatment that should be directed to acertain definite aim, the therapeutic effect may be more satisfactory.

Lupus erythematosis

Lupus erythematosis is a kind of connective tissue disease. Its chief clinical manifestations are typical skin lesions, fresh red colored macular patches with sticky scales, mostly found over the nasal and cheek region, may be fused into butterfly shaped, and other regions such as frontal and mandibular region, car margins, limbs and trunk may be affected. The accompanied systemic symptoms are fever, arthralgia, and heart, kidney, liver and other visceral organs may be simultaneously involved. In traditional Chinese medicine it belongs to the category of 'red butterfly', 'sun-exposure' or 'cat eye' skin disease or '*xu lao*' (consumptive disease).

I. TCM syndrome differentiation and treatment

Pathogenesis in brief: Bi syndrome due to wind, toxic and heat pathogen, prolonged stay in *yin* and blood system with exhaustion of *qi* and *yin* and involvement of heart and kidney and other viscera.

(I) Exuberance of heat and toxic pathogen

Key points of pathogenesis: Wind, toxic and heat pathogen invasion of *yin* and blood system, with adverse flow of blood and, impeded function of joints.

Chief manifestations: High fever, red macules over face and other parts of the body, general aching of the joints, vexation, insomnia, thirsty, like to drink cold, malaise, in a trance or absent minded, even delirium and coma. Tongue proper deep red, tongue coat yellow and slimmy. Pulse slippery and rapid.

Therapeutic principle: To clear away heat and toxic material, to cool the blood and remove the obstruction in the collaterals and make them patent.

1. Patent drug:

(1) *Xi Ling Jie Du Pian* 10~20 tablets, t.i.d.

(2) *Niu Huang Qing Xin Wan*, one bolus, t.i.d.

2. Decoction recipe: *Qing Wen Bai Du Yin* with modifications:

Rehmannia root 30g, Red peony root 15g, Moutan bark 12g, Buffalo horn 30g, Stellaria root 30g, Gypsum 30g, Anemarrhena rhizome 12g, Honeysuckle flower 30g,

Globethistle root 15g, Black tailed snake 12g, Scorpion 12g, Licorice 6g, for oral administration after being decocted in water, one dose a day.

Plus-minus: Exuberance of heat and toxic material plus scutellaria, coptis root, rhubarb; coma and oonvulsion add uncaria stem with hooks, hawksbill shell, and antelope horn powder; with external pathogen, plus pueraria root, schizonepeta.

3. Acupoints: *Quchi, Waiguan, Hegu, Dazhi, Xiangu* (all reducing technique). Excess heat and unconsciousness add *Shixuan, Weizhong* (all puncture to bleed).

(II) *Qi* and *yin* deficiency on account of heat

Key points of pathogenesis: Prolonged action of heat and toxic material with the result of exhaustion of *qi* and *Yin*.

Chief manifestations: Low grade fever of long standing, dysphoria with feverish sensation in chest, palms and soles; general malaise, spontaneous perspiration or night sweat, chest oppression and shortness of breath, spiritless, red patches over face, arthralgia, palpitation, hair falling. Tongue coat thin and white. Pulse thin, rapid and without strength.

Therapeutic principle: To replenish *qi* and nourish the *yin* and associated with heat clearing.

1. Patent drug: *Bu Zhong Yi Qi Wan* and *Zhi Bai Di Huang Wan*, one bolus, t.i.d.

2. Decoction recipe: *Qin Jiao Bie Jia San* and *Bao Yuan Tang* with modifications:

Astragalus root 30g, Ginseng 10g, Large-leaf gentian root 10g, Turtle shell 20g, Wolfberry fruit 15g, Glehnia root 15g, Ophiopogon root 20g, Licorice 6g, Mulberry twigs 24g, for oral administration after being decocted in water, one dose a day.

Plus-minus: The involvement of cardiac spirit plus fragrant solomonseal rhizome, lotus seed; toxic heat in excess plus honeysuckle flower, coptis root; joint pain add black tailed snake, scorpion; functional disorder of spleen add coix seed, cereal sprout (stir-fried).

3. Acupoints: *Feishu*, *Pishu*, *Shenshu*, *Sanyinjiao* (all reinforcing technique), *Guanyuan* (moxibustion), *Chize*, *Xingjian Dazhui* (all reducing technique).

(III) *Yin* deficiency of liver and spleen

Key points of pathogenesis: Retained toxic heat and exhaustion of kidney essence, and the depletion of nutrition of liver, and the heart fire devoid of control.

Chief manifestations: Red butterfly shaped patches over face, aching pain of loin and knee, burning pain or causalgia of both hypochondria, persistant low grade fever, listless, ulceration in buccal mucosa or tongue, dysphoria with feverish sensation in chest, palms and soles, dizziness, insomnia, abdominal distension and anorexia. Tongue proper red with ecchymosis. Pulse deep, thin and rapid.

Therapeutic principle: To replenish the kidney and liver essence, to clear the heat and dissolve blood stagnation.

1. Patent drug: *Liu Wei Di Huang Wan*, one bolus, t.i.d.

2. Decoction recipe: *Zhi Bai Di Huang Tang* with modifications:

Anemarrhena rhizome 10g, Phellodendron bark 10g, Rehmannia root 24g, Eclipta 15g, Lucid ligustrum 15g, Moutan bark 12g, Dogwood fruit 15g, Red sage root 15g, Red and white poeny root each 10g, Coptis root 10g, Black tailed snake 12g, Coix seed 30g, for oral administration after being decocted in water, one dose a day.

Plus-minus: Arthralgia plus siegesbeckia, *tougucao* (speranskia tuberculata); in case with *qi* deficiency, add astragalus root, white atractylodes rhizome, ledebouriella root; with *yang* deficiency add epimedium, morinda root; with abdominal distension and hypochondriac pain add bupleurum, bitter orange, tangerine peel.

3. Acupoints: *Shenshu, Ganshu, Sanyinjiao, Taixi* (all reinforcing technique), *Chize, Xingjian* (both reducing technique), With associated *qi* deficiency plus *Guanyuan* (Moxibustion); in associated arthralgia add *Quchi, Yanglingquan* (both reducing technique); with abdominal distension add *Zusanli, Neiting* (both reducing technique).

II. Case report

Miss Lui, 21 years old, worker, came to the clinic on June 18, 1972. Complained of fever, red rash over face for more than 20 days, she had received treatment in a hospital, with lupus cell found in blood, prednisone given without improvement, she still had temperature 39.5°C on admission, and red macular rash over face, joint pain, general discomfort, dysphoria in the afternoon, thirsty, like to drink cold, malaise, urination short and dark colored, slightly constipated. Tongue proper red, tongue coat thin and yellow. Pulse thin and rapid. It belonged to deficiency of *qi* and *yin*, with toxic heat stagnation in skin and joints, the therapeutic principle was to replenish *qi* and *yin*, to clear away heat and toxic material.

Recipe: Astragalus root 45g, Pseudostellaria root 30g, Rehmannia root 24g, Phellodendron bark 12g, Eclipta 15g, Coptis root 10g, Red sage root 15g, Stellaria root 21g, Moutan bark 12g, Siegesbeckia herb 15g, Coix seed 30g, Black tailed snake 12g, Licorice 6g, for oral administration after being decocted in water.

The second visit on June 25: After the above six doses fever lower 38.3°C, aching discomfort over joints. Stool normal, urine still yellow, mouth and throat dry. Tongue proper red, tongue coat thin and yellow, pulse thin and rapid.

The above same recipe with the reduction of coptis

root, with the addition of 15g wolfberry bark, 21g spatholobus stem, 20g honeysuckle flower decoction as before.

The third visit on August 24: Another five herb doses. When 15 doses taken, complete stoppage of prednisone. All symptoms disappeared. Body temperature was 36.8°C. General malaise, impaired appetite, tongue proper light red, tongue coat thin and white, pulse sluggish and weak.

Bu Zhong Yi Qi Wan 5g t.i.d. and *Xiang Sha Liu Jun Zi Wan* 5g t.i.d. taken after meal. Continuous in-take of above drugs for two months to reinforce the therapeutic results.

Follow up after 7 years, she married and gave birth two sons, quite healthy.

III. Personal experience

At the beginning, the disease is characterized with exuberance of toxic heat, followed by exhausion of fluid and the appearance of *yin* deficiency, thus the therapeutic principle is to clear away heat and toxic material, to replenish the kidney and nourish the *yin*. Yet it's important not to neglect the aspect of *qi* deficiency. With the proverb 'Where the pathogen accumulates, there must be deficiency of vital energy'. 'The fierce fire will impede the vital energy' in mind, thus drugs for replenishing the vital energy usually adopted, such as astragalus root, ginseng, pseudo-stellaria root, American ginseng are added.

Alopecia areata

Alopecia areata is a kind of functional disease, its causes are still not well known. The chief clinical manifestation is patchy falling of hairs without sign of inflammation. Eyebrows and beard or whisker hair may also fall in patches. In severe cases, the hair fall may be so complete that it extends to the entire head—the bald head or the whole body. This belongs to the category of '*you feng* (oily wind)' or '*gui ti tou* (ghosty hair cut)' in TCM.

I. TCM syndrome differentiation and treatment

Pathogenesis in brief: The malnutrition of skin due to heart and kidney deficiency and the asthenia of yin and blood. The invasion of exogenous wind and the dryness resulted thereby renders the fall of hair just like to be shaved.

Chief manifestations: Hair falls in patches, even the eyebrows, associated with dizziness, tinnitus, insomnia, plenty of dreams, dysphoria with hotness in the chest, palms, and soles, palpitation and forget-fulness. Tongue proper red and dry. Pulse thin and rapid.

Therapeutic principle: To replenish the kidney and nourish the heart, to promote blood circulation and expel the wind.

1. Pre-made preparations:

(1) Drynaria rhizome 30g, Dittany bark 30g, Biota tops 30g, Chinese angelica root 30g, the above drugs soaked in 500ml white wine with frequent agitations or sway. Half month later, after filtration, to the filtrate add 2g Camphor. Apply to the bald area two or three times a day.

(2) Fleece flower root 60g, Chinese angelica root 45g, Tribulus fruit 30g, Chuanxiong rhizome 45g, the above drugs made into coarse powder immersed in 1000ml white wine for half a month, 15ml t.i.d. p.c. After medication rub the affected site with hands.

2. Decoction recipe: *Shen Ying Yang Zhen Dan* with modifications:

Fleece flower root (prepared) 15g, Eclipta 15g, Rhemmania (raw and prepared) each 10g, Asparagus and ophiopogon root each 12g, Chinese angelica root 12g, Red and white poeny root each 10g, Dodder seed 15g, Chuanxiong rhizome 12g, Tribulous fruit 12g, Dittany bark 12g, Pueraria root 15g, Schizonepeta 10g, Gastrodia tuber 10g, for oral administration after being decocted in water, or to make water pills as follows.

Five times the above dosage to be made into fine powder, with addition of water to make pills the size of parasol seed, each time 15g, with white wine 15ml, twice a day.

Plus-minus: Dysphoria and insomnia plus fleece flower vine, aroborvita seed, capejasmine fruit; *yin* deficiency with internal heat, plus moutan bark, wolfberry bark, honeysuckle flower.

3. Acupoints:*Shenshu, Ganshu, Pishu, Xinshu* (all reinforcing technique), *Fengchi, Fengfu, Waiguan* (all reducing technique).

Besides, light tapping on affected area with plum-blossom needle once daily.

II. Case report

Mr. Yang 35 years old, cadre, came to our clinic on June 6, 1975. With patchy fall of hair for 3 months. Since last year on account of heavy burden of learning he often had dizziness and tinnitus, insomnia and plenty of dreams, dysphoria, palpitation and amnesia. In recent three months most of his hair fall in patches, even eyebrow also involved. Tongue proper red, tongue coat thin and white. Pulse taut, thready and rapid. This pertains to deficiency of *yin* and blood, and with wind formation. The therapeutic principle is to nourish the *yin* and blood, and get rid of the wind.

Recipe: Prepared fleece flower root 15g, Herba eclipta 12g, Rehmannia 15g, Ophiopogon root and asparagas root each 10g, Chinese angelica root 12g, Chuanxiong rhizome 12g, Wild jujube seed (stir-fried) 15g, Fleece flower stem 24g, Pueraria root 15g, Tribulus fruit 12g, Schizonepeta 12g, for oral administration after being decocted in water. In the same time light tap on affected area with plum-blossom needle once daily.

The second visit on July 8: After 30 doses, sleep sound, dizziness and tinnitus disappeared. There were yellow thready hair grew out on the alopecia area, and other symptoms also improved. Tongue proper light red, tongue coat thin and white. Pulse thready.

Recipe: In the above prescription with schizonepeta removed and with the addition of Lucid ligustrum 12g, Scrofularia root 12g. Astragalous root 15g, Safflower 10g, for oral administration after being decocted in water, one dose a day. Continued the light tap with plum-blossom needle.

The third visit on September 10: Another 30 recipe dosages taken. The symptoms disappeared almost completely. The hair grew out, only not so black and shinny as his original, eyebrows also grew out. Tongue proper light red, tongue coat thin and white, pulse moderate and forceful.

The treatment consisted of pills prepared as follows: 5 times the above recipe formula dosage, made up refined powder and flooded with water, the pill thus made the size of Chinese parasol seed, each dose 10g, three times a day to strengthen the therapeutic results.

Follow up 6 months later, after the course of pill therapy, the hair black and shinny, even better than his original before illness.

III. Personal experience

Besides medication mentioned above. Topical application of medicated alcohol in combination with light tap with plum blossom needle also had good therapeutic effect. In light cases no medication needed and spontaneous recovery may ensue.

Myasthenia gravis

Myasthenia gravis is a comparatively commonly met chronic disease of neuromuscular transmission disturbance, its etiology and pathogenesis are still not entirely known, its main manifestation is characterized by easy fatigue of affected striated muscles, and relieved after rest. Its clinical manifestations are ptosis of eyelids, chewing and swallowing difficulty, flaccidity of muscles of limbs. In severe cases, it may cause death. It belongs to the 'wei syndrome (flaccidity syndrome)' in TCM.

I. TCM syndrome differentiation and treatment

Pathogenesis in brief: Weak constitution on account of chronic illness, the visceral vital energy is injured, the vital energy and blood, the essence and fluid of liver, kidney, spleen, lung are all affected. Spleen loses its chief responsibility to muscles, kidneys its chief responsibility to bones, and thus the symptoms of this disease.

(I) The damp heat of spleen and lung, the impaired circulation of *qi* and blood

Key points of pathogenesis: The loss of pulmonary fluid due to heat, and the embarrassment of spleen due to dampness, Without removal of the damp heat, the impairment of vital energy and blood circulation will bring about invasion of skin, muscles, and tendons.

Chief manifestations: At onset fever usually present. After fever the occurrence of flaccidity of four limbs, lassitude, ptosis of eyelids, exaggerated in the afternoon, there may be cough, yellow sputum, dryness of mouth and throat, or epigastric oppression and impaired appetite, urination short and dark. Tongue proper red, tongue coat yellow and slimmy. pulse thready and rapid.

Therapeutic Principle: To clear away heat and dampness, to moisten the tendon and channels.

1. Patent drug: *Long Dan Xie Gan Wan* 6g, t.i.d. *Yang Yin Qing Fei Wan*, one bolus, t.i.d.

2. Decoction recipe: *Er Miao San* with modifications: Atractylodes rhizome 12g, Phellodendron bark 10g, Scutellaria root 10g, Hypoglouca yam 12g, Tetrandra root 12g, Coix seed 30g, White poeny root 15g, Chaenomeles fruit 15g, Glehnia root 15g, Silkworm excrement 20g, for oral administration after being decocted in water, one dose a day.

Plus-minus: Heat damage of pulmonary *yin* with cough and yellow sputum, minus atractylodes rhizome, plus gypsum, ophiopogon root, mongolian snakegourd, thunberg fritillaria bulb; in cases of exuberance of dampness with epigastric oppression and anorexia, add magnolia bark.

3. Acupoints: *Jianyu, Quchi, Hegu, Shousanli, Lieque, Zusanli, Jiexi, Yanglingquan, Huantiao* (with exuberance of evil pathogen the reducing technique selected, with decline of evil pathogen, reinforcing technique selected).

(II) Deficiency of spleen and kidney, malnutrition of muscles and bones

Key points of pathogenesis: Sustained disease, enfeebles the spleen and kidney. Kidney and spleen deficiencies influence their support to bones and muscles. Malnutrition of bones and muscles results flaccidity and weakness of limbs.

Chief manifestations: Limbs flaccid, loin and spinal column aching and weak, easily fatigued. There may be impaired appetite and loose stool, loss of facial brilliance; or blurred vision and falling of hair, dryness of phargnx and tinnitus, even inability to walk, atrophic changes of muscles gradually occur. Tongue proper light red, with white coat. Pulse thready and weak.

Therapeutic principle: To replenish spleen and kidney, to strengthen the tendons and bones.

1. Patent drug:

(1) *Bu Zhong Yi Qi Wan* and *Fu Zi Li Zhong Wan*, each time one bolus, t.i.d. (indicated for *yang* deficiency of spleen and kidney).

(2) *Hu Qian Wan*, one bolus t.i.d. *Long Ma Zi Lai Dan* one bolus daily, with gradual increase of dosage in case without effect, up to the state of mild intoxication (indicated for *yin* deficiency of spleen and kidney).

(3) *Jin Suo Gu Jing Wan* and *Ren Shen Jian Pi Wan*, each time one bolus t.i.d.

2. Decoction recipe: *Bu Zhong Yi Qi Tang* with modifications:

Ginseng 12g, White atractylodes 12g, Astragalus root 60g, Prepared fleece flower root 15g, Wolfberry fruit 15g, Prepared aconite 15g, Cimicifuga rhizome 12g, Bupleurum root 12g, Pueraria root 30g, Chinese angelica root 15g, Ephedra (stir-fried with honey) 10g, Licorice (stir-fried with honey) 6g, to be decocted in water, the fluid obtained divided into three portions taken in a day.

Plus-minus: With inclination to kidney *yang* asthenia plus cinnamon bark, pilose deer horn, indian mulberry root; with inclination to kidney *yin* deficiency such as throat dryness, tinnitus, blurred vision and hair falling, *Hu Qian Wan* may be added.

3. Acupoints: *Shenshu, Pishu, Ganshu, Xinshu* may be added (all using reinforcing technique).

II. Case report

Mr. Tan, 19 years old, student. He came to our clinic on April 25, 1972, with chief complaint of flaccidity and weakness of four limbs for 25 days. The onset of the present illness gave a history of common cold and fever. After the subsidence of fever, he felt gradual increase of flaccidity and weakness of four limbs, better in the morning, and worse in the afternoon. He was diagnosed myasthenia gravis in a hospital, and treated with prostigmin and ambestigmin without improvement: The four limbs all flaccid and weak, he could not hold with hands, and could not walk. At supper, he could not chew on account of without strength, and the food intake small in quantity. On examination loss of facial brilliance, general malaise. Tongue proper light red, coat thin and white. Pulse deep thready and weak.

TCM syndrome differentiation and treatment: It pertains to asthenia of *zhongqi*, devoid of lifting power. The principle of treatment should be to reinforce *qi* and replenish the spleen, to recover the power of ascending and lifting.

Recipe: Pilose asiabell root 20g, Astragalus root 45g, White atractylodes 20g, Pueraria root 24g, Licorice (stir fried with honey) 6g, Immature bitter orange (stir fried) 10g, Chinese angelica root 15g, to be decocted in water, one dose a day.

The second visit on May 10: After 14 days, the gradual increase of strength of limbs and the increase in amount of food intake were prominent, he was capable to walk more than 10 meters far, he only complained of prominent lumbar aching and weakness of legs. The tongue and pulse findings the same as the previous visit.

Recipe: The above prescription with further addition of 15g wolfberry fruit, 15g prepared fleece flower root, 12g prepared aconite root, and 15g of achyranthes root, to be decocted with water, one recipe dose daily.

The third visit was on June 11. The above prescription one dose daily for 30 doses. The symptoms almost disappeared, only when the duration of activity was somewhat long, some feeling of lumbar aching, and leg weakness. The appetite, the defecation and urination were all normal: Tongue proper light red, tongue coat thin and white. Pulse deep and moderate.

Recipe: *Ren Shen Jian Pi Wan*, *Jin Gui Shen Qi Wan*, each time one bolus twice a day, to strengthen the curative effect.

Follow up after 2 years, the recovery was complete.

III. Personal experience

Myasthenia gravis is a complicated disease, the deficiency of *qi* and *yang* of spleen and kidney pertains to the commonly met type. And thus *Bu Zhong Yi Qi Tang*, *Fu Zi Li Zhong Tang* are commonly used prescriptions. In cases using the former, besides the dosage of astragalous root should be big, it should be noticed that the addition of pueraria root and immature bitter orange should be emphasized. Especially the use of immature bitter orange as using corrigent to increase the therapeutic effect. In cases using *Fu Zi Li Zhong Tang*, the amount of aconite should be emphasized. Prepared aconite root 30~60g may be used. It's important to decoct it beforehand for more than two hours, and after medication wine and hot water bath are contraindicated.

Recurrent aphtha

Recurrent aphtha is most frequently met in diseases of buccal mucous membrane. At onset, there may be blisters, usually light yellow in color, rapidly ruptured with formation of round or oval ulcers, single or multiple in number, inducing causalgic pain without foul odor, there may be associated with mild fever. Apparent cure and easy recurrence are the feature. It pertains to '*kou gan*' (referred to aphtha in children), '*kou chuang*' (the aphtha or wound in mouth) in TCM.

I. TCM syndrome differentiation and treatment

Pathogenesis in brief: The exuberance of heart evil fire goes upward along the channels to mouth, with result of *yin* damage and a lingering course.

(I) Flare up of cardiac evil fire

Key points of pathogenesis: The exuberance of heart fire goes upward to the mouth, with canker formation usually at the apex of tongue.

Chief manifestations: Recurred episode of buccal ulcerations, redness, swelling, hotness and pain mostly at the tongue apex usually accompanied by dryness of mouth and pharynx, dysphoria, easy to lose temper. Dark urination and constipation. Tongue apex red, tongue fur thin and yellow. Pulse slippery and rapid.

Therapeutic principle: To clear the heat and purge the fire.

1. Patent drug:

(1) *Niu Huang Shang Qing Wan*, one bolus t.i.d. and *Xi Lei San* a little applied to the lesion, twice a day.

(2) *Niu Huang Jie Du Pian*, 5 tablets t.i.d. Topical application with *Xi Lei San* the same as above.

2. Decoction recipe: *Dao Chi San* with additional ingredients:

Coptis root 10g, Rehmannia root 30g, Lophatherum 10g, Moutan bark 12g, Ophiopogon root 20g, Akebia stem 6g, Licorice 3g, for oral administration after being decocted in water, one dose a day.

Plus-minus: Heat in excess, plus honeysuckle flower, forsythia fruit, isatis leaf; yin deficiency due to exuberance of fire, add anemarrhena rhizome, scrophularia root; upward aversion of damp heat, add cabin pachouli, capejasmine fruit and gypsum.

3. Acupoints: *Ganshu, Danshu, Taichong, Xingjian,*

Laogong (all reducing technique).

(II) Yin deficiency and exuberance of fire

Key points of pathogenesis: Exuberance of fire leads to deficiency of *yin*, and the up burst of asthenic fire results aptha formation in mouth and over tongue, with pain more severe in the afternoon.

Chief manifestations: Recurrent episodes of buccal ulcerations is easily induced after fatigue, pain more severe in the afternoon, accompanied by dysphoria, insomnia, hotness over palms and soles. Tongue proper red. Pulse thready and rapid.

Therapeutic principle: Nourishing *yin* to reduce the pathogenic fire.

1. Patent drug: *Zhi Bai Di Huang Wan*, one bolus t.i.d.

2. Decoction recipe: *Liu Wei Di Huang Wan* and *Zi Shen Wan* with modifications:

Rehmannia root 24g, Scrophularia root 15g, Dogwood fruit 10g, Moutan bark 12g, Alismatis rhizome 21g, Poria 12g, Capejasmine fruit 10g, Anemarrhena 12g, Phellodendron 10g, Cinnamon bark 3g, for oral administration after being decocted in water, one dose a day.

Plus-minus: *Yin* deficiency prominent with tidal fever and night sweat, plus prepared rehmannia, tortoise plastron; in cases of the perverse excess of heart evil fire add coptis root; moreover with additional damp heat add atractylodes rhizome, cyathula root.

(3) Acupoints: *Xinshu, Shenshu, Taixi, Sanyinjiao* (all reinforcing technique), *Laogong* (reducing technique).

II. Case report

Mr. shu, 40 years of age, cadre, came to clinic on March 7, 1972, with chief complaint of recurrent buccal ulcerations for 3 years. More than ten buccal ulcers found over mucous membrane of oral cavity and surface of tongue, the bigger one as the size of yellow bean, the smaller one the size of pin head, light red in color. Pain severe in the afternoon and night accompanied with dysphoria with hotness in the chest, palms and soles, insomnia, plenty of dreams, palpitation and listlessness, easy to get angry, stool slight dry. Short and dark urination. Tongue proper red with a little coat. Pulse thready and rapid. VitB$_2$ and oryzanol had been used. This pertains to *yin* deficiency and exuberance of evil fire, the up burst of asthenic fire. The principle of treatment should be to nourish the *yin* and to reduce the pathogenic fire.

Recipe: Rehmannia root 24g, Ophiopogon fruit 24g, Scrophularia root 15g, Dogwood fruit 10g, Moutan bark 12g, Poria 12g, Capejasmine fruit 10g, Anemarrhena rhizome 10g, Phellodendron 10g, Cinnamon bark 3g, Lotus seed 3g, Licorice 3g, to be decocted in water, one dose a day. Topical application of *Xi Lei San* three times a day.

After six days, all the symptoms disappeared. He was

told to continue intake of *Zhi Bai Di Huang Wan* one bolus b.i.d. continued for one month to strengthen the therapeutic effect. Follow up one year later, no recurrence.

III. Personal experience

The excess syndrome of this disease usually presents repeated episodes and has lingering course. Yin deficiency and exess of pathogenic fire or with damp heat are often obstinate to treatment. The simultanuous use of topical medication, acupuncture and moxibustion may help.

Regular living order, sufficient sleeping hour, the abstention of acrid, wine and tobacco smoking, and stimulating food, good sentiments, to avoid anger, as the stagnation of *qi* may induce production of pathogenic fire and the later as an inducing factor of aphtha formation.

Cerebral vascular accident

Cerebral vascular accident, or apoplexy is a common cerebral vascular disease mainly due to hypertension, cerebaral arterioscleresis, and others. In accordance with the variant nature of the lesion, the disease may be classified into two eatagories, the haemorrhagic and the ischemic cerebral vascular disease. The clinical features of this disease are sudden onset, rapid development, with sudden fall and loss of consciousness, accompanied by deviation of mouth, hemiplegia, epigastric fulness and distension, constipation. In mild cases, there may be only hemianesthesia, hemiplegia, wry mouth with distorted eyes, slurred speech or dysphasia. It pertains to the category of windstroke in TCM.

Once the disease ensues, the mortality rate and the disability rate are high, thus vigorous measures should be adopted.

I. TCM syndrome differentiation and treatment

Pathogenesis in brief: The sthenic incidental and the asthenic fundamental. The incidental excess pertains to wind, fire, phlegm and heat. The fundamental deficiency pertains to deficiency of *qi*, blood, *yin* and *yang*.

(I) Windstroke of channel and collateral

1. The invasion of wind and phlegm into collaterals

Key points of pathogenesis: hepatic wind and phlegm getting into the channel and collateral.

Chief manifestations: Wry mouth with distorted eye, tongue stiffness and slurred speech, hemianesthesia salivation from angle of mouth. In severe cases there may be contrature pain. Tongue coat white and glimmy. Pulse taut and slippery.

Therapeutic principle: To arrest wind and resolve sputum. To stimulate the sensitive orifices and make the channels and collaterals patent.

(1) Patent drug: *Zhi Mi Fu Ling Wan*, 10g t.i.d.

(2) Decoction recipe: *Qian Zheng San* and *Dao Tan Tang* with modifications:

Stirfried batryticated silkworm 12g, White mustard seed 12g, Dried scorpion powder 6g (to be taken with fluid), Pinellia tuber 12g, Arisaema tuber 10g, Gastrodia tuber 12g, Uncaria stem with hooks 24g, Grassleaved sweetflag rhizome 10g, Curcuma root 12g, Polygala root (stirfried) 10g, for oral administration after being decocted in water, one dose a day.

Plus-minus: Liver wind from interior, plus seaear shell, oyster shell; the contracture pain of affected side, add white poeny bark 20g, siegesbeckia herb 20g.

(3) Acupoints: *Fengchi, Jianyu, Quchi, Hegu, Huantiao, Yanglingquan, Juegu, Fenglong, Lianquan, Yamen, Jiache, Dicang* (all with reducing technique).

2. Qi deficiency and blood stagnation

Key points of pathogenesis: Impaired transportation due to *qi* deficiency, and collateral blockage due to stagnated blood.

Chief manifestations: Tongue stiffness and speech slurred, spiritless and malaise, hemiplegia, hemianesthesia, palpitation. Tongue proper dark red, coat white, pulse thready and uneven.

Therapeutic principle: To replenish *qi* and to promote blood circulation, and remove channel obstruction.

(1) Patent drug: *Bu Zhong Yi Qi Wan*, one bolus t.i.d. and *Fu Fang Dan Shen Pian* 5 tablets t.i.d.

(2) Decoction recipe: *Bu Yang Huan Wu Tang* with modifications:

Astragalus root 120g, Tail of Chinese angelica root 10g, *Chuanxiong* rhizome 6g, Peach kernel 6g, Carthami flower 6g, Red poeny root 10g, Earthworm 10g, Spatholobus stem 30g, for oral administration after being decocted in water, one dose a day.

Plus-minus: Blood stasis severe, plus stir-fried cockroach, parched pangolin scales; when *qi* asthenia prominent, plus pilose asiabell root, white atractylodes rhizome, minus earthworm.

(3) Acupoints: *Guanyuan, Qihai Zusanli* (all reinforcing technique). Other points selected the same as the type of windstroke of channel and collateral devoid of *Fengchi*(using reinforcing and reducing balanced technique).

3. *Yin* deficiency of liver and kidney

Key points of pathogenesis: Deficiency of blood and essence, malnutrition of muscles.

Chief manifestations: Hemiatrophy of muscles, hemiplegia, hemianesthesia, flaccid tongue and aphonia, accompanied with dizziness, tinnitus, lumbar aching and flaccidity of legs, muscular twitching of hands and feet. Tongue proper red, pulse thready.

Therapeutic principle: To reinforce kidney and liver, to nourish muscles.

(1) Patent drug: *Qi Ju Di Huang Wan*, one bolus t.i.d.

(2) Decoction recipe: *Di Huang Yin Zi* with

modifications:

Rehmannia 18g, Prepared fleece flower root 24g, Chinese angelica root 12g, Epimedium 12g, Dogwood fruit 10g, Lucid ligustrum fruit 12g, Wolfberry fruit 15g, Achyranthes root 18g, Stir-fried mulberry twig 20g, for oral administration after being decocted in water, one dose a day.

Plus-minus: Stirring up of interior asthenic wind, plus uncaria stem with hooks, clam shell; deficiency of heart *yin* in cases of palpitation and dysphoria, add ophiopogon root, dendrobium, capejasmin fruit; in cases with the perversion towards deficiency of kidney *yang* such as chilliness, cold limbs, incontinence of urine, add prepared aconite root, morinda root.

(3) Acupoints: *Taixi, Shenshu, Guanyuan* (all reinforcing technique), *Jianyu, Quchi, Shousanli, Hegu, Huantiao, Fengshi, Zusanli, Jiexi* (all even reinforcing and reducing technique). Wry mouth with distorted eyes add *Jiache, Dicang, Hegu, Taichong* (even reinforcing and reducing technique). Tongue stiffness and slurred speech, add *Yamen* (shallow puncture), *Lianquan, Zusanli* (all reinforcing technique) *Tongli, Guanchong, Fenglong* (all reducing technique).

(II) Apoplectiform attack on *yang* visceral organs

Key points of pathogenesis: Six *yang* visceral organs attacked and *fuqi* blocked.

Chief manifestations: Besides the symptoms involving the attack of channels and collaterals, epigastric distension and fullness, constipation, foul breathing, anorexia, tongue coat yellow thick and slimmy, pulse slippery and rapid.

Therapeutic principle: To purge the bowels and clear away heat, to resolve phlegm and make sensitive orifices patent.

1. Patent drug: *Niu Huang Qing Xin Wan*, one bolus t.i.d. and *Da Huang Pian*, four tablets three times a day.

2. Decoction recipe: *San Hua Tang* with modifications:

Prepared Rhubarb 10g, Stir-fried immature bitter orange 12g, Fruit and pericarp of mongolian snakegourd 30g, Grass-leaved sweetflag rhizome 12g, Notopterygium root 6g, for oral administration after being decocted in water, one dose a day.

Plus-minus: After medication still no defecation, rhubarb add to 12g, and further addition of 6g mirabilite (to be taken with water). Phlegm-heat in excess, plus bile prepared arisaema tuber, red poeny root, radish seed. Yin deficiency and tongue dry plus scrophularia root, anemarrhena rhizome.

3. Acupoints: *Dadun, Hegu, Fenglong, Neiting, Tianshu, Daheng, Fengfu* (all reducing technique).

(III) Apoplectiform attack on *yin* visceral organs

Key points of pathogenesis: Internal block with pathogen, and *yang* collapse manifested. Clinically there are tight syndrome (excess syndrome of stroke) and collapse syndrome.

1. Tight syndrome

Key points of pathogenesis: Blockage with pathogens in exces, and the impaired sensitivity of the nine sensitive orifices.

Chief manifestations: Sudden fall and loss of consciousnes, lockjaw or trismus, clenched fists, without urination and defecation, cramp of limbs or body. In clinical practice, further division into tight syndrome of *yang* and tight syndrome of *yin*.

(1) Tight syndrome of *yang*

Key points of pathogenesis: Blockage of clean orifices with pathogens of wind, fire, phlegm and heat.

Chief manifestations: Besides those mentioned above with flush of face, body hot, noisy and foul breathing, dysphoria. Tongue coat yellow and slimmy. Pulse taut and slippery.

Therapeutic principle: To clear liver and quench the wind. To recover consciousness with purgent and cold drugs.

① Patent drug: *Zhi Bao Dan*, one bolus or *An Gong Niu Huang Wan*, one bolus. Or *Qing Kai Ling* injection 40~60ml in 10% glucose solution 250~500ml intravenous drip, once daily.

② Decoction recipe: Modified *Ling Yang Jiao Tang*: Antelope's horn powder 2g (taken after mixing it with water), Uncaria stem with hooks 20g, Chrysanthemum flower 15g, Prunella spike 12g, Scutellaria root 12g,

Sea-ear shell 30g(to be previously decocted), Hematite 15g (to be previously decocted), Tortoise plastron 15g, White poeny root 12g, *Tianzhuhuang* 10g, Moutan bark 15g, Rehmannia root 20g, Grass-leaved sweetflag rhizome 10g, for oral administration after being decocted in water, either by nasal feeding or by route of rectal drip.

In cases with muscular twitching or cramp add scorpion or centipede powder each dose 3g; with plenty sputum, add bamboo shaving, bile treated arisaema tuber; with hiccough, add bamboo shaving, pinellia tuber.

③ Acupoints: *Shoushierjing, Renzhong, Baihui Daling, Laogong, Fengchi, Fengfu, Jiache, Quchi, Yanglingquan, Fenglong* (all reducing technique).

(2) Tight syndrome of *yin* nature

Key points of pathogenesis: Blockage of clean orifices in the interior with wind dampness or phlegm.

Chief manifestations: Besides the general manifestations of tight syndrome, the presence of pale facial appearance, darkness of lips, lying silently. Without vexation, but with exuberance of phlegm and salivation. Tongue coat white slimmy. Pulse deep slippery and relaxed.

Therapeutic principle: To remove phlegm and arrest the wind with pungent and warm orifice stimulants.

① Patent drug: *Su He Xiang Wan*, one bolus fed by mouth or by nasal tube or intrarectal drip.

② Decoction recipe: *Di Tan Tang* with modifications:

Prepared arisaema tuber 12g, Pinellia tuber 12g, Tangerine peel and pericarpium 12g, Poria 15g, Gastrodia tuber 12g, Uncaria stem with hooks 30g, Earthworm 10g, Stir-fried immature bitter orange 10 g, Grass leaved sweetflag rhizoma 10g, to be decocted in water fed by mouth, or through nasal tube, or rectal drip.

③ Acupoints: *Shoushierjing, Renzhong, Baihui, Yongquan, Lieque, Zusanli, Fenglong, Jiache, Hegu* (all reducing technique).

2. Collapse syndrome

Key points of pathogenesis: Collape of vital energy and mental confusion.

Chief manifestations: Sudden fall with loss of consciousness, with eyes closed, mouth open, snoring sound weak, respirations feeble, fist open, limbs cold, profuse sweating, incontinence of urine and stool. Flaccid paralysis of limbs. Flaccidity of tongue. Pulse feeble and thready with impending stoppage.

Therapeutic principle: To reinforce the *qi* and recuperate the extremely depleted *yang*, to rescue the exhausted *yin* from collape.

(1) Patent drug: *Shen Fu* injection 20ml added to 50% glucose solution 40ml intravenous drip. Or in alteration with *Shen Mai Zhen* twice daily.

(2) Decoction recipe: *Shen Fu Tang* and *Sheng Mai San* with modifications:

Red ginseng 20g, Prepared aconite root 15g, Ophiopogon root 30g, Schisandra fruit 10g, to be decocted in water and taken by mouth or through nasal tube.

Spontaneous sweating add astragalus root, dragon's bone and oyster shell.

(3) Acupoints: *Shenque, Guanyuan, Qihai, Zusanli* (all using moxibustion with big mox cones till the stoppage of sweating and the recuperation of pulse), *Yongquan, Sanyinjiao, Zhongwan, Mingmen* (acupuncture with reinforcing technique).

Ⅱ. **Case report**

Mr. Zhang, 63 years old, worker, hospital No.41571. This patient was admitted to hospital on March 20,1987 with complaints of right hemiplegia and slurred speech for 6 days. 6 days prior to admission while riding bicycle he suddenly found the loss of function of right limb. Accompanied with slurred speech, headache, vomiting He was treated with drugs to lower the intracranial pressure for three days. When his ill condition stabilized, he came to our hospital. The manifestations of present illness were right hemiplegia, deviation of mouth and tongue, slurred speech, epigastric fulness and distension, constipated. Foul breathing, anorexia. Tongue proper red, tongue coat slight yellow, thick slimmy. Pulse taut.

Examination on admission: T: 37.8℃, P: 72/min, R 20/min, B. P. right upper limb 155/100 mmHg, left upper limb, 165/105, mmHg.

A senile male, mentally clear, right hemiplegia, left pupil smaller than right, renchong groove deviated to left, right nasolabial groove shallow. Tongue deviated to right, right upper limb muscle strength grade 0, right lower limb muscle strength grade 1. Heart sound low, regular rhythm. In both sides of lungs full of rhonchi. Liver and spleen not palpable. Physiological reflexes Right bicep tricep and brachioradialis reflexes all diminished, patellar and Achillis tendon reflexes hyperactive. Babinski sign positive. Laboratory examination CT hemorrhage of internal capsule, external capsule of left thalamus, rupture into left ventricule, size of hematoma $3 \times 2\,cm^2$. Plasma β-lipoprotein 560 mg.

Diagnosis: TCM: windstroke (stroke of *yang* viscera)

Modern medicine: Cerebral hemorrhage bronchopneumonia

TCM syndrome differentiation: Upburst of wind and fire. Internal blockage with phlegm and heat and blocked *qi* of *yang* viscera.

Course of treatment: Modified *San Hua Tang*: Rhubarb 9g (put in and decocted late), Fruit and pericarp of mongolian snakegourd 15g, Cockroach 9g, Bile treated arisaema tuber 9g, Grassleaved sweetflag rhizome 9g, Curcuma root 12g, Pueraria root 30g, White peony root 30g, Red sage root 30g, decocted with water, and divided into two portions, oral intake. After nine doses of daily recipe, the tongue coat become thin, the tongue proper red, mouth dry and like to drink, general malaise, pulse thready rapid and weak. Left upper limb B.P. 150/95 mmHg. The integration of pulse and symptoms, gave the impression of deficiencies of both *qi* and *yin*. The therapeutic principle altered to reinforce *qi*, replenish *yin* and remove the blockage of collaterals. The daily recipe consisted of the following drugs, i.e. Astragalus root 30 g, Scrophularia root 15 g, Ophiopogon root 30 g, Glehnia root 21g, Red peony root 12 g, Chinese angelica root 12 g, Safflower 9 g, Cockroach 9 g, Spatholobus stem 30 g, Prepared fleeceflower root 21 g, Wolfberry fruit 12 g, Club mass 15 g, to be decocted with water. After thirty doses, patient's muscular strength recovered evidently the right upper and lower limb both attain 4th grade. Speech clear. Blood β-lipoprotein dropped to 250mg. Left upper limb B.P. 150/90 mmHg. Pathological reflexes disappeared. Discharged on clinical cure state.

II. Personal experience

(I) Windstroke may be divided into three phases, wind stroke attacking the channel and collateral with manifestation of hemianethesia, wry mouth and distorted eyes, slurred speech. The *yang* viscera (*fu*) phase with further addition of epigastric fulness, constipation, and hemiplegia. At the *yin* viscera (*zang*) phase, with the presence of mental confusion or coma.

(I) At the phase or stage attacking only the channel and collateral, the disease superficially located and being mild. Development toward the *zang fu* stage means increase in severity, development from *zang fu* stage toward *jingluo* stage tends to recovery.

(II) The stages or phases may be overlapped, and may be transferred from one to another stage. Once the stage or phase altered, the corresponding change of its treatment accordingly.

(IV) The tight and collapse syndrome are critical, the former being excess in incidental status, the later deficiency in fundamental status. The tranference from tight to collape syndrome means increase in severity. The full and complete consideration of excess and deficiency during treatment is extremely important.

(V) In comatous patient (stroke of *yin* viscera) avoid unnessesary shift, especially the head, let the patient lie on side. The sputum and saliva should be sucked out on time. In case with lock-jaw, rub teeth with borneol and arisaema tuber may loosen the jaw.

Coma

A state of loss of consciousness is called coma. Coma is most frequently met in many diseases, such as cerebro-vascular disease, traumatic brain injury, cerebral and meningeal infections and general infections, metabolic disorder, various intoxications, epilepsy, and others in severe critical condition. In TCM *'shen hun'*, *'hun meng'*, *'hun jue'*, *'zhan hun'* are synonyms of coma. This may occur in epidemic infectious disease, windstroke, syncope, epilepsy, phlegm syndrome, diabetes mellitus and asthmatic seizures in severe critical stage. This usually has an acute onset, and rapid changes, and rather complicated course and types. With correct diagnosis and differentiation, suitable management, the critical condition can be tide over in most cases.

I. TCM syndrome differentiation and treatment

Pathogenesis in brief: Either of pestilence the interior invasion of toxic pathogen, or other pathogens tends to invade the upper part of body to cause mental cloudiness or confusion with blockage of clean orifices and the impairment of mentality.

(I) Pericardium invasion with noxious heat

Key points of pathogenesis: Invasion of toxious heat to the interior, perversive transmission to the pericardium, and the impaired mental activities lead to the blockage of clean orifices.

Chief manifestations: Impaired consciousness and delirium, high fever, burning hotness of the palpation hand, eruptions of the body, epistaxis, hematochezia, convulsion, opisthotonus. Tongue proper deep red, tongue coat yellow with scanty salivation. Pulse thready and rapid.

Therapeutic principle: To clear away heat and remove intoxication, to stimulate the sensitive orifices and recover consciousness (to cause resuscitation).

1. Patent drugs:

(1) *An Gong Niu Huang Wan* or *Zhi Bao Dan*, one bolus t.i.d. or q.i.d. to pour into mouth, or nasal feed or intra-rectal drip.

(2) *Xing Nao Jing* injection 10~20ml dissolve in isotonic glucose solution 500ml intravenous drip, 1~2 time daily.

2. Decoction recipe: Modified *Qing Gong Tang*:
Rehmannia 30g, Moutan bark 15g, The central portion of scrophularia root 20g, Hindu lotus plumule 10g, Bamboo leaf 3g, Ophiopogon root (without removal of center) 30g, Honeysuckle flower 30g, Grass-leaved sweetflag rhizome 12g, Curcuma root 10g, Isatis leaf 30g, Reed rhizome 45g, Rhinoceros horn powder 1.5g, for oral administration after being decocted in water, 1~2 doses a day.

Plus-minus: Convulsion or opisthotonus add antelope's horn, uncaria stem with hooks, sea-ear shell carthworm, batryticated silkworm, scorpion, or with additional use of *Zi Xue San*. In case of constipation add rhubarb, immature bitter orange, mirabilite.

3. Acupoints: *Shaoshang, Hegu, Yongquan, Quchi Dazhui, Kunlun, Renzhong, Suliao* (all reducing technique).

(Ⅰ) Mental confusion due to phlegm

key points of pathogenesis: Long standing asthma, the mislaid cleaning and descending pulmonary function, the stagnation and obstruction of phlegm, and the shading of cardiac orifices.

Chief manifestations: Dementia, sometimes mind clear and sometimes cloudy, cough and dyspnea, the exuberation of phlegm and salivation, low grade fever. Tongue coat thick and slimmy. Pulse slippery and rapid.

Therapeutic principle: To dispel phlegm and render the orifices sensitive. To clear away heat and to arouse the mind.

1. Patent drug: *Chang Pu Yu Jin* injection 10~20ml infusion fluid in 10% glucose solution 250 ml intravenous drip once daily.

2. Decoction recipe: *Chang Pu Yu Jin Tang* with modifications:

Grass leaved sweetflag rhizome 10g, Ginger treated pinellia tuber 10g, Poria 12g, Tangerine peel 10g, Stir-fried capejasmine fruit 10g, Perilla fruit 12g, White mustard seed 10g, Bamboo juice 30g (to be added to the decoction fluid), Licorice 3g, to be decocted with water, the decoction fluid given by mouth, or through nasal feeding or intrarectal drip.

Plus-minus: In cases with high fever, plus paris rhizome, rhinoceros horn powder; in severe comatous patient, add *Su He Xiang Wan* or *Yu Shu Dan*, each time one pill, three times a day. The way to administer the same as above.

3. Acupoints: *Hegu, Yongquan, Zhongwan, Fenglong, Laogong, Zhongchong* (all reducing technique).

(Ⅲ) The accumulation of constipated excreta in *fu*-organs

Key points of pathogenesis: Accumulated excreta in large intestine, with mislaid transportation, noxious heat exuberated in the interior, with upward disturbance of mentality.

Chief manifestations: Coma and delirium, vexation and irritability, abdominal fulness and constipation, late afternoon tidal fever, tongue proper deep red, tongue coat yellow and dry, with prickles on the tongue. Pulse deep and sthenic with force.

Therapeutic principle: To purge off the internal heat, to restore consciousness with stimulants.

1. Patent drug: *Zi Xue San* 3g two or three times a day, to be administered orally or through nasal tube, or by intra-rectal drip.

2. Decoction recipe: *Da Cheng Qi Tang* with additional ingredients:

Rhubarb 12g, Mirabilite 10g (dissolved in water and add to the decoction fluid), Stirfried immature bitter orange 15g, Magnolia bark 10g, Gypsum 30g, Anemarrhena 15g, Licorice 6g, to be decocted and the method to be used the same as above.

3. Acupoints: *Shierjing Dadun, Hegu, Zusanli* (all

with reducing technique).

(Ⅳ) Collateral obstruction of stagnation and heat

Key points of pathogenesis: The invasion of pestilence virulence to the interior, the exuberance of noxious fire in *qi* and *ying* phases, the collateral obstruction of stagnated blood, and the obliteration of cardiac orifices.

Chief manifestations: Cloudiness of mind and mania, fever high at night, the fulness and pain of lower abdomen, purpura over the body, cyanosis of lips and nails, dark urination and constipation. Tongue proper dark red or cyanotic. Pulse deep and replete.

Therapeutic principle: To clear off heat and remove stagnation, to recover consciousness with stimulants.

1. Patent drug: *Shen Xi Dan*, each dose 3 g, two or three times a day, dissolved in water and administered by pouring into mouth, nasal feed, or through intra-rectal drip.

2. Decoction recipe: *Xi Jiao Di Huang Tang* with modifications:

Rhinoceros horn powder 6g, Rehmannia root 30g, Moutan bark 15g, Red peony root 15g, Peach kernel 10g, Safflower 10g, Amber powder 3g (taken after pouring hot water into it) Grass leaved sweetflag rhizome 12g, Curcuma root 12g, to be decocted with water and given as mentioned above.

Plus-minus: In cases of constipation, plus rhubarb and mirabilite; prominent blood stagnation, add compound mixture of red sage root injection 10~20ml, added to 5% glucose solution 500 ml, intravenous drip once daily.

3. Acupoints: *Shierjing, Baihui, Yongquan* (puncture to bleed), *Xuehai, Hegu, Quchi* (all reducing technique).

(V) Sudden extension of liver *yang*

Key points of pathogenesis: The deficiency of hepatic and renal *yin*, up burst of liver *yang*, and with wind production. The movement of phlegm due to wind, and the shading of upper orifices.

Chief manifestations: Sudden fall into unconsciousness, hemiplegia, rattling of phlegm in the throat, vexation, biting of teeth and clench of fists, fever and flush of face. Tongue coat yellow and dry. Pulse taut slippery and rapid.

Therapeutic principle: To tranquilize the liver and allay the wind. To subdue the *yang* and restore consciousness.

1. Patent drug: *Qing Kai Ling* injection 20~40 ml added to 10% glucose solution 250 ml intravenous drip.

2. Decoction recipe: *Ling Jiao Gou Teng Tang* with modifications:

Antelope's horn powder 3g (to be taken alone with fluid), Uncaria stem with hooks 30g (to be put in late during decoction), Tortoise plastron 30g, White poeny root 15g, Rehmannia 30g, Moutan bark 15g, Prunella spike 12g, Sea-ear shell 30g, Chrysanthemum flower 12g, Mulberry leaf 10g, to be decocted with water, and given by mouth or through nasal tubes or intrarectal drip.

Plus-minus: With exuberant phlegma and salivation, minus tortoise plastron and white poeny root, add pinellia tuber, tangerine peel, poria, stir-fried immature bitter orange and bile treated arisaema tuber; in case with high fever, add *Zhi Bao Dan.*

3. Acupoints: *Baihui, Hegu, Yongquan, Ganshu, Taichong, Xingjian, Yanglingquan* (all with reducing technique).

(Ⅵ) The upward invasion of heat and dampness

Key points of pathogenesis: The sinking of noxious heat to interior, accumulated in liver and gallbladder, the smoking and steaming of damp heat, the up disturbance of mind.

Chief manifestations: Coma and delirium, or with seizure of loss of consciousness interrupted with awakenness, yellowish skin bright as orange, nausea and tends to vomiting. Rashes over the body, epistaxis, abdominal distension typanic as drum. Fever high at night. Dark urination and constipation. Tongue proper dark red, tongue coat yellow and slimmy. Pulse taut rapid.

Therapeutic principle: To clear heat and remove dampness, to restor consciousness with stimulants.

1. Patent drug:

(1) *Shen Xi Dan*, 3g three or four times a day. Or *Xing*

Nao Jing injection 20 ml added to 10% glucose solution 500 ml intravenous drip, twice a day.

(2) *Da Huang* injection 4~5 ml each time intramuscular injection, or add to 10% glucose 500 ml intravenous or intrarectal drip.

2. Decoction recipe: *Yin Chen Hao Tang* with modifications:

Oriental wormwood 30g, Capejasmine fruit 10g, Rhemmania root 30g, Water buffalo horn 15g (ground into coarse powder), Bupleurum root 15g, Scrophularia root 30g, Moutan bark 12g, Grass leaved sweetflag rhizome 12g, Curcuma root 12g, Lophatherum 10g, to be decocted with water, given by mouth with soupful pour, or by nasal feed, or by intrarectal drip.

Plus-minus: In cases with dark yellow colored jaundice, no fever but with chilliness, minus rehmmania, scrophularia, waterbuffalo horn, lophatherum, plus prepared aconite root, dried ginger, coix seed; in case with constipation, add stirfried immature bitter orange, magnolia bark; for the occurrence of epistaxis, add imperata rhizome, rubia root, lotus node, agrimony.

3. Acupoints: *Shierjing, Shuigou, Yongquan, Ganshu* (all with reducing technique), *Pishu, Zusanli* (uniform reinforcing and reducing technique).

Ⅱ. Case report

Mis. Qi, 68 years old, first visit on Oct. 9, 1986,

with sudden fall and loss of consciousness for 9 hours. At 4 O'clock this morning while getting up from bed, she had a sudden fall and loss of consciousness, wry mouth with distorted eye, right hemiplegia, accompanied by vomiting, snoring, incontinence of urine and stool, facial flush, foul breathing, abundant sputum and salivation, pulse taut and slippery.

On examination: T 37.3℃; P 80 times/min; R 24/min; B.P. 180/110 mmHg. Comatous, with disappearance of supraorbital reflexes, pupils of equal size, reflexes to light sluggish, right eyeball gazed fixedly to the right temporal side. Right nasolabial groove shallow, angle of mouth deviated to the left, tongue unable to protrude out. Neck slight resistent, heart rhythm regular, heart rate 80/min, without murmur. Rhonchi in both sides of lungs, with no rales. Right upper and lower limb, muscle strength 0 grade with much lowered muscular tension. Hoffmann sign (−), Babinski sign of both sides (+). CT examination: Left cerebellar hematoma 2×2.5 cm size, cerebral atrophy. Electrocardiographic examination showed left axis deviation, coronary arterial deficiency,

Diagnosis: TCM: apoplexy (*yin* viscera attack). Western medicine: Essential hypertension, cerebral hemorrhage, coronary arterial insufficiency.

TCM syndrome differentiation and treatment: *Yin*

deficiency with fire exuberance, endogenous formation of phlegm, with up-burst of phlegmnous fire and the retarded function of clean orifices. The therapeutic principle is to clear heat and resolve phlegm, to extinguish the wind and stimulate orifices. The emergent use of *An Gong Niu Huang Wan* one bolus melted by nasal feed. 20% mannital 250 ml intravenous drip, three times a day, for consecutive three days.

Recipe: Rehmmnia root 30g, Moutan bark 15g. Uncaria stem with hooks 30g (put in late after other drugs), Chrysanthemum flower 12g, Mulberry leaf 12g, Grass-leaved sweetflag rhizome 12g, Curcuma root 9g, Bile treated arisaema tuber 10g, Rhubarb 10g, Antelope's horn powder 3g (to be swallowed with fluid), Red sage root 12g, for oral administration after being decocted in water, one dose a day.

Oct. 10, 1986, the patient mentally clear, speech distinct, right upper and lower limb movement improved. The diappearance of foul breathing and phlegm upsurge. Tongue proper red, with light yellowish thick slimmy coating. Pulse taut and fine. B. P. 140/80 mmHg. Right upper muscle strength grade Ⅱ°, right lower muscle strength grade Ⅲ°, neck resistent, Babincki's sign positive on both sides.

To treat the fundamental when the critical condition tided over, to nourish the *yin* and extinguish the wind, to clear off the heat and resolve phlegm.

Recipe: Scrofularia root 30 g, White peony root 20 g, Tortoise plastrone 20 g, Sea-ear shell 30 g, Uncaria stem with hooks 30 g (to be put in after other drugs during decoction), Grass-leaved sweetflag rhizome 12g, Prepared polygala root 10 g, Bile treated arisaema tuber 10 g, Antelope's horn powder 3 g (to be swallowed with boiled water or decocted fluid), for oral administration after being decocted in water, one dose a day.

Oct. 29, 1988: After medication, the limb movement gradually recovered, other symptoms alleviated. She could walk, drinks and meal, sleep, urination and defecation all up to normal. Tongue proper dark red, with thin yellow coat, pulse thready. B.P. 140/90mmHg. Right upper and lower limb muscle strength grade 2. Babinski sign of both sides negative. The evil qi gone, yet the propriel energen still not restored. The therapeutic principle should be then to tonify the kidney and reinforce the marrow, to strengthen the spleen and stomach. With the purpose to consolidate the therapeutic results.

Recipe: Prepared fleece flower root 30g, Dogwood fruit 10 g, Chinese yam 12 g, Poria 15 g, Red sage root 20g, White atractylodes rhizome 12g, Alismatis rhizome 15 g, Amomum fruit 10 g, Tangerine peel 10 g, Pinellia tuber 6 g, Hawthorn fruit 15 g, to be decocted with water, one recipe dose daily continuous for two months.

Follow up in 3 months time, patient capable to

manage the live himself, without any discomfort.

II. Personnal experience

In treating comatous patient with herb medicine, nasal feed is better than spoonful feeding by mouth. And the nasal feed is less efficient than intrarectal drip. To administer medicine by mouth may induce inhalation of foreign body into trachea and cause inhalation pneumonia. Nasal feed may interfere the respirations, and especially harmful in gastric hemorrhage. Intrarectal drip is simple and easy to manage, medicinal absorption complete, and the intoxication and side effects of medicine less, so is a good way or route of medicinal administration.

The onset of this disease is acute and sudden, with rapid course of development, in clinic, the management must be prompt and the diagnosis exact, thus to rescue life from margin of death. The simultanuous use of traditional and western medicine, acupuncture and moxibustion, massage, acupoints pressing and others may be necessary for life saving and more complete recovery.

Brain atrophy

Brain atrophy is resulted from localized circulatory disturbance and long standing ischaemia and anoxemia of brain. clinically various functional disturbances of brain may occur. In TCM it pertains to the categories of 'windstroke', 'flaccidity syndrome', 'melancholia' and 'phlegm syndrome'.

I. **TCM syndrome differentiation and treatment**

Pathogenesis in brief: The deficiency of kidney essence, the malnutrition of brain and spinal cord, the deficiency of brain, the dicline and fall of mentality, the disharmony of *yin* and *yang*, the disturbance of viscera and *qi* functions, various symptoms appear.

Chief manifestations: The melancholia and depressive mentality, reactions sluggish, restrained eyesight, amnesia, even dementia, or loss of consciousness and speech, or dysphoria and insomnia, or hemilateral tremor, parathesia, and even paraplegia, or deviation of mouth and distorted eyes, or hemianopia, strabismus; strange vision, such as two objects with only one visualized, or double vision (one object looks as two), or stiffness of tongue and sluggishness of speech, aphasia, or epigastric fulness and distension, abnormality of urination and defecation, or disordered mentality, incoherent speech (divagation or allophasis). Tongue coat white and slimmy. Pulse thready and weak, especially prominent over the *'chi'* position.

Therapeutic principle: To tonify the vital energen and to refill the essence and marrow. In case of impaired consciousness and phlegm exuberance, to be assisted with resolving phlegm and removing blood stasis, to restore consciousness with stimulants. Hepatic wind stirred up from the interior, to be assisted with nourishing the liver essence and extinguishing the wind. With the decline of vital gate fire, to be assisted with tonifying the fire of vital gate and reinforcing the kidney yang. In cases with constipation, to be assisted with the confluent passage of *fu* organ and purge off the waste in intestine; in case with *qi* deficiency, to be assisted with tonification of vital energen.

1. Patent drug: *Mai Wei Di Huang Wan*, one bolus t.i.d.

2. Decoction recipe: *Bu Sui Jian Nao Tang* with additional drugs:

Prepared fleece flower root 30 g, Siberian solomonseal rhizome or Rehmannia 24 g, Ophiopogon root 20 g, Ginseng 6 g (or Pseudostellaria root 30 g), Glue of pilose antler 10 g, Oriental wormwood 20 g, Alismatis rhizome 20 g, Pueraria root 20 g, Lotus plumule 3 g, Cinammon bark 3 g, for oral administration after being decocted in water.

Plus-minus: For comatous patient, minus glue of pilose antler and lotus plumule, plus grass leaved sweetflag rhizome, curcuma root, musk (to be enveloped with tough silk), cow-bezoar, or plus *Su He Xiang Wan*; vexation and insomnia, add rhemmania, ophiopogon, coptis root, stirfried wild jujuba seed; dizziness, vexation and tendency to anger, add dragon's bone and oyster shell, cinnabar mixed poria with hostwood, capejasmine fruit; phlegm and stagnated blood obstruction of collaterals, minus antler's glue, siberian solomon seal rhizome, plus red tangerine peel, pinellia tuber, white mustard seed *tianzhuhuang* (the coagulated mass of wound juice from bamboo septa due to bee-bite), red sage root, spatholobus stem; retention of water and fluid, add prepared aconite root, poria, white atractylodes rhizome, acanthopanax bark, stir-fried immature bitter orange; obdominal distension and constipation, minus dogwood fruit, add stir-fried immature bitter orange, sichuan magnolia bark, rhubarb.

3. Acupoints: *Shenshu, Mingmen, Qihai, Guanyuan, Zusanli, Yongquan* (all reinforcing).

Plus-minus: Hemianesthesia or hemiplegia, plus *Jianyu, Quchi, Hegu, Huantiao, Yanglinquan, Xuanchong*; in comatous patients, add *Shierjing, Renzhong*; for deviation of mouth and distorted eye, add *Jiache, Dicang, Hegu, Yingxiang, Sibai*; for exacerbated fire, add *Laogong*; for exuberation of phlegm, add *Tiantu, Zhongwan, Neiguan*.

II. Case report

Mr. Cheng, 57 years old, retired worker.

Sudden onset of left hemiparesis, accompanied by slurred speech. He was admitted into our hospital on May 20, 1987, with a history of present illness of left upper and lower limb paresis, deviation of mouth and tongue, slurred speech, mouth and tongue dry, he felt thirsty and drank a lot. Dark urination, and stool constipated. Tongue proper red, tongue coat thin and yellow. Pulse taut and slippery. On physical examination: T 37°C, P 68 /min, R 18/min, B.P. 150/100 mmHg, patient an old man, with clear mentality, and active posture, cooperative, right nasolabial groove shallow left upper and lower limb paresis, muscle strength Ⅱ-Ⅲ grade, with normal muscular tonicity and sensations normal. Physiological reflexes normal. No pathological reflexes. On CT examination: Right frontal lobe atrophy, and left parital lobe suspected infaction β-lipoprotein 620mg%, cholesterol 278mg %, glycerine triesterase 225mg %. Microcirculatory disorder of Ⅲ grade. Blood rheology RBC hematocrit 53%. E.S.R. 14 mm/hour. Plasma specific viscosity 1.88; E.S.R equation K value 84~85; whole blood reduction specific viscosity 9.43/11.08. Rheogram of brain demonstrate pulsative vascular insufficiency of brain. Patient had history of diabetes mellitus for 20 years. In combination with tongue and pulse manifestations. TCM diagnosis was 'windstroke' (at the stage of attack or stroke of channel and collateral), and in western medicine, cerebral thrombosis.

TCM syndrome differentiation and treatment: The insufficiency of kidney essence, the asthenia of brain (the accumulated sea of marrow), the malnutrition of muscles. The therapeutic principle is to fill up the marrow and essence, to nutrite the muscles and make the collaterals patent. The decoction selected is a modified recipe of *Bu Sui Jian Nao Tang*: Prepared fleece flower root 30 g, Rehmannia root 30 g, Scrofularia root 18 g, Ophiopogon root 30 g, Lucid ligustrum fruit 24g, Honey-suckle stem 30 g, Red sage root 24g, Pueraria root 30 g, Chinese trichosanthes root 18g, the ingredients altered in accordance with the change of symptoms. In the condition with the appearance of yellow slimmy tongue coat to remove rehmannia and add Atractylodes rhizome 9 g, Oriental wormwood 20 g, Alismatis rhizome 15 g, Phellodendron bark 10 g. Shortness of breath and malaise add Astragalous root 30 g. Lumbar aching and weakness of knee, add Achyranthes root 15 g, Mulberry mistletoe 15 g. In all 50 recipe doses taken, the speech more fluent and coherent, muscular strength of upper and lower limbs of affected side restored to grade Ⅳ. For the ordinary house hold work he could help himself. Clinical symptoms essentially disappeared. Cholesterol lowered to 240mg%, glycerine triesterase to 177mg%, β-lipoprotein remained unchanged. Blood rheology RBC hematocrit 39%, E.S.R. 10mm/hour. Plasma specific viscosity 1.59. He was discharged at cure state on July 27, 1987.

Ⅲ. Personal experience

(Ⅰ)In cases with manifestations of 'Windstroke' at stage of channel-collateral stroke, the corresponding treatment in accordance with windstroke should be followed. When the condition becomes steady, then the modified decoction to reinforce the brain and marrow should be chosen.

(II) The so-called brain atrophy is quite the same as in TCM the insufficiency of brain and marrow, and the impaired mentality. In case the CT examination give this diagnosis, the TCM syndrome differentiation mentioned above may be followed.

Dementia senilis

Dementia senilis is mainly due to multi-infarctional foci or multiple focal lesions in the lacunae and is also related with psychic or emotional stimulation, infection, intoxication and other exogenic etiologic factors. The fundamental pathologic changes are disseminated atrophy and degenerative changes of brain tissue. The chief clinical manifestations are prominent orientation disturbance, time and place orientations mainly involved; memory disturbance, the recent memory mainly involved. And calculation disorder, personality change, behavior abnormalities, slurred speech, blurred phonation etc. This pertains to the scope of 'dian syndrome' (melancholia), 'chi dai syndrome' (aphrenia), 'windstroke' or its postsequele in TCM.

I. TCM syndrome differentiation and treatment

Pathogenesis in brief: The decline and asthenia of vital gate, the disharmony of *yin* and *yang*, the deficiency of five viscerae, the distorted and disordered *qi* function, mental derangement, mental confusion due to phlegm.

(I) Stagnation of phlegm and *qi*

Key points of pathogenesis: The psychic depression and stagnation of liver *qi*, dysfunction of the spleen in transport, phlegm stagnation and upper sensitive orifices hood-winked.

Chief manifestations: Mentally depressed, apathetic expression, dementia, irrational speech, joy and anger of no time, subject to changing moods. No appetite. Tongue coat white and slimmy. Pulse taut and slippery.

Therapeutic principle: To regulate the flow of *qi*, to remove mental depression. To resolve phlegm and restore consciousness with stimulants.

1. Patent drug: *Mu Xiang Shun Qi Wan*, each dose 6 g, three times a day. Bamboo juice 15 ml t.i.d.

2. Decoction recipe: *Shun Qi Dao Tan Tang* with modifications:

Tangerine peel 12 g, Pinellia tuber 12 g, Bile treated arisaema tuber 10 g, Poria 12 g, Cyperus tuber 10 g, Curcuma root 12 g, Prepared polygala root 10 g, Grass-leaved sweetflag rhizome 12 g, Capejasmine fruit 6g, for oral administration after being decocted in water, one dose a day.

Plus-minus: Dull appearance with gazed eyes, take *Su He Xiang Wan* (storax pill) as fragrant stimulant; long standing stagnation with tranformation into heat, plus stir-fried immature bitter orange, bamboo shaving, coptis root; for impaired consciousness, *Zhi Bao Dan* may be added to resolve dampness and stimulate the sensitive orifices.

3. Acupoints: *Xinshu, Shenmen, Renzhong, Fenglong, Xingjian, Daling* (all with reducing technique), *Dazhong, Shenshu* (both with reinforcing technique).

(Ⅱ) Deficiency of heart and spleen

Key points of pathogenesis: Weak constitution on account of advanced age, spleen damage due to contemplation, depletion of both *qi* and blood, devoid of nutrients of psychic mentality.

Chief manifestations: Be in a trance, palpitation and easily frightened, incoherent speech, prone to melancholy and cry, general malaise, or hemiesthesia, hemiplegia, anorexia, tongue proper light, pulse thready and strengthless.

Therapeutic principle: To reinforce kidney and replenish spleen, to nourish heart and sedate the brain.

1. Patent drug: *Bai Zi Yang Xin Wan*, one bolus, t.i.d.

2. Decoction recipe: *Bao Yuan Tang* with modifications:

Ginseng 10 g, Astragalus root 15 g, Prepared fleece

flower root 15 g, Chinese angelica root 12 g, Chuanxiong rhizome 10 g, Poria 12 g, Prepared polygala root 10 g, Arborvitae seed 10 g, Wild jujube seed 15g, Schisandra fruit 6 g, Cinnamon bark 3g, for oral administration after being decocted in water, one dose a day.

Plus-minus: Slurred speech, minus schisandra fruit, plus curcuma root, grass leaved sweetflag rhizome; in case of hemiplegia, remove schisandra fruit, stirfried wild jujube seed, add siegesbeckia herb, spatholobus stem; with prominent symptoms of melancholia and cry, add albizia flower, rose flower.

3. Acupoints: *Guanyuan, Qihai, Xinshu, Yongquan, Xuehai, Shenmen* (all reinforcing technique). For hemiplegia cases add *Quchi, Jianyu, Yanglingquan, Huantiao* (all reducing technique). Deviation of mouth with distorted eyes add *Jiache, Dicang, Hegu* (all reducing technique).

(Ⅲ) Deficiency of brain, the marrow sea

Key points of pathogenesis: The deficiency of kidney essence and its inability to fill in the marrow, the vacancy of marrow sea, and the loss of control of mentality by the brain.

Chief manifestations: Dull and apathetic, dizziness and tinnitus, lumbar aching and leg weakness, insomnia, forget-fulness or amnesia, irrational speech. Tongue proper light red, pulse deep, thready and without force.

Therapeutic principle: To reinforce the kidney and

replenish the brain, to fill in the marrow and reinforce the mentality.

1. Patent drug: *Jian Nao Bu Shen Wan*, one bolus, t.i.d.

2. Decoction recipe: *Liu Wei Di Huang Tang* with additional ingredients:

Prepared rehmannia 15 g, Prepared fleece flower root 15 g, Siberian solomonseal rhizome 12 g, Chinese yam 12g, Poria 12 g, Moutan bark 12 g, Alismatis rhizome 15 g, Dogwood fruit 10 g, Tortoise plastron 20 g, Amomum fruit 5 g, Grass leaved sweetflag rhizome 10 g, for oral administration after being decocted in water, one dose a day.

Plus-minus: For general malaise, plus pilose asiabell root 15 g, astragalus 15 g; chilliness with cold limbs, plus prepared aconite root 10 g, cinnamon bark 3 g; with incontinence of urine and stool, add galangal fruit 9 g, mantis egg case 9 g.

3. Acupoints: *Mingmen, Shenshu, Kunlun, Taixi Zhishi, Shenmen* (all reinforcing technique). With *yang* asthenia and cold limbs, add *Guanyuan, Baihui* (both moxibustion). With *qi* deficiency, add *Qihai, Zusanli, Guanyuan* (all reinforcing technique).

II. **Case report**

Mr. Xu, 59 years old, cadre, came to our clinic on April 3, 1986. In the past he had essential hypertension and coronary artery disease. Recently he had sudden onset of mental dulness and apathy, amnesia. He forgot things, letters, names even his own surname, dull, lazy, dislike to move, sometimes he talked to himself. In take of food and drinks, the urination and defecation were all normal. Tongue proper light, thin and white coat. Pulse taut and slippery. CT multiple focal infarction of lacunae B.P. 175/100 mmHg, EKG showed chronic coronary insufficiency. This pertains to *qi* stasis and phlegm stagnation, phlegmatic shading of sensitive orifices. The therapeutic principle should be to disperse the depressed liver and resolve the phlegm and stimulate the sensitive orifices.

Recipe: The Red tangerine peel 12 g, Pinellia tuber 12 g, Poria 12 g, Bile treated arisaema tuber 10 g, *Tianzhuhuang* 10 g (the occult powder from the bamboo juice from bee-bite wound over the nodes), Bupleurum root 10 g, Curcuma root 10 g, Rose flower 10 g, Stir-fried immature bitter orange 10 g, Grass-leave sweetflag rhizome 12 g, Prepared polygala root 10 g, to be decocted with water, one recipe dosage daily.

In the same time, acupuncture points selected *Xinshu, Pishu, Shenshu* (all reinforcing technique), *Fenglong, Xingjian, Daling* (all reducing technique) once daily.

41 days after treatment, all symptoms got better, spirit turned better, he could describe things, the recall of old memories many years ago, the recent memory, the very day past still forgotten. He was told to take

medicine frequently of the *Ren Shen Jian Pi Wan*, *Xiao Yao Wan* to fortify the therapeutic results.

Ⅲ. Personal experience

This disease is a frequent complication of windstroke or cerebral apoplexy. In case the coexistence of both, the choice is to adopt the scheme to treat the cerebral apoplexy first, usually adopt the TCM syndrome differentiation and treatment. When the diseased condition becomes steady, then adopt the method mentioned under this category.

To severe dementia patient, the nursing care of life is very important. On account of the incontinence of urination and defecation and the prolonged course and time to confine to bed, it's important to emphasize the prophylaxis of bed sore and infection. Patient is not allowed to go outside the home household without accompanied person, just the same as to take care of children.

Rhythmic palatopharyngo laryngeal muscular clonus

The chief manifestations of this disease are fine rhythmic clonic contractions of muscles of soft palate, uvula, pharynx or larynx, and involuntary phonation of croup sound. The affected part is chiefly at the brain stem, especially the inferior olivary body. The pathogenesis of this disease is at present not well known. There is no such corresponding term in TCM. From thoretical point of view, larynx has the distributions of lung, liver and kidney channels and collaterals and this disease is treated accordingly.

I. TCM syndrome differentiation and treatment

Pathogenesis in brief: The insufficiency of the liver and kidney; the failure of dispersion of pulmonary *qi*; the loss of wetness of pharynx and larynx; the clonic spasm of muscles.

(I) The deficiency of kidney *yin*, and the internal agitation of hepatic wind

Key points of pathogenesis: The deficiency of kidney *yin*, the kidney fluid can't nourish the hepatic wood, the agitative flow of endogenous hepatic wind, the wood-fire injures the metal, the failure of dispersion of lung-*qi*, and the loss of wetness of pharynx and larynx.

Chief manifestations: 'Ge-Ge' sound produced in larynx, slurred speech, tremble of Adam's apple, the 'Ge-Ge' sound alleviated during talking, feeding or sound sleep, dryness of mouth and pharynx, vexation and hotness over palms, soles and the heart, insomnia and dreaminess, muscular twitching, trembling of hands or feet. Aching and flaccidity of loin and knee; Tongue proper red with little fur. Pulse taut and thready.

Therapeutic principle: To nourish the kidney and liver essence, to moist the lung and extinguish the wind.

1. Patent drug: *Liu Wei Di Huang Wan*, one bolus, t.i.d., scorpion and centipede powder each 2 g.

2. Decoction recipe: *Yang Yin Qing Fei Tang* with modifications:

> Rehmannia root 24 g, Ophiopogon root 24 g, Platycodon root 6 g, Licorice 3 g, Scorpion powder 6 g, Centipedes powder 4 g, to be decocted in water and the powdered drug mixed with the decocted fluid and taken by mouth.

Plus-minus: With prominent vexation and insomnia plus stir-fried wild jujube seed, and capejasmine fruit; with pronounced muscular twitching or trembling of hands and feet add dragon's bone, oyster shell, earthworm (dried); pronounced dryness of mouth and pharynx vexation and anger tendency, add bupleurum, oroxylum seed, anemarrhena, capejasmine fruit; with constipation add Rhubarb, Anemarrhena.

3. Acupoints: *Shenshu, Ganshu, Taixi* (all with reinforcing technique), *Taichong, Xingjian, Tiantu, Lianquan* (all with reducing technique).

4. Ear acupoints: Kidney, Liver, Heart, Sympathetic.

(Ⅱ) Insufficiency of kidney *yang*, with upward disturbance of wind and phlegm

Key points of pathogenesis: The insufficiency of

kidney *yang*, the failure of transference of fluid which accumulated and resulted phlegm. The up-surge of wind-phlegm; the dysfunction of lung in cleansing and descending the *qi*, and thus with the pharynx and larynx affected.

Chief manifestations: Thyroid cartilage clonus, production of 'Ge-Ge' sound, continuous and persistent, temporary remissions while eating or drinking or during sleep, spitting of saliva or sputum, oppressive sensation in chest, chilliness over the lumba and back, muscular twitching, urination clear and not short, stool soft; exacerbated after exposure to cold. Tongue body plump with tooth indentations over the margin, tongue coat white and moist. Pulse deep and relaxed.

Therapeutic principles: To warm up the kidney and assist the *yang*; to resolve the phlegm and extinguish the wind.

1. Patent drug: *Jin Gui Shen Qi Wan*, one bolus t.i.d. Earthworm, centipede, scorpion powder each 3 g three times a day.

2. Decoction recipe: *Zhen Wu Tang* and *Er Chen Tang* with modifications:

Prepared aconite 12 g, White atractylodes rhizome 15 g, Poria 24 g, Red tangerine peel 12 g, Pinellia tuber 12 g, Thunberg fritilliary bulb 10 g, Lily bulb (stirfried with honey) 30 g, Batryticated silkworm 12 g, Earth worm 12 g, Oyster shell 24 g, for oral administration after being decocted in water, one dose a day.

Plus-minus: Clonus of thyroid cartilage with prominent 'Ge-Ge' sound, plus scorpion and centipede powder; aversion to cold, loose stool pronounced, plus dried ginger; profuse salivation and sputum, add evodia fruit, round cardamon seed.

3. Acupoints: *Guanyuan, Mingmen, Shenshu, Zusanli* (all moxibustion), *Zhongwan, Fenglong, Tiantu, Lianquan* (all with reducing technique).

4. Ear acupoints: Kidney, Spleen, Heart, Liver, Sympathetic.

II. **Case report**

Mr. Zhang, 38 years old, cadre, first visit on May 25, 1980.

Larynx clonus, with 'Ge-Ge' sound production, associated with tightness in the pharynx for 5 months. The diagnosis of rhythmic clonus of palate, pharynx, larynx made and received treatments in many hospitals in Shandong province, Beijing and Shanghai. Oryzanol, Diazepamum, Perphenazine, Calcium bromide, and patent herb drug pill *Zhi Bai Di Huang Wan, Long Dan Xie Gan Wan* without evident effect, and went back to Shandong for TCM therapy. The onset of disease after thundering anger and loss of sleep for a whole night, and he felt tightness over the pharynx and larynx, and then gradual occurrence of clonus of larynx, and slight 'Ge-Ge' sound produced, vexation and anger tendency, insomnia and easily frightened, hotness over palms and soles, all the symptoms aggravated in the afternoon and night, soreness and weakness of loin and knee. Tongue proper red with a little coat. Pulse thready and rapid. This pertained to deficiency of kidney *yin*, and impaired nutrition of liver-wood, with endogenous agitation of asthenic wind. The therapeutic principle was to nourish the kidney and soften the liver, to extinguish the wind and moisten the larynx.

Recipe: Rehmannia root 30g, Ophiopogon root 30g, Scrofularia root 24 g, White peony root 21 g, Thunberg fritilliary bulb 12 g, Platycodon root 12 g, Licorice 6g, Capejasmine fruit 6 g, The whole scorpion powder, Centipede powder, Earthworm powder each 3g, for oral administration after being decocted in water, one dose a day.

On the second visit after six recipe doses the larynx clonus alleviated, the 'Ge-Ge' sound of larynx disappeared. In the night he could sleep for five hours. The soreness and weakness of loin and knee and vexation, easily frightened still persisted. The tongue and pulse findings were the same as the previous visit. The previous recipe used with addition of prepared fleece flower root 24 g, dragon's bone 20 g, oyster shell 20 g.

On the third visit, another 31 recipe doses taken, all symptoms disappeared. Tongue proper light red, tongue coat thin and white. Pulse moderate only a little bit soreness and weakness of loin and knees. *Liu Wei*

Di Huang Wan, one bolus t.i.d. continuous for another month to strengthen and consolidate the therapeutic effect. Follow-up 5 years later, he remained healthy without recurrence.

III. Personal experience

To any TCM type of this disease, herb medicine with the effect of putting off the wind and relieve cramp should be used in order to get satisfactory results, such as earthworm, the whole scorpion, centipede, the batryticated silkworm and others. In the same time, the addition of herb drugs to sooth and soften the liver, to regulate lung and moist the larynx such as white peony root, bupleurum root, thunberg fritilliary bulb, platycoden root, licorice and others. During period of medication, pungent and irritating, greasy, fishery food should be forbidden in order to prevent damage of spleen and stomach and exhausion of lung *qi*.

Meniere's syndrome

Meniere's syndrome, or vertigo of inner ear, the labyrinth hydrop, with clinical manifestations of paroxysmal vertigo, often accompanied by nausea, vomiting; tinnitus and gradual impairment of hearing. It pertains to the category of 'vertigo', 'vomiting' and others.

I. TCM syndrome differentiation and treatment

Pathogenesis in brief: The stagnation of the liver-*qi* and deficiency of the spleen; the up-surge of phlegm-fluid retention, with involvement of stomach and the blockage of the sensitive orifices of ear.

Chief manifestations: Vertigo or dizziness, as if in the boat; nausea, vomiting, dazzled vision, tinnitus, vexation, dreamfulness, oppression in chest and epigastrium. All the symptoms aggravated by motion, alleviated by silent sleep. Tongue proper light red, tongue coat white and slimmy, pulse taut and slippery.

Therapeutic principle: To disperse the liver and replenish the spleen; to resolve phlegm and descend the upward *qi*.

1. Patent drug: *Xiao Yao Wan*, 10g t.i.d. *Shu Gan He Wei Wan*, 6 g t.i.d.

2. Decoction recipe: *Ban Xia Bai Zhu Tian Ma Tang* with modifications:

Ginger prepared pinellia 12 g, Bighead atractylodes 15 g, Poria 24 g, Gastrodia tuber 12 g, Bupleurum root 12 g, Magnolia bark 10 g, Alismatis rhizome 30 g, Red ochre (hematite) 20 g, Ginger prepared bamboo shaving 6 g, for oral administration after being decocted in water.

Plus-minus: With prominent vexation, insomnia; plus capejasmine fruit, white peony root, stir-fried wild jujube seed; mouth bitter tasted and throat dry, vexation and restlessness, flush of face, pulse taut rapid, stagnant heat of liver and gall bladder, add scutellaria root, gentian root, pearl shell; soreness and weakness of loin and legs, dryness of mouth and throat, tongue red with little coat, with evident *yin* deficiency, add eclipta, prepared fleece flower root, dendrobium; dizziness, malaise, palpitation, shortness of breath, tongue proper light in color, pulse weak, with evident deficiency of *qi* and blood add Dangshen, Chinese angelica root, Chuanxiong rhizome, Longan aril, Licorice.

3. Acupoints: *Fengchi, Hegu, Zhongwan, Fenglong, Jiexi, Neiguan, Yifeng, Tinggong.*

4. Ear acupoints: *Shenmen*, Sympathetic, Adrenal, Spleen, Stomach, Liver.

II. Case report

Mr. Wang, 44 years old, worker, the first visit on May 20, 1988. With a history of paroxysmal attack of vertigo, tinnitus and vomiting for 6 years, the recent paroxysm was due to fatigue and exposure to cold. During the attack, vertigo, inability to stand, repeated vomiting, noisy tinnitus of both ears, vexation, chest oppression and palpitation, epigastric fulness and anorexia, insomnia and dreamfulness, tongue proper red, coat thin and slimmy. Pulse taut and slippery. A diagnosis of meniere's syndrome was made, the attack was not controlled with many times western medicine treatment, thus referred to traditional Chinese medicine. The TCM syndrome, diagnosis pertained to the stagnancy of liver-*qi* and deficiency of the spleen, the upward disturbance of phlegm and fluid, the upward aversion of gastric *qi*, and the therapeutic principle should be to soothe the liver-*qi* and remove the stagnancy, to resolve phlegm and descend the up-averted *qi*.

Recipe: Bupleurum root 12 g, Scutellaria root 10 g, Red tangerine peel 12 g, Ginger prepared pinellia tuber 12 g, White atractylodes rhizome 30 g, Alismatis rhizome 30 g, Ginger prepared bamboo shaving 10 g, Stir-fried immature bitter orange 10 g, Pueraria root 15 g, Dalbergia wood 6 g, Capejasmine fruit 6 g, Uncaria stem with hooks 15 g, for oral administration after being decocted in water, one to two dose a day. Acupuncture points of *Fengchi, Hegu, Zhongwan, Fenglong, Neiguan, Yifeng, Tinggong* selected and all with reducing technique. After relief of symptoms, then decoction given.

The second visit on May 28,1988. After six doses, all symptoms alleviated except some dizziness, malaise, tinnitus like ciccada chirping, soreness and weakness of loin and knee. Dreamfulness, dryness of mouth, and vexation. Tongue proper red, tongue coat thin and white. Pulse taut and thready. This indicated the clearance of phlegm and fluid, the kidney and liver *yin* deficiency still left.

Recipe: Chrysanthemum flower 10 g, Wolfberry fruit 12 g, Prepared fleece flower root 24 g, Eclipta 15 g, Dogwood fruit 12 g, Poria 12 g, Lily bulb (stir-fried with honey) 21 g, Grass-leaved sweetflag rhizome 10 g, Magnetite 15 g, Bupleurum root 6 g, Tangerine peel 10 g, to be decocted in water, the above recipe one dose daily.

The third visit on June 20,1988, after 20 recipe doses of the above prescription, all symptoms disappeared. Tongue and pulse normal. *Qi Ju Di Huang Wan* was taken twice a day for another month in order to consolidate the therapeutic effects.

Follow-up 6 months later. He had caught cold twice, but no recurrence of meniere's syndrome.

III. Personal experience

The pathogenesis of meniere's syndrome is the exuberance of dampness due to spleen insufficiency, and the up-surge of phlegm and fluid, the principle of replenishing spleen and removing dampness with diuretics should be emphasized, and drugs like alismatis rhizome, poria, white atractylodes rhizome chosen. During period of lysis, because of involvement of liver and kidney, the therapeutic principle should be to soothe the liver and nourish the kidney essence, and to replenish the spleen.

In acute phase, on account of severe vomiting, to be relieved with difficulty, to the recipe on the basis of TCM syndrome differentiation red ochre, inula flower, magnetite and other heavy or sedative material, in the mean while acupuncture or ear acupuncture to be used simultaneously to control the giddiness and vomiting, then frequent intake of herb medicine decoction.

As the spleen considered to be the source of phlegm production, during period of lysis, in case the *yin* deficiency of liver and kidney not prominent, the fundamental therapeutic principle should be put on to reinforce the spleen and regulate the gastric activity, thus to abolish the sources of phlegm production.

Trigeminal neuralgia

Trigeminal neuralgia is manifested by paroxysmal attacks of transient but very sharp pain along the branches and sensory distributions of trigeminal nerve with frequent recurrences. The pain distribution is strictly in accordance with the sensory nerve supplies of trigeminal nerve, with clear demarcations, without dissemination to the posterior part of head. Its etiology is not yet well known, and lack of ideal treatment. This disease pertains to the category of 'headache', 'toothache' in TCM and satisfactory therapeutic effects usually obtained according to the principle of TCM syndrome differentiation and treatment.

I. **TCM syndrome differentiation and treatment**

Pathogenesis in brief: The exuberance of evil fire in liver channel with wind production; the flare up of wind and fire, with muscular contracture. In long standing cases, the damage of *yin* leads to the transference from sthenic to asthenic conditions.

(I) Wind-fire of liver channel

Key points of pathogenesis: Exuberance of fire of liver channel with production of wind, the flare up of wind-fire resulting in muscular contracture.

Chief manifestations: Sudden paroxysmal attack of lightning pain, stabbing or needling or burning over one side of face, continuous for several seconds, as frequent as several times in a minute, or only several times in a whole day, accompanied by muscular twitching, congested eyes and lacrimation, saliva flowing out from angle of mouth, vexation and easy to lose temper, deep colored urination and constipation. Even a light touch of the affected side may induce the siezure. Tongue proper red, tongue coat thin and yellow. Pulse taut and rapid.

Therapeutic principle: To allay the liver and purge off the fire; to relieve the spasm and arrest the pain.

1. Patent drug:

(1) *Long Dan Xie Gan Wan*, 10 g t.i.d. or *Niu Huang Shang Qing Wan*, 5 g t.i.d. and *Yuan Hu Zhi Teng Pian* 5 tablets t.i.d.

(2) Equal portions of whole scorpion, centipede and batryticated silkworm ground into fine powder, 6 g t.i.d.

2. Decoction recipe: *Xiong Zhi Shi Gao Tang* with modifications:

Chuanxiong rhizome 15 g, Dahurian angelica root

12g, Gypsum 30g, Chrysanthemum flower 12g, Bupleurum root 10g, Scutellaria root 12g, Moutan bark 12g, Capejasmine fruit 12g, Peppermint 10g, Gentian root 10g, White peony root 24g, Licorice 6g, for oral administration after being decocted in water, one dose a day.

Plus-minus: For acute pain with muscle cramp, add whole scorpion, centipede, batryticated silkworm, earthworm; for exuberant heat with exhaustion of body fluid add anemarrhena rhizome dendrobium, Chinese trichosanthes root; constipation, ulcerations in mouth and over tongue, add rhubarb, magnolia bark, mirabilite.

3. Acupoints: *Zanzhu, Yuyao, Taiyang, Yangbai, Jiache, Juliao, Chengjiang, Zhiyin, Neiting, Hegu, Waiguan* (all with strong manipulation of reducing technique).

(Ⅱ) Hyperactivity of *yang* due to *yin* deficiency

Key points of pathogenesis: Due to long standing fire exuberance with exhaustion of *yin* fluid, the kidney water can't nutrite the liver wood, with the upward disturbance of wind *yang*.

Chief manifestations: Paroxysmal distending hemicrania, contracture of the cranial angle, with referred pain to teeth, twitching of facial muscle, dryness of mouth and throat, dysphoria and insomnia, urine scanty in amount and deep colored. Tongue proper red, tongue coat dry and yellow, Pulse taut, thready and rapid.

Therapeutic principle: To cultivate the kidney-water and nourish the liver-wood; to subdue the liver *Yang* and arrest the pain.

1. Patent drug: *Qi Ju Di Huang Wan*, one bolus t.i.d. and magnetite powder 3g, cinnabar powder 1g (to be swallowed with water), three times a day.

2. Decoction recipe: *Tian Ma Gou Teng Yin* with modifications:

Gastrodia tuber 12g, Uncaria stem with hooks 24g, Prepared fleece flower root 30g, Rehmannia 15g, Sea-ear shell 30g, Magnetite 24g, Chrysanthemum flower 12g, Tribulus fruit 12g, Cicada slough 12g, Whole scorpion 12g, for oral administration after being decocted in water, one dose a day.

Plus-minus: Exuberance of liver-fire, dysphoria and easy to lose temper, plus gentian root, capejasmine fruit. With prominent insomnia add stir-fried wild jujuba seed, Fleece flower stem. For severe twitching of facial muscle, add earthworm, batryticated silkworm, scorpion.

3. Acupoints: *Shenshu, Ganshu, Houxi, Zusanli, Neiting* (all with reinforcing technique), *Zanzhu, Yuyao, Taiyang, Yangbai, Jiache, Chengjiang* (all reducing technique).

4. Ear acupoints: Kidney, Gall bladder, Liver, Sympathetic.

II. Case report

Mr. Cui, 48 years old, cadre, came to the clinic on February 21, 1979. Complained of paroxysmal left hemicrania for three years. The recent attack was induced by loss of temper. The seizure attack characterized by sharp pain like needling, associated with muscular twitching, congested eye with lacrimation, dysphoria, dryness of mouth and tongue, deep colored urine and constipation. Tongue proper red, tongue coat thin and yellow. Pulse taut and rapid. A diagnosis of trigeminal neurlgia made with involvement of maxillary branch mainly, with repeated treatment in western hospital without control.

This pertained to exuberance of fire in liver channel, with upward disturbance of wind-fire. The therapeutic principle should be to clear the liver and purge the fire, to extinguish the wind and arrest the pain.

Emergent disposal: Acupuncture *Zanzhu, Yuyao, Taiyang, Yangbai, Jiache, Hegu, Waiguan* (with reducing technique, strong manipulation) or using pulsating electrice needle.

Recipe: *Chuanxiong* rhizome 12 g, Tribulus fruit 12 g, Dahurian angelica root 12 g, Gypsum 30 g, Anemarrhena rhizome 12 g, Bupleurum root 10 g, Scutellaria root 12 g, Capejasmine 12 g, Gentian root 12 g, Whole scorpion 12 g, Cicada slough 12 g, White poeny root 15g Licorice 3 g, to be decocted in water, one dose a day.

The second visit on February 26. After three recipe doses, and acupuncture three times, the pain much less, only felt dull pain. Vexation and easy to lose temper, insomnia, dryness of mouth, had stool, urine still deep yellow in color. Tongue proper red, tongue coat thin yellow. Pulse taut, thready and rapid. This indicated the subsidence of liver fire, the depletion of *yin* and body fluid. The acute phase is over, it's time to treat the basic condition.

Recipe: Chrysanthemum flower 12g, Mulberry leaf 12g, Chuanxiong rhizome 12g, Prepared fleece flower root 24g, Dogwood fruit 10g, White peony root 15g, Moutan bark 12g, Poria 15g, Capejasmine fruit 10g, Stirfried wild jujube fruit 24g, Earthworm 12g, to be decocted in water, one recipe dose daily.

The third visit on March 15, another 18 doses taken, all symptoms disappeared, tongue and pulse normal. He was told to continue the intake of *Qi Ju Di Huang Wan* one bolus t.i.d. for another month to consolidate the therapeutic results.

3 months later the follow-up showed no relapse.

II. Personal experience

During interval of remission, regardless the asthenic or sthenic type, it's important to cultivate the kidney water and nourish the liver-wood, to restore the dispersal function of liver as the fundamental disposal, to remove the cause of the disease, thus to prevent relapses.

In cases with frequent episodes of headache and long courses, the pain rather acute, those drugs with the function to search for and expell the wind, and to make the collaterals patent, such as whole scorpion, centipede, batrificated silkworm, black tailed snake. Those with attack occurred after exposure to cold, sichuan aconite root, wild aconite root beginning with the dose of 2g and gradually increasing to 12g, previously decocted for two hours and then other drugs.

Facial neuritis

Facial neuritis is an acute nonpyogenic facial nerve inflammation while the nerve passes through the stylomastoid foramen or Tarin's foramen (hiatus fallopii or hiatus canalis nervi facialis) and induces peripheral facial paralysis. Usually the condition appears after getting up in the morning while washing face or brushing teeth. The condition includes the deviation of angle of mouth, paralysis of facial muscle, lack of expression. The etiology is still not well known. This disease pertains to the category of 'side wind', 'mouth deviation' in TCM.

I. TCM syndrome differentiation and treatment

Pathogenesis in brief: Wind phlegm obstruction of collateral, stagnation of qi and blood, blood insufficiency and collateral obstruction, muscular paralysis.

(I) Wind phlegm invasion of collateral

Key points of pathogenesis: Imprudent living, collateral stroke by wind phlegm, collateral obstruction and blood stagnation, paralysis of facial muscle.

Chief manifestations: Sudden appearance of mouth deviation and distorted eye, tenderness at Jiache point, inability to close eyes, accompanied by chill and fever, numbness of tongue root, tongue coat thin and white. Pulse floating and relaxed.

Therapeutic principle: To expel the wind and resolve phlegm; to activate circulation and collateral.

1. Patent drug: *Xiao Huo Luo Dan* one bolus t. i. d. and *Fu Fang Dan Shen Pian*, 4 tablets t.i.d.

2. Decoction recipe: *Qian Zheng San* with additional ingredients:

Prepared typhonium tuber 12g, Batryticated silkworm 12g, Whole scorpion 12g, Dahurian angelica root 12g, Chuanxiong rhizome 12g, Dried earthworm 12g, Bupleurum root 6g, Smilax glabra rhizome 20g, Cicada slough 12g, for oral administration after being decocted in water, one dose a day.

Plus-minus: Exopathogenic cases, add ledebouriella root, schizonepeta, dahurica gentian root, pueraria root, cinnamom twig, notopterygium root; associated with wind heat, minus dahurian angelica root, plus peppermint, honeysuckle flower, chrysanthemum flower; profuse sputum and salivation, add bamboo juice, bile treated arisaema tuber, pinellia tuber, *Tianzhuhuang* (crystallized bamboo juice from the wound of the node bite by yellow bee).

3. Topic medication: Croton seed two pieces (after removal of the pericarpium) ground into fine powder, mylabris (removal of head, feet and wings) stirfried and

ground into fine powder, fresh ginger 15g pound into paste and thoroughly mixed with the above drug, applied to 2cm below the maxilla of the affected side, with 1 cm in diameter for 20~30 minutes, scorching with carbon fire, and correct to the right position in the meantime.

4. Folk prescription or simple remedy with only a few drugs:

(1) Blood from living finless eel applied to affected side, once daily.

(2) Arisaema tuber suitable dose ground into powder, and mixed with fresh ginger juice applied to affected side, changed once in two days.

5. Acupoints: Perforating puncture from *Dicang* to *Jiache, Xiaguan, Yingxiang, Hegu, Lieque* (moderate reinforcement and reduction). In cases due to wind cold, indirect moxibustion with ginger slice in between, *Dicang, Jiache* selected. Or in combination with acupuncture, mox stick may be used once daily, each time 10 minutes, 7 days for a course.

(Ⅱ) Wind agitation due to blood deficiency.

Key points of pathogenesis: Collateral blockage due to blood insufficiency, agitation of asthenic wind.

Chief manifestations: Wry mouth and distorted eye for long time without recovery; paroxysmal tightness of face, with some twitching. Dizziness and blurred vision, palpitation, insomnia. Tongue proper red with little coat. Pulse thready and rapid.

Therapeutic principle: To nourish the *yin* and blood,

to remove wind and make collateral harmonic.

1. Patent drug: *Liu Wei Di Huang Wan*, one bolus t.i.d. and *Ji Xue Teng Pian* 5 tablets t.i.d.

2. Decoction recipe: *Si Wu Tang* with additional drugs: Prepared rehmannia root 15g, Chinese angelica root 12g, Chuanxiong rhizome 10g, Red and white peony root each 10g, Spatholobus stem 15g, Tribulus fruit 12g, Batryticated silkworm 12g, Earthworm 10g, for oral administration after being decocted in water, one dose a day.

3. Acupoints: *Shenshu, Sanyinjiao, Xuehai* (all with reinforcing technique), *Jiache, Dicang, Hegu, Fengchi, Yingxiang, Yifen, Sibai, Taichong* (moderate reinforcement and reduction).

II. Case report

Mr. Liu, 40 years old, worker. Came to attend clinic on May 6,1981. A sudden onset of wry mouth and distorted eye occured this morning. At the same time there were inability to close his right eye, right palpebra and face puffiness, salivation from right angle of mouth, with leakage of water while drinking, accompanied by chill, fever, headache, numbness of tongue root, rigidity of hind neck, and tongue proper light red, tongue coat thin and white. Pulse superficial and tense. Right *Jiache* point tenderness. B.P. 130/85 mmHg. TCM diagnosis: Wind-stroke-like disease (the invasion of channel and collateral).

TCM syndrome differentiation and treatment: The external invasion of wind-cold, the obstruction of collaterals with phlegm stagnation. The therapeutic principle to expel wind cold, to resolve phlegm and remove collateral obstructions.

Recipe:

1. Emergent disposal: Croton seed, mylabris, fresh ginger, prepared as above for topic application.

2. Decoction recipe: Prepared typhonium tuber 12g, Batryticated silkworm 12g, Whole scorpion 12g, Dahurian angelica root 12g, Pueraria root 15g, Honey treated ephedra 10g, Chuanxiong rhizome 12g, Earthworm 12g, Cicada slough 12g, Smilax glabra rhizome 15g, Fresh ginger three slices licorice 3g, to be decocted in water, one dose a day.

The second visit on May 9. Half an hour after application of topic medication blisters found locally. Today the fluid in blister already absorbed. Wry mouth and distorted eye alleviated. Chill, fever, headache and other exopathic symptoms disappeared. Tongue proper light red, tongue coat white. Pulse thready.

Recipe:

1. Acupuncture *Dicang* perforating *Jiache*, *Xiaguan*, *Yingxiang*, *Taiyang*, *Yangbai* perforating *Yuyao*, *Hegu*, *Lieque* (all with reducing technique), once daily.

2. Decoction recipe: The above recipe with removal of pueraria root, ephedra, dahurian angelica root, and Chinese angelica root, red peony root added, to be decocted

in water, one dose a day.

The third visit on May 15. 6 recipe doses taken, all symptoms essentially disappeared, only felt some discomfort over right face, tongue and pulse normal. The patient was told to massage himself the points of *Yingxiang, Xiaguan, Jiache* three times a day to fortify the therapeutic results.

II. Personal experience

This disease is chiefly due to the invasion of collaterals with wind and phlegm and resulting in stasis and obstruction of collaterals. At the onset usually with exopathic syndrome, in the late stage usually with exhaustion of *ying* and blood, and obstruction of phlegm and stagnation. Therefore besides the use of resolving phlegm and activating the function of collateral, in the beginning the associated use of dispelling wind and diaphoretic drug. After the lysis of exopathic disease, assistant drugs to nourish blood and activate circulation and resolve stagnation should also be used. Since topic medication has ideal therapeutic effects, thus to use it the earlier the better. After the blister formation at local area, it's suitable to wait for the absorption of the blisters, and the second application needs 15 minutes quite enough (the topic application indicates the recipe of croton seed, mylabris, and fresh ginger).

Acute infectious polyneuritis

Acute infectious polyneuritis (Guillain-Barre' syndrome) may occur in any age, most frequently from 20~40 years of age. There are many doctrines about its etiology such as 'hypersensitivity', 'auto-immunization', 'virus toxin' and others. Previous to the appearance of nervous symptoms there is frequent history of general or local infections. It may occur sometimes after vaccination or surgical operation, or during the course of leukemia or lymphoma. Usually a feeling of soreness, heaviness and loss of strength over the lower limbs, and 1~2 days later, various degrees of paralysis occur, rapidly spreading to the upper limbs, and the occurrence of symenetrical tetraplegia, with more severity over the lower limbs. In cases with involvement of intercostal muscles, there may be dyspnea, and it may endanger life. The physiological tendon reflexes diminished or abolished. The abdominal muscle reflexes disappear. In majority cases there are usually associated with cranial nerve lesions causing facial paralysis or oculomotor nerve disturbance, swallowing and phonation difficulty may occur. There may be various degrees of sensory disturbances. CSF examination frequently gives protein and cell count dissociation, namely increase of protein amount without corresponding increase of cells. This disease pertains to the category of 'wei syndrome' or 'bi syndrome'.

I. TCM syndrome differentiation and treatment

Pathogenesis in brief: Noxious heat invasion of interior, accumulation of damp heat with damage of five viscera, depletion and exhaustion of essence and blood, the flare up of the asthenic fire and result in disuse of muscles.

(I) The initial stage

Key points of pathogenesis: Virulent heat in lungs, with damage of essence and vital energy, the scald of lung leafs resulting in the malnutrition of muscles.

Chief manifestations: After the lysis of high fever, with sudden appearance of weakness of limbs, dryness of skin, choking cough with scanty sputum, dryness of pharynx, dark urination and constipation. Tongue proper red, tongue coat yellow and dry. Pulse thready and rapid.

Therapeutic principle: To clear off the heat and moisten the dryness, to nourish the lung and enhance salivation.

1. Patent drug: *Yang Yin Qing Fei Wan*, one bolus t.i.d. *Xi Ling Jie Du Pian*, each time 12 tablets, two or three times a day.

2. Decoction recipe: *Qing Zao Jiu Fei Tang* with modifications:

American ginseng root 12 g, Ophiopogon root 30g,

Gypsum 30g, Mulberry leaf 12g, Bitter apricot kernel 10g, Honeysuckle flower 30g, Forsythia fruit 12g, Stirfried mulberry twig 21g, Licorice 3g, for oral administration after being decocted in water, one dose a day.

Plus-minus: High fever plus *Xi Jiao Wan* one bolus daily, or add bupleurum root, anemarrhena rhizome, pueraria root. Severe choking cough with scanty sputum add mulberry bark, thunberg fritillaria bulb, loquat leaf; in cases of severe dryness of throat add Chinese trichosanthes root, fragrant solomonseal rhizome, reed rhizome.

3. Acupoints: *Shaoshang, Hegu, Shousanli, Quchi, Zusanli, Jiexi, Yanglingquan, Huantiao* (moderate reinforcement and reducement).

(II) The middle stage

Key points of pathogenesis: Spread of damp heat, with impaired motility of *qi* and blood, the malnutrition of muscles, and the disuse of four limbs.

Chief manifestations: Flaccidity and weakness of four limbs, bound heaviness of the body, or numbness, slight puffiness, especially of the lower limb, or with fever, chest and epigastric fulness, painful dysuria with scanty and dark urine, tongue coat yellow and slimmy. Pulse thready and rapid.

Therapeutic principle: To clear up heat and remove dampness by diuresis, to activate channels and restore function of muscles.

1. Patent drug: *Zhi Bai Di Huang Wan*, one bolus

t.i.d. with *Er Miao San* 10g t.i.d.

2. Decoction recipe: *Er Miao San* with additional ingredients:

Phellodendron bark 12g, Atractylodes rhizome 12g, Hypoglauca yam 15g, Tetrada root 12g, Coix seed 45g, Silkworm droppings 30g, Chenomeles fruit 15g, Smilaz glabra rhizome 20g, Achyranthes root 15g, for oral administration after being decocted in water, one dose a day.

Plus-minus: Epigastric fullness and anorexia due to excess of dampness, plus magnolia bark, alismatis rhizome, agastache, eupatorium; exuberance of heat with *yin* exhaustion, minus atracty-lodes rhizome, smilaz glabra rhizome, add rehmannia root, tortoise plastron, asparagus root; omplicated with stagnation and numbness of limbs, impaired joint motion, add red sage wood, red peony root, peach kernel, safflower.

3. Acupoints: Besides those used in the early phase, add *Pishu, Xuehai, Sanyinjiao* (all with reducing technique).

(Ⅲ) The late stage

Key points of diagnosis: The deficiency of liver and kidney, the insufficiency of blood and essence, the loss of nutrition of muscles and bones, the withering of marrow and atrophy of muscles.

Chief manifestations: The flaccidity and atrophy of the lower limb, the soreness and weakness of loin and knee, unable to endure long standing, the associated symptoms are blurred vision, hair falling, throat dryness and tinnitus, nocturnal emission or incontinence of urine, or menoxenia. In severe cases, inability to walk and atrophy of leg muscles. Tongue proper red with little coat. Pulse superficial forceless and rapid.

Therapeutic principle: To nourish the kidney and fill in the marrow, to strengthen the muscles and bones.

1. Patent drug:
(1) *Hu Qian Wan*, one bolus t.i.d.
(2) *Placenta humanis power* 10g t.i.d.
(3) Bone marrow of pig or cow cooked 500g, mashed and mixed with stirfried rice powder 2000g, each time 20g, with adequate quantity of sugar, two or three times a day.

2. Decoction recipe: *Liu Wei Di Huang Tang* with modifications:

Prepared rehmmania root 15g, Tortoise plastron 15g, Dogwood fruit 12g, Achyranthes root 12g, Chinese yam 15g, Moutan bark 12g, Poria 15g, Alismatis rhizome 18g, Chaenomeles fruit 15g, White peony root 15g, Tangerine peel 6g, for oral administration after being decocted in water, one dose a day.

Plus-minus: With withered yellow complexion, palpitation with or without external stimuli, pulse thready and weak, plus ginseng, astragalus root, spatholobus stem. In cases *yin* damage expanding to *yang*, with the appearance of cold limbs, impotence, urine clear, not scanty in amount. Pulse deep and forceless, add antler slice, psorales fruit, morinda root, cinnamon bark, prepared aconite root and others.

3. Acupoints: Besides those used in initial phase, further addition of *Guanyuan, Shenshu, Qihai, Sanyinjiao, Mingmen* (all with reinforcing technique).

I. Case report

Mr. Yu, 45 years old, cadre, came to clinic on July 10, 1971. With a history of damp cold exposure 20 days ago, chill and fever, headache, general aching and others. After treatment the fever subsided, yet on the next morning with sudden appearance of weakness of four limbs, unable to walk and wear clothing, respiratory distress, slight dyspnea, feverish, slight aversion to wind cold, slight mouth dryness and thirsty, choking cough with scanty sputum, urine yellow, stool a little bit dry. Tongue proper red, tongue coat thin and yellow. Pulse thready and rapid. A diagnosis of acute infectious polyneuritis made and the disease became steady after treatment with penicillin and cortisone preparations, yet the improvement of symptoms not obvious. This disease was considered from TCM syndrome differentiation and treatment to be the case of failure of diaphoresis of external cold, its transference into heat and the invasion to interior, with the exhaustion of body fluid due to pulmonary heat, and the loss of moistening activity and nourishment of the muscles. The corresponding treatment should be to treat the exterior syndrome with diaphoretic drugs and clear off the heat, to nourish the lung and enhance body fluid formation.

Recipe: Honey prepared ephedra 6g, Cinnamon twig 30g, Forsythia fruit 15g, Gypsum 30g, Anemarrhena rhizome 12g, Stir-fried bitter apricot kernel 10g, Ophiopogon root 15g, White peony root 12g, Prepared fleece flower root 20g, to be decocted in water, the oral dosage for a day. Acupuncture *Dazhui, Shaoshang, Hegu, Quchi, Juegu, Yanglingquan, Huantiao* (all with reducing technique).

The second visit on August 2, 1971. After 21 recipe doses, the flaccidity weakness of four limbs improved, he was capable to wear clothing himself, still unable to walk. He felt the heaviness of body, respirations not embarassed, no fever, no cough. Some chest oppression and epigastrium distension, anorexia, mouth thirsty but drink not much. Tongue proper red, tongue coat yellow and slimmy. Pulse soft and rapid. This indicated the superficial exopathogen already cleared, still the embarassment of interior with damp heat. Thus to clear off the heat and remove dampness with diuretics, to replenish spleen and recover muscular weakness.

Recipe: Atractylodes rhizome 15g, Phellodendron bark 10g, Coix seed 45, Smilaz glabra rhizome 24g, White peony root 24g, Chenomeles fruit 10g, Fleece flower root 15g, Honeysuckle stem 45g, Tangerine peel 10g, Achyranthes root 15g, Licorice 3g, to be decocted in water, one dose daily. Acupuncture *Pishu, Ganshu, Zusanli*, besides *Zusanli* using reinforcing, the other points reducing technique.

The third visit on October 5, 1971. After 63 recipe

doses, most symptoms disappeared, only thin in constitution, he could walk 300 meters, but no further, on account of flaccidity and weakness of lower limbs, soreness and weakness of loin and spinal column, dizziness and blurred vision. After rest for a while, with the support of hand crane, he could walk slowly. Dryness of mouth, blurred vision, impotence, tongue proper red with little coat. Pulse deep, thready, weak and rapid. The therapeutic principle then was to nourish the kidney and fill in the marrow, to strengthen the muscle and bones.

Recipe: Prepared rehmannia root 100g, Prepared fleeceflower root 100g, Tortoise plastron 100g, Dogwood fruit 40g, Achyranthes root 60g, Chinese yam 100g, Eucommia bark 50g, Moutan bark 30g, Chinese angelica root 45g, Dioscorea rhizome 50g, Astragalus root 60g, Finger citron 25g, Amomum fruit 15g, the above drugs ground into fine powder, mix with water to make pill, as the size of parasol seed. Each time 10g, three times a day. Acupuncture *Shenshu*, *Ganshu*, *Pishu*, *Zusanli*, *Juegu*, *Yanglingquan* (all with reinforcing technique).

The fourth visit on March 5, 1972. After finishing the above pill three times, all symptoms gone, he resumed his normal work, Only he felt weakness of lower limbs in the afternoon, tongue proper slight red, tongue coat thin and yellow. Pulse thready, slightly rapid. He was told to take bolus of *Hu Qian Wan* and *Liu Wei Di Huang Wan* alternatively one bolus b.i.d. to fortify the therapeutic results. Stop the use of acupuncture.

II. Personal experience

Clinically the acute infectious poly-neuritis is usually divided into three stages by TCM syndrome differentiation and treatment. In cases with proper treatment, the disease will be cured in first or second stage, and generally not to reach the third stage. In the early stage the exhaustion of body fluids with evil heat, with the burning of lung leaflets, and the use of heat clearing drugs with sweet and cold property. The abuse use of bitter cold, or pungent drug should be forbidden in order to avoid further exhaused sion of body fluids, otherwise the five viscera burned, with deficiency of Kidney and liver, then reaching the late stage.

There is the old saying to treat *Wei* syndrome the *yang ming* channels should be selected". In the early stage the essential principle is to clear the lung and nourish the *yin*, should be assisted with nourishing the stomach and clearing up the heat to obtain better therapeutic effect, as clearing the stomach fire attained, the cleaning and descending function of *qi* will be resumed. In middle stage, the chief role is to replenish the spleen, as one point is to cultivate the 'earth' (spleen and stomach) and promote the growth of 'metal' (lung). Secondly spleen is chiefly responsible for the four limbs, only if the *qi* of spleen earth, become strong and the supply of *qi* and blood and body fluids will become sufficient, the lung leaflet will get suitable moisture and nutrition, and the proper feeding of the four limbs, resulting in gradual recovery of the illness. The late or third stage pertains to *yin* deficiency of liver and kidney, to nourish and tonify the liver and kidney must be couped with drugs to replenish spleen and strengthen the stomach, in order to attain better absorption of tonic drugs without retardation of digestive function.

Epilepsy

Epilepsy is a common nervous disease. The clinical manifestations are sudden episode of transient cerebral dysfunction such as impaired consciousness, convulsions and others, with inclination to relapses. This disease pertains to the category of *'xian zheng'* or *'yang xian feng'*, considered its etiology due to phlegm. In western medicine, in order to control the disease, it is necessary to take medicine continuously, and about 30% the seizure cannot be completely set under control, especially difficult to deal with in cases with impairmemt of liver or kidney function. In TCM its therapeutic measure pretty safe and reliable and the therapeutic effects fairly satisfactory.

I. **TCM syndrome differentiation and treatment**

Pathogenesis in brief: Visceral dys-function and phlegm stagnation in the interior, up-set of *qi*, with internal agitation of wind-*yang*.

(I) Wind-phlegm obstruction

Key points of pathogenesis: The agitation of liver-wind in the interior, and the phlegm follows its ascending course, the impaired mentality resulting from the obstruction by wind phlegm.

Chief manifestations: Prior to the episode there may be dizziness, oppressive sensation in the chest, general malaise and others. The episode is characterized by a sudden fall, and loss of consciousness, convulsion and spitting saliva, or with a scream or other strange sound and incontinence of urine and stool. There may be only transcient loss of consciousness or fall into a trance without convulsion. Tongue coat white and slimmy. Pulse taut and slippery.

Therapeutic principle: To expel the sputum and extinguish the wind; to stimulate the sensitive orifices and allay convulsions.

1. Patent drug: *Ding Xian Wan* or *Wu Xian Zai Sheng Wan* each dose 10g, two or three times a day.

2. Decoction recipe: *Ding Xian Wan* with modifications:

Bamboo juice 30g (added to the decoction), Grass leaved sweetflag rhizome 12g, Pinellia tuber 12g, Bile treated arisaema tuber 10g, Gastrodia tuber 12g, Scorpion 12g, Batryticated silkworm 12g, Poria with hostwood 15g, Prepared polygala root 10g, Cinnabar and amber powder each 1g (to be swallowed with fluid), for oral administration after being decocted in water, one dose a day.

3. Acupoints: *Ganshu, Xinshu, Yongquan, Shenmen* (all with reinforcing technique), *Juque, Fenglong* (all with reducing technique).

(II) Exuberance of phlegm-fire in the interior

Key points of pathogenesis: The exuberance of liver fire with wind production, and the production of phlegm from the burning of the body fluid, the agitation of the wind phlegm and its obstruction of the sensitive orifices of heart with the result of impeded consciousness.

Chief manifestations: Hot tempered, dysphoria and insomnia, bitter taste in mouth, and dryness of pharynx, cough with sputum, not fluent, dark urine and constipated, During the episode, the sudden fall and loss of consciousness, convulsion and saliva spitting, or with screaming.

Therapeutic principle: To clear and purge the liver fire, to resolve phlegm and induce resuscitation.

1. Patent drug: *Long Dan Xie Gan Wan*, each dose 10g, two or three times a day. Or *Yang Jiao Feng Wan* each dose 10g two or three times a day. In case with constipation, *Zhu Li Da Tan Wan* each dose 10g t.i.d.

2. Decoction recipe: *Di Tan Tang* with modifications:

Pinellia tuber 12g, Bile treated arisaema tuber 12g, Stir-fried immature bitter orange 10g, Grass leaved sweetflag rhizome 12g, Gentian root 10g, Akebia stem 6g, Capejasmine fruit 12g, Sea-ear shell 30g, Uncaria stem with hooks 30g (put in late), Earthworm 10g,

Rhubarb 6g, for oral administration after being decocted in water, one dose a day.

3. Acupoints: *Ganshu*, *Xinshu* (both with reinforcing technique), *Shaoshang*, *Laogong*, *Juque*, *Fenglong* (all with reducing technique).

II. Case report

Miss Wang, 18 years old, peasant, came to clinic on March 21, 1969. With a history following fright the development of frequent seizures of sudden loss of consciousness, salivation, biting lips and tongue for three years, and was diagnosed epilepsy-grand mal in a hospital. Usually she had one such seizure every third day, yet the seizure became frequent recently, each day might have 4~5 seizures. At the beginning of the seizure you could hear a loud cry followed by loss of consciousness and fall, convulsions, with eyes gazing upward, white frothy foam from the mouth, the lips and tongue bitten. Each seizure lasted about twenty minutes and then the consciousness recovered. After a seizure, she felt dizzy, very fatigued and the soreness of limbs. The tip and margin of tongue reddened, the tongue coat was white and greasy, the pulse was taut and slippery. After the use of phenytoin sodium for two months there was no control of the seizure.

A diagnosis of *xian* syndrome was made. The pathogenesis was the retardation of mind with wind-phlegm. The therapeutic principle was to expel the phlegm and extinguish the wind, to control the *xian* syndrome with aromatic stimulants.

Recipe: Pinellia tuber 12g, Bile treated arisaema tuber 12g, Gastrodia tuber 12g, Poria 12g, Curcuma root 12g, Grass leaved sweetflag rhizome 10g, Polygala root 10g, Bamboo juice 30g (to be added into the decocted fluid), Scorpion 12g, Batryticated silkworm 12g, Sea-ear shell 30g, Cinnabar and amber powder each 1g (to be swallowed with fluids), for oral administration after being decocted in water, one dose a day.

During the seizure acupunctured *Renzhong, Shixuan* to arose the patient. After the seizure acupunctured *Ganshu, Xinshu, Yongquan* (all with reinforcing technique), *Shaoshang, Laogong, Juque, Fenglong* (all with reducing technigue).

Therapeutic effect: The seizure stopped after two months medication, and then one recipe dose every other day for consecutive three months. Follow-up study one year later still no seizure.

II. Personal experience

(I) In long-standing cases, with weak constitution, palpitation, dizziness, malaise, it is adequate to prescribe *Xiang Sha Liu Jun Zi Wan*, 10g two or three times a day, and simultaneously use *Zhi Bai Di Huang Wan*, one bolus a day, to replenish spleen to wall off the source of phlegm formation, to nourish the kidney essence just like to moisten the wood and extinguish the fire.

(II) In the recipe of treating epilepsy, the simultaneous

intake of the scorpion, centipede and batryticated silkworm in equal portions, ground into fine powder, each time 1.5g t.i.d. to extinguish the wind and arrest the spasm, thus to relieve epileptiform attack.

Schizophrenia

The concept of schizophrenia is founded on the basis of clinical manifestations characterized by variety of disorders of emotional activities, but generally marked as the failure of coordination (so-called seperation or dissociation phenomenon) between thinking, emotion, behaviour and environment. Though studies from many aspects have been carried out, the mechanism of the disease has not yet been made clear. It is considered that the defect is on the gene of patient's fifth chromosome. It is this gene, which is passed on generation after generation, that constitutes the latent cause of schizophrenia. In TCM, the disease belongs to the catagory of 'insanity', 'melancholia', etc. TCM has gained rich experience and obtained remarkable effect in the treatment of the disease.

I. TCM syndrome differentiation and treatment

Pathogenesis in brief: Stagnacy of qi (vital energy) of the liver, stagnation of phlegm in the interior, and impairment of consciousness, transformation into fire in long-standing cases, the disturbance of heart with phlegm fire and resulting in exhaustion of heart *yin*.

(I) Stagnancy of phlegm and vital energy

Key points of pathogenesis: The stagnation of the liver *qi*, the accumulation of phlegm in the interior with the result of impeded consciousness.

Chief manifestations: Emotional depression, dementia, apathy, incoherent speech, frequent sadness or cry, visual or auditory hallucination, over-suspicious or paranoiac, ignorance of being dirty or clean, strange behaviour, tongue proper pale with whitish greasy coating, pulse taut and slippery.

Therapeutic principle: To sooth the liver and disperse the depressed vital energy, to dissipate phlegm to induce resuscitation.

1. Patent drug:

(1) *Su He Xiang Wan*, one bolus, b.i.d. or t.i.d.

(2) *Xiao Yao Wan*, 5g, t.i.d.

2. Decoction recipe: *Dao Tan Tang* with modifications:

Prepared pinellia tuber 12g, Red tangerine peel 12g, Bile treated arisaema tuber 10g, Poria with hostwood prepared with cinnabar 12g, Nutgrass flatsedge 12g, Stir-fried immature bitter orange 12g, Curcuma root prepared with alum 12g, Grass leaved sweetflag rhizome 12g, Bupleurum root 6g, for oral administration after being decocted in water, one dose a day.

3. Acupoints: *Xinshu, Shenmen, Renzhong, Daling, Yifeng, Tinggong, Fenglong* (all with reducing technique),

Dazhong, *Zusanli* (both with reinforcing technique).

4. Ear acupuncture points: *Shenmen*, Sympathetic, Brain, Spleen.

(Ⅱ) Insufficiency of both the heart and the spleen

Key points of pathogenesis: Dysfunction and insufficiency of the heart and the spleen due to long-standing mental stress, malnourishment of *shen* (spirit).

Chief manifestations: Disturbance of mentality and thinking, absentminded, palpitation with irritability, less sleep with more dreams, mental fatigue, loss of appetite, dim complexion, deficiency of *qi* and disinclination to talk, pale tongue proper with thin whitish coating, pulse thready and weak.

Therapeutic principle: To reinforce the heart and the spleen, and to tranquilize the mind.

1. Patent drug:

   (1) *Gui Pi Wan* one bolus t.i.d.

   (2) *Yang Xin An Shen Wan* one bolus t.i.d.

2. Decoction recipe: *Yang Xin Tang* with modifications: Dangshen 12g, Bighead atractylodes rhizome 12g, Poria with hostwood 12g, Chinese angelica root 10g, Prepared fleece-flower root 20g, Stir-fried wild jujuba seed 30g, Honey-fried lily bulb 15g, Honey-fried polygala root 10g, Grassleaved sweetflag rhizome 12g, Licorice root 3g, for oral administration after being decocted in water, one dose a day.

Plus-minus: Astragalus root is supplemented in case with obvious deficiency of *qi*; honey-fried licorice root, floating wheat, and Chinese date supplemented in case with deficiency of blood and hysteria; raw dragon's teeth and magnetite for those with palpitation and restlessness; prepared aconite root, morinda root, and epimedium for those with deficiency of spleen-*yang* and kidney-*yang* due to chronic illness.

3. Acupoints: *Xinshu, Pishu, Shenmen, Shenshu, Zusanli, Dazhong* (all with reinforcing technique).

4. Ear acupoints: Kidney, Heart, Spleen, *Shenmen*, Sympathetic, *Naogan*.

(III) Mental disturbance due to phlegm-fire

Key points of pathogenesis: Long-standing phlegm stagnation with transformation into fire invading the heart, giving rise to mental disturbance.

Chief manifestations: Maniac and restlessness, flushed face and irritability, frequent cry or laugh for no apparent reason, constant scolding and beating people, and destroying utensils at will, scanty dark urine and constipation, tongue proper red with yellowish greasy coating, pulse taut, slippery and rapid.

Therapeutic principle: To clear up fire and remove phlegm; to allay the heart and tranquilize the mind.

1. Patent drug:

(1) *Meng Shi Gun Tan Wan* 6g t.i.d. or *Kong Xian Dan* 6g t.i.d.

(2) *Niu Huang Qing Xin Wan* one bolus t.i.d.

(3) *Long Hu Wan* one bolus b.i.d.

2. Decoction recipe: *Sheng Tie Luo Yin* with modifi-

cations:

Pig iron cinder 60g (decocted prior to others), Scutellaria root 12g, Coptis root 10g, Capejasmine fruit 12g, Gentian root 10g, Red tangerine peel 12g, Bile treated arisaema tuber 12g, Fritillary bulb 12g, Forsythia fruit 12g, Chlorite-schist 24g, Stir-fried wild jujuba seed 30g, for oral administration after being decocted in water, one dose a day.

Plus-minus: Rhubarb root, stir-fried immature bitter orange and dried glauber's salt are supplemented to treat constipation due to *fu*-organ excess; gypsum and anemarrhena rhizome supplemented to treat intense heat in *Yangming* Channel, thirst with predilection for drinks; further addition of *Zi Xue Dan* (purple snowy powder) to treat mental disturbance due to phlegm and fire.

3. Acupoints: *Renzhong, Shaoshang, Laogong, Xingjian, Taichong, Neiguan, Hegu, Yongquan, Juque, Fenglong, Fengfu* (all with reducing technique).

4. Ear acupoints: *Shenmen, Jiaogan, Naodian, Naogan,* Spleen, Kidney, *Pizhixia*.

(Ⅳ) Impairment of *yin* caused by excessive fire

Key points of pathogenesis: Overabundance of phlegm and fire for long time with impairment of *yin*, hyperactivity of fire due to *yin* deficiency, with upward disturbance of mental activities.

Chief manifestations: Mental confusion at a certain time, and mental clarity at others, restlessness and irritability, flushed face, low grade fever in the afternoon, emaciation, scanty dark urine, constipation, red tongue proper with little coating, pulse thready and rapid.

Therapeutic principle: To nourish *yin*; to purge down and clear the intense heat from the heart, and to tranquilize the mind.

1. Patent drug:
(1) *Zhu Sha An Shen Wan*, 6g, t.i.d.
(2) *Qian Jin San* 0.9g t.i.d.
(3) *Zhi Bai Di Huang Wan* one bolus t.i.d.

2. Decoction recipe: *Er Yin Jian* with modifications: Dried rehmannia root 24g, Ophiopogon root 24g, Scrophularia root 20g, Coptis root 6g, Sichuan clematis stem 3g, Poria with hostwood prepared with cinnabar 12g, Stirfried wild jujuba seed 30g, Schisandra fruit 6g, Honey-fried licorice root 6g, for oral administration after being decocted in water, one dose a day.

Plus-minus: Bile-treated arisaema, *Tianzhuhuang* (crystallized bamboo juice from the wound of the node bite by yellow bee), bamboo shavings, and immature bitter orange are employed in case with phlegm-fire; for the case with sever impairment of *yin*, Sichuan clematic stem is taken out of the recipe, while tortoise plastron, donkeyhide gelatin and white peony root are added to recipe.

3. Acupoints: *Shenshu, Xinshu, Houxi, Yongquan, Sanyinjiao, Zusanli* (all above with reinforcing technique), *Laogong, Danshu, Taichong* (all above with reducing technique).

I. Case report

Mr. Wang, 31 years old, farmer, first visit on May 20, 1978.

After anger, he had a sleepless night. The second day, he suddenly became mentally deranged, maniac and restless. With his bared body, he climbed up the wall to the top of the house, running on the wall without difficulty. He beat people, destroyed utensils, had no desire for sleep all the night, no bowel movement for three days with urine scanty dark, tongue proper deep red with little fur, and pulse taut, slippery and rapid.

TCM syndrome differentiation and treatment: Stagnation of *qi* turning into fire, transformation of body fluid into phlegm, disturbance of the heart with phlegm-fire, loss of control of the mentality. The treatment should be aimed at clearing up heat from the heart, purging the fire, eliminating phlegm for resuscitation. Acupuncture was administered priorly: *Renzhong, Laogong, Xingjian Juque, Fenglong* (reducing technique by strong stimulation).

Recipe: pig iron cinder 30g, Chrorite schist 30g (decocted prior to others), Bile treated arisaema tuber 12g, Pinellia tuber 12g, Curcuma root 12g, Rhubarb root 15g, Capejasmine fruit 12g, Gentian root 9g, Grassleaved sweetflag rhizome 9g, Prepared polygala root 9g, Cinnabar powder 1.5g (taken with water), to be decocted in rust water, one dose a day.

The second visit on May 21. After taking a dose of medicine, the patient vomited out some mucoid thick sputum twice, diarrhea three times, mentality clear, capability of falling into sleep, tongue proper red, tongue coat white, pulse taut rapid and slightly slippery. Continued the above medication and acupuncture.

The third visit on May 22. After another dose, vomiting once of undigested food, diarrhea three times, spirit bitter, thought normal, diet and sleep well, only spells of vague pain in the belly. Tongue proper red with thin and white coating, pulse thready and rapid.

Recipe: Pinellia tuber 12g, Bitter cardamon 15g, Red tangerine peel 9g, Ginger-treated bamboo shavings 9g, stir-fried immature bitter orange 6g, Curcuma root 6g, Grassleaved sweetflag rhizome 6g, Coptis root 4.5g, Licorice root 3g. Each dose, after being decocted in water, and with its residue removed, was seperated into three portions for three times' administration. One dose a day.

The fourth visit on May 26. Another three doses of medicine had been taken. All the symptoms disappeared except general lassitude and weakness, tongue proper with light red thin whitish coating, pulse thready and moderate.

Recipe: The same recipe as the above with the exclusion of grassleaved sweetflag rhizome, polygala root, and with the addition of *dangshen* 15g, poria 9g and bighead atractylodes rhizome 15g, One dose every other day. Five doses in succession for the sake of good recovery.

Follow-up 6 months later, the patient was well.

II. Personal experience

The pathological factor of the disease is phlegm. At the beginning of the disease, the primordial *qi* is not exhausted and phlegm-damp is dominant, especially when phlegmatic fire is overabundant, the method of inducing vomiting or purgation may be adopted. In the case report, the method of purgation is involved in the treatment. With the purging of stool, phlegm-fire is carried out of the body and all the symptoms are reduced accordingly.

As rust water has very good tranquilizing action, the decoction with it can increase the therapeutic effect.

If the patient has deep purple tongue or ecchymosis on the tongue and his mental disturbance occurs now and then, especially for woman patients when these signs are aggravated before menstruation, it is suggested that stagnated blood is accumulated in the interior. The drugs for adjusting *qi* and promoting blood circulation to remove blood stasis can be administered to assist the treatment, such as bupleurum root, nutgrass flatsedge, peach kernel, red sage root and others. Electrotherapy is effective for the disease, developing fewer complications and not any sequelae. Over the acupoints mentioned above, two corresponding points are selected each time. The filiform needle (No.28) are inserted 35mm deep into the body. After insertion, on to the manubrium of the needle, a transistor electric-impulse therapeutic instrument is connected. When electric circuit is set up, both the amount of electric current and the frequency of impulse should be gradualy increased. Strong stimulation (for reduction) is required to treat patients of type one and type three. The frequency during stimulation is 40~60 times per second, the output value of impulse is about 20~30 volt. Weak stimulation (for reinforcement) is for patients of type two and type four. The output amount of electric current is within the range of patient's tolerance, the circuit time being longer, as long as 20~30 minutes, 2~3 times a day, half an hour after meals, 1~2 months as a therapeutic course. In the course of therapy, the method for reinforcement and that for reduction can be utilized interchangeably, or reinforcement follows reduction or reinforcement and reduction simultaneously.

Though this therapy is safe, the patient's condition should be put under close observation so as to avoid accidents. Especially for patients with organic pathologic change, such as patients with angiocardiopathy or with cerebrovascular disease, it is not advisable to practise the method of strong stimulation (for conduction).

While various therapies are being carried out, the guidance to patient's thought should not be ignored. In accordance with the different stages of cause and development of the disease, different ways and means can be adopted to inspire and guide patients, being good at exposure of contradictions, and facing up to them, urging patients to transform their mental contradictions into right way. So long as mental advice is integrated with the proper method of therapy, better therapeutic effect can be expected.

Nervous tinnitus and deafness

The pathological change of nervous tinnitus and deafness is at the receptors of intracohlear nerve ending or at the cerebral cortex. Its etiology is still not well known. The clinical manifestation is subjective ringing in the ear, simulating the sound of cicada, or tide, high or low, strong or mild with impeded hearing. The impairment of hearing may interfere with conversation. In severe cases the auditory power may be entirely lost, in that case it is called nervous deafness.

I. TCM syndrome differentiation and treatment

Pathogenesis in brief: The upward invasion of ear sensory orifices with wind-phlegm-fire, the exhaustion of essence and vital energy with the result of malnourishment of brain.

(I) The flare up of phlegm-fire

Key points of pathogenesis: The upward disturbance of ear sensitive orifices with wind fire of liver and gall-bladder, and the obstruction of ear sensitive orifices with phlegm-fire.

Chief manifestations: Sudden appearance of tinnitus or deafness, ringing like cicada, blocking of hearing like deafness, usually exacerbated by anger, mild or severe at times, bitter taste of mouth and dryness of throat, dizziness, dysphoria with inclination to anger, oppressive sensation in chest, and much sputum. Tongue proper red, tongue coat thin, yellowish and greasy. Pulse taut slippery and rapid.

Therapeutic principle: To resolve phlegm and purge fire, to extinguish wind and stimulate the sensitive orifices.

1. Patent drug:
(1) *Long Dan Xie Gan Wan*, each dose 10g, three times a day, and take bamboo juice in the meanwhile, each time 15g three times a day.
(2) *Niu Huang Shang Qing Wan* one bolus t.i.d.

2. Decoction recipe: *Long Dan Xie Gan Tang* and *Er Chen Tang* with modifications:

Gentian root 10g, Capejasmine fruit 10g, Bupleurum root 12g, Alismatis rhizome 12g, Coptis root 6g, Red tangerine peel 12g, Pinellia tuber 12g, Stir-fried immature bitter orange 10g, Grass leaved sweetflag rhizome 10g, Curcuma root 10g, Sea-ear shell 20g, for oral administration after being decocted in water, one dose a day.

Plus-minus: Heat accumulated in bowel and constipation, plus rhubarb, rehmmania root, scrofularia root; severe phlegm heat, add *Meng Shi Gun Tan Wan*.

3. Acupoints: *Fenglong, Hegu, Daling, Neiguan, Zhongdu, Tinghui, Xingjian* (all with reducing technique).

(Ⅱ) Insufficiency of kidney essence

Key points of pathogenesis: Ear is the sensitive orifice of kidney, the insufficiency of kidney essence, the deficiency of brain, the malnutrition of ear orifice.

Chief manifestations: Gradual increase of severity of tinnitus or deafness, persistent and lingering, dizziness, soreness of loin and softness of leg, aggravated in the afternoon and night. Plenty dreams and nocturnal emission. Tongue proper red with little coating. Pulse thready and weak.

Therapeutic principle: To replenish kidney and enhance the essence, to fill in the marrow and subdue the yang.

1. Patent drug: *Du Qi Wan*, one bolus three times a day, and magnetite 3g, cinnabar 1g, three times a day.

2. Decoction recipe: *Er Long Zuo Ci Wan* with modifications:

Prepared rehmannia root 15g, Chinese yam 15g, Dogwood fruit 12g, Moutan bark 12g, Poria 12g, Alismatis rhizome 12g, Magnetite 30g, Stir-fried wild jujuba seed 15g, Honey-fried lily bulb 15g, Schisandra fruit 6g, Walnut flesh 15g, for oral administration after being decocted in water, one dose a day.

Plus-minus: With deficiency of kidney *yang*, plus indian mulberry root, wolfberry fruit, cinnamon bark; for the unconsolidation of kidney essence, add respberry fruit, cherokee rose hip, scald oyster shell, lotus seed.

3. Acupoints: *Shenshu, Mingmen, Pishu, Taixi, Zusanli* (all with reinforcing technique).

(II) Deficiency of spleen *qi*

Key points of pathogenesis: The deficiency of spleen *qi*, and the failure of the clear *qi* to ascend, the insufficiency of *qi* and blood, the vacancy of ear orifices.

Chief manifestations: The tinnitus low, lingering, or deafness with increase of severity after fatigue, malaise and anorexia, the stool not solid. Tongue proper light colored, with tooth imprint, tongue coat thin and white, pulse thready and weak.

Therapeutic principle: To replenish spleen and reinforce *qi*, to ascend *yang* and nourish the ear.

1. Patent drug:

(1) *Ren Shen Jian Pi Wan*, one bolus t.i.d.

(2) *Bu Zhong Yi Qi Wan*, one bolus t.i.d.

2. Decoction recipe: *Yi Qi Cong Ming Tang* with modifications:

Ginseng 10g, Astragalus root 20g, Chinese angelica root 12g, White peony root 12g, Cimicifuga rhizome 12g, Pueraria root 20g, White atractylodes rhizome 12g, Chastetree fruit 10g, Germinated barley sprout 20g, Honey fried licorice 3g, for oral administration after being decocted in water, one dose a day.

Plus-minus: With prominent deficiency of spleen, plus Chinese yam, poria; in case prominent deficiency of blood add prepared fleece flower root, eclipta, glossy privet fruit.

3. Acupoints: *Qihai, Guanyuan, Zusanli, Pishu, Baihui, Tinggong* (all with reinforcing technique).

II. Case report

Mis. Wang, 48 years old, cadre, came to the clinic on May 21, 1978, with the chief complaint of deafness for three days. Three days ago she lost temper and had roaring sound of both ears, followed by deafness of left ear, accompanied with stuffy sensation, vexation and inclination to anger, headache, insomnia, dryness of mouth and throat, constipation, urination short and dark colored. Tongue proper red, with thin and yellowish coating. Pulse taut and rapid. This was considered to be due to upper invasion of ear orifices with wind-fire of liver and gallbladder. The principle of treatment was to clear and purge the fire of liver and gall-bladder, to allay the wind and make the orifices patent.

Recipe: Gentian root 10g, Capejasmine fruit 12g, Scutellaria root 12g, Rehmmania root 30g, Scrofularia root 24g, Chrysanthemum flower 12g, Bupleurum root 12g, Grass-leaved sweetflag rhizome 12g, Rhubarb 6g, Alismatis rhizome 12g, Plantain seed 12g, Licorice root 3g, to be decocted in water, one recipe dose daily. After three recipe doses, the bowel moved, and the deafness gone, the other symptoms disappeared gradually.

III. Personal experience

In general, the acute tinnitus and deafness pertain to excess. In cases due to wind-phlegm-fire invasion of the upper part, namely the sensitive orifices of the ear, it is proper to treat with clearing and purging method of liver and gall bladder, and to extinguish the wind and resolve the phlegm. A prompt recovery will usually ensue. In cases with gradual development of long standing tinnitus and deafness usually pertains to asthenia of essence, blood, and vital energy, it is suitable to use the principle to replenish essence and blood, to reinforce spleen and promote *qi*, yet slow recovery is usually the case, so the therapeutists have to be patient in treating such cases. And it is advisable to combine the use of acupuncture therapy. In difficult and knotty cases, drugs to activitate the circulation and collaterals such as insects or scurry penetrating drug such as chuanxiong rhizome, safflower, peach kernel, red peony root, pangolin scales, sweetgum fruit, earthworm, batryticated silkworm, to enhance the replenishing and stimulant action.

No matter the disease is sthenic or asthenic, it is important to add bupleurum root, cimicifuga rhizome, grassleaved sweetflag rhizome, curcuma root, pueraria root and others as guiding drug to lead to the proper channel and other stimulants of the sensitive orifices to enhance the therapeutic effects.

Hydrocephalus after intracranial operation

Intracranial postoperative hydrocephalus is due to retardation of cerebrospinal fluid absorption secondary to subarachnoid adhesion resulting from trauma of brain tissue during operation. This belongs to the type of communicating hydrocephalus. Its clinical manifestations consist of headache, vomiting, limb paralysis, strabismus, and mentality changes. It pertains to the catagory of headache, vomiting, windstroke in TCM.

I. TCM syndrome differentiation and treatment

Pathogenesis in brief: The brain damage and blood stasis after intracranial operation, the accumulation of phlegm and body fluids will be responsible for the impaired mentality and various manifestations.

(I) Phlegm and stagnated blood obstruction in brain

Key points of pathogenesis: The trauma of channels and collaterals, with phlegm and blood stasis obstructing the brain, with involvement of mental and visceral changes.

Chief manifestations: Headache, projectile vomiting, deviation of mouth and distortion of eyes, hemiplegia, listlessness, incontinence of urine and stool or uroschesis, phlegm rattling in the throat, slurred speech or aphasia. Tongue proper light colored with white and slimmy coat. Pulse taut and slippery.

Therapeutic principle: To resolve phlegm and remove stagnation; to stimulate the sensitive orifices and arouse the patient.

1. Patent drug:

(1) *Fu Fang Dan Shen* injection 15 ml added to 5% glucose solution 250 ml intravenous drip, and in the mean while drink fresh bamboo juice 15g t.i.d.

(2) *Qing Kai Ling* injection 15 ml added to 10% glucose solution 250 ml intravenous drip.

2. Decoction recipe: *Tong Qiao Huo Xue Tang* and *Er Chen Tang* with modifications:

Chuanxiong rhizome 12g, Red peony root 10g, Peach kernel 6g, Red tangerine peel 10g, Safflower 6g, Pinellia tuber 10g, Grass leaved sweetflag rhizome 10g, Curcuma root 10g, Prepared polygala root 10g, Alismatis rhizome 21g, Pueraria root 21g, Scallion 3 pieces, Fresh ginger 10g, Musk 1g (silk enveloped), decoct the above 13 drugs (counting from the anterior) in 500g yellow rice wine for 25 minutes, remove the residue, then add musk into the wine, and decocted to boiling twice, divided into two portions for drinking two times.

Plus-minus: For uroschesis, plus plantain seed, lindera root; for headache, convulsion, add earthworm, scorpion, centipede; for constipation, add trichosanthes root, rhubarb and ground beetle.

3. Acupoints: *Baihui* penetrating to *Sishencong, Fengchi, Dazhui, Shenshu, Shuifen, Sanyinjiao, Fenglong* (all with reducing technique).

(Ⅱ) Brain insufficiency

Key points of pathogenesis: The phlegm and stagnated blood accumulation, the stasis of collaterals, and the malnourishment of brain.

Chief manifestations: Hemicrania, blurred vision, mouth deviation and distorted eyes, hemi-anesthesia, hemiplegia, emaciation, or with slurred speech, soreness and aching of loin and knees. Tongue proper red, with thin yellow greasy coating. Pulse fine and rapid.

Therapeutic principle: To reinforce kidney and replenish the marrow, to resolve phlegm and remove stasis.

1. Patent drug: *Qi Jiu Di Huang Wan*, one bolus t.i.d. and notoginseng powder 2g t.i.d.

2. Decoction recipe: *Liu Wei Di Huang Tang* with modifications:

Prepared rehmannia root 12g, Prepared fleece flower root 15g, Chinese yam 12g, Moutan bark 12g, Chuanxiong rhizome 15g, Poria 20g, Alismatis rhizome 20g, Bile treated arisaema tuber 10g, Trichosanthes fruit 12g, Leech 10g, Pueraria root 24g, Asarum herb 3g, for oral administration after being decocted in water, one dose a day.

Plus-minus: Slurred speech plus grass-leaved sweetflag rhizome, curcuma root, polygala root; stiffness of affected limb add scorpion, centipede, batryticated silkworm; emaciation, malaise, weak pulse, add *Dangshen*, White atractylodes rhizome and licorice.

3. Acupoints: *Shenshu, Pishu, Zusanli* (all with reinforcing technique), *Baihui, Shangxing, Fengchi, Taiyang, Hegu, Sanyinjiao, Xuehai, Fenglong* (uniform reinforcing and reducing technique).

I. Case report

Mrs. Zhang, 48 years old, worker, came to our clinic on November 12, 1987 with a history of over-fatigue, dizziness, left limb paresis, repeated vomiting, gazing of both eyes, and through CT examination in a hospital revealed hemorrhage of right basal ganglion, the internal and external capsule, the parietal lobe and the subarachnoid space. An operation to remove the blood clot from right temperoparietal lobe, about 100 ml. blood clot removed and followed by antibiotics, hormone, mannitol, and drugs to lower the blood pressure. This scheme of treatment continued for two weeks without apparent effect, and thus transfered to our hospital. The present ill condition, the mentality state clear for a while and confusion for another, left limb paralysis, right hemicrania, strabismus to the right, no bowel motion for three days, some incontinence of urine. CT examination revealed hydrocephalus. On examination, the tongue proper red, with yellow and thick coating. Pulse taut and slippery. B.P. 120/85 mmHg. Listlessness, right palpebral fissure narrowed, gaze of both eyes to the right. The pupils unequal, right bigger than left, right nasolabial groove shallow. Muscle strength, left upper and lower limb grade 0, right upper and lower limb grade III. Muscular tonus lowered on both sides. Pathological reflexes Gordon's sign (+) on left side, Babinski sign (±). A diagnosis of cerebral hemorrhage and postoperative hydrocephalus made.

TCM syndrome differentiation and treatment: Damage of brain collaterals, obstruction of collaterals with phlegm and stagnation, the loss of sensitivity of sensitive orifices, and the paralysis of limbs. The suitable principle of treatment should be to resolve phlegm and remove stagnation to stimulate the sensitive orifices and to arouse the mentality.

Recipe: Trichosanthes fruit 30g, Bile treated arisaema tuber 6g, Rhubarb 6g, Prepared fleece flower root 24g, ground beetle 10g, Hawthorn fruit 30g, Notoginseng powder 3g (to be swallowed with fluid), to be decocted in water, one dose daily.

The simultaneus use of *Qing Kai Ling* injection 40 ml, added to 10% glucose solution 500 ml intravenuous drip, once daily.

On November 20, after seven days medication, the symptoms not relieved, stool changed from constipation to incontinence, 5~6 times a day, the fluid consistency of stool, black colored. Tongue proper deep red and dry, thin yellow coating, pulse thready and rapid. This indicated the accumulation of phlegm and stagnation, and the insufficiency of brain, thus the proper disposal should be to reinforce the kidney and replenish the brain, to resolve the phlegm and remove the stagnation.

Recipe: Eclipta 15g, Prepared fleece flower root 20g, Rehmannia root 24g, Ophiopogon root 24g, Glehnia root 24g, Moutan bark 12g, Red peony root 12g, Chuanxiong rhizome 12g, Chinese yam 12g, Dogwood fruit 6g, Poria 10g, Alismatis rhizome 18g, Hawthorn fruit 18g, to be decocted in water, one dose daily.

On December 4, 14 the above recipe doses taken. All the symptoms gradually better. Spirit better, speech clear, food and drinks normal, stool self control. Tongue proper tip red, tongue coat thin and white. Pulse fine and rapid. Right upper and lower limbs muscle strength normal, left upper and lower limb still grade 0. Muscular tonus slightly low. B.P. 130/100 mmHg. She was told to continue the above prescription.

On March 5, 1988, she went back home and continued the above prescription with some modifications for 68 recipe doses. She could walk with the help of sticks or crutches, no other complaints. Tongue proper light red, with thin and white coating. Pulse taut and fine. B.P. 150/100 mmHg. She was told to take *Qi Ju Di Huang Wan* or *Zhi Bai Di Huang Wan* one bolus t.i.d. and to strengthen the functional training, in order to promote the recovery of affected limbs. Follow-up half year later, the patient could live on herself, and she could walk with cripple gait.

Ⅲ. Personal experience

Hydrocephalus after intracranial operation is an emergent critical disease with manifold complicated changes. The fundamental pathogenesis is phlegm-stagnant obstruction of brain collaterals and the gradual depletion of brain. The therapeutic principle is to resolve phlegm and remove stagnation, to reinforce the kidney and refill the marrow. In early stage the chief role is to resolve phlegm, and at the lysis of disease the main thing should direct to reinforce the kidney and refill the marrow.

Coronary atherosclerotic heart disease

Coronary atherosclerotic heart disease (abbreviated to coronary artery disease or CAD) is the result of atherosclerosis of coronary artery leading to the reduction of coronary blood flow, myocardia ischemia and hypoxia, and other pathologic changes. In mild cases there may appear angina pectoris, while in serious cases there may appear myocardial infarction, even sudden death. The incidence of the disease is very high. In most western countries, angiocardiopathy is the first among the list of causes of death, covering half of total mortality, more than half of which is caused by coronary artery disease. For instance, over 600 thousands out of 20 billions people in the United States die from CAD every year. According to the analysis records of postmortem examination, the same degree of atherosclerosis of coronary artery in our country is 15~20 years later than that in western countries. Latent coronary artery disease covers 70~90% of coronary artery disease found in our country. In 1972, a general check-up was carried out among 3474 residents over 40 years old in Shijiazhuang district. The number of the people who were found to suffer from coronary artery disease was 233, 6.71% of the all residents in the district. Of all the cases, 79.4% pertained to latent coronary artery disease. Here, we only deal with the syndrome differentiation and treatment of the chronic CAD, which, in TCM, is categorized as 'obstruction of vital energy in the chest', 'heartache', etc.

I. TCM syndrome differentiation and treatment

Pathogenesis in brief: *Ben Xu* means deficiency of the fundamental, *biaoshi* means excess of the incidental, deficiency includes *yin*, *yang*, *qi* and blood, phlegm, blood stasis, fire and stagnancy belong to 'excess'.

(I) Blood stasis due to *qi* deficiency

Key points of pathogenesis: Insufficiency of the heart-*qi*, weakness of the promotive force in maitaining the circulation of the blood, blood obstruction in the heart collaterals, and the seizure of chest pain.

Chief manifestations: Pain in the chest, shortness of

breath, lassitude and fatigue, listlessness, severe palpitation, aggravation by movement, dark colour of tongue proper with ecchymosis, thready and hesitant pulse.

Therapeutic principle: To replenish *qi* and promote blood circulation; to nourish the heart and sedate the mind.

1. Patent drugs: *Bu Zhong Yi Qi Wan*, one bolus a day, t.i.d. Along with the administration of *Fu Fang Dan Shen Pian*, 4 tablets each time, t. i. d. Or together with the administration of *Xin Ling Wan*, 1 bolus each time, t.i.d.

2. Decoction recipe: *Bu Yang Huan Wu Tang* with modifications:

Astragalus root 60g (or Ginseng 10g), Peach kernel 6g, Safflower 3g, Chinese angelica root 3g, Stir-fried ground beetle 6g, Curcuma root 6g, Red peony root 10g, Pueraria root 24g, Arborvitae seed 24g, for oral administration after being decocted in water, one dose a day.

Plus-minus: Dogwood fruit 15g should be supplemented in case with fatigue and obvious spontaneous perspiration; notoginseng powder and amber powder for the case with stabbing pain, severe palpitation and restlessness; red sage root, sandal wood and amomum fruit for the case with epigastric fullness and anorexia.

3. Acupoints: *Qihai, Zusanli, Xinshu* (all with moxibustion technique), *Jianshi, Shanzhong, Tongli* (all with moderate reinforcing-reducing technique).

4. Ear acupuncture points: Heart, *Shenmen*, Sympathetic.

(II) Deficiency of both *qi* and *yin*

Key points of pathogenesis: Long-standing illness of the heart, consumption of *qi* and *yin*, want of nourishment of the heart collaterals, resulting in heart damage.

Chief manifestations: Chest pain with dyspnea, shortness of breath, fatigue, restlessness and insomnia, thirst with predilection for hot drinks, a tendency to hunger with no desire for more food, tongue proper red, tongue coat white and dry, pulse thready and weak, intermittent or slow and uneven.

Therapeutic principle: To replenish *qi* and nourish *yin*; to activate pulse and tranquilize the mind.

1. Patent drug: *Bu Xin Dan* and *Gui Pi Wan*, 1 bolus of each, t.i.d.

2. Decoction recipe: *Bao Yuan Tang* and *Sheng Mai San* with modifications:

Astragalus root 30g, Pseudostellaria root 15g, Red sage root 24g, Ophiopogon root 15g, Schisandra fruit 10g, Dendrobium 15g, Stir-fried wild jujuba seed 20g, Hawthorn fruit 15g, for oral administration after being decocted in water, one dose a day.

Plus-minus: In case with remarkble chest pain, cinnamon twig and peach kernel are to be added to the recipe; for thirst with likeness of drink, dried rehmannia root and anemarrhena rhizome added; for listlessness, root of American ginseng added.

3. Acupoints: *Qihai, Xinshu, Xuehai, Sanyinjiao, Zusanli* (all with reinforcing technique), *Neiguan, Jianshi, Shanzhong* (all with moderate reinforcing-reducing technique).

(Ⅲ) Hyperactivity of fire due to *yin* deficiency

Key points of pathogenesis: *Yin* deficiency of the heart and the kidney, fire of deficiency type in the interior, lack of moistening the heart channel, contracture pain results.

Chief manifestations: Sudden hot pain in the chest, restlessness and irritability, palpitation and insomnia, dysphoria with feverish sensation in chest, palms and soles, soreness of the loin, flushed cheeks, deep-coloured urine and constipation, deep red colour of tongue proper with little coating, pulse taut thready and rapid.

Therapeutic principle: To nourish body fluid and clear off fore, to replenish the heart and promote the circulation of blood.

1. Patent drugs: *Zhi Bai Di Huang Wan*, 1 bolus each time, t.i.d.

2. Decoction recipe: *Zi Shui Qing Huo Tang* with modifications:

Anemarrhena rhizome 12g, Scrophularia root 30g, Dried rehmannia root 30g, Red sage root 24g, Loranthus mulberry mistletoe 20g, Arisaema tuber 15g, Ophiopogon root 15g, Stir-fried wild jujuba seed 90g, Capejasmine fruit 10g, Moutan bark 10g, for oral administration after being decocted in water,

One dose a day.

Plus-minus: In case with low-grade fever and night sweat salted anemarrhena rhizome, salted phellodendron bark and cinnamon bark are to be included in the recipe; in case with remarkble palpitation and insomnia, lotus plumule and flavescent sophora root included.

3. Acupoints: *Shenshu, Xinshu, Yongquan* (all with reinforcing technique), *Laogong, Xingjian, Ganshu* (all with moderate reinforcing-reducing technique).

4. Ear acupuncture points: Kidney, Heart, *Shenmen*, Sympathetic.

(Ⅳ) Stagnation and obstruction of chest-*yang*

Key points of pathogenesis: Loss of warmth in chest-*yang*, cold formation in the interior, cold phlegm obstruction, and stagnation of heart channels.

Chief manifestations: Pectoral pain radiated to the back, oppressed feeling in chest, with dyspnea, productive cough, restlessness, even coma, sweating, coldness in the limbs, tongue proper whitish, thick and greasy, pulse deep, slippery and thready.

Therapeutic principle: To remove obstruction in *qi* and blood circulation and activate *yang*, to resolve phlegm and induce resuscitation.

1. Patent drug: *She Xiang Bao Xin Dan*, 2 pills each time, b.i.d. or t.i.d. or *Guan Xin Su He Wan*, 1 bolus each time, t.i.d.

2. Decoction recipe: *Gua Lou Xie Bai Ban Xia Tang* with additional ingredients:

Trichosanthes fruit 30g, Macrostom onion 15g, Pinellia tuber 12g, Red sage root 30g, Peucedanum root 12g, Curcuma root 12g, Lepidium seed 12 g, Cinnamon twig 12g, for oral administration after being decocted in water, one dose a day.

Plus-minus: with obvious palpitation and edema, plus poria and white atractylodes rhizome; with expectoration of white phlegm and perspiration and cold limbs, trichosanthes fruit should be withdrawn, prepared aconite root, ginseng, poria and mulberry bark supplemented; to treat coma, cold limbs and weak pulse, the following ingredients added: ginseng, prepared aconite root, schisandra fruit and musk (wrapped for decoction): to treat severe chest pain, further administration of *She Xiang Bao Xin Dan* and *Huo Xin Dan* (melted for intake), 2 pills of each.

3. Acupoints: *Guanyuan*, *Xinshu*, Tanzhong (all with moxibustion technique), *Zhongwan*, *Fenglong*, *Neiguan* (all with reducing technique).

(V) Stagnancy of *qi* and blood stasis

Key points of pathogenesis: Emotional upset, impaired flow of *qi*, disability to take the guiding role of blood, obstruction of the heart collateral.

Chief manifestations: Severe chest pain, twisting and stabbing, distension and fullness in the hypochondrium, oppressive sensation in chest with dyspnea, contracture of the limbs, profuse sweating, deep red tongue proper marked with ecchymosis, tongue coat thin and white, pulse taut and rapid.

Therapeutic principle: To relieve the depressed liver and regulate the circulation of *qi*, to promote blood circulation and stop the pain.

1. Patent drugs:

(1) *Shu Gan He Wei Wan*, 6g each time, t.i.d. Concurrently, *Fu Fang Dan Shen Pian*, 4 tab. t.i.d.

(2) *Huo Xin Dan*, 1 bolus each time, t.i.d.

2. Decoction recipe: *Chai Hu Shu Gan San* with modifications:

Bupleurum root 15g, Curcuma root 15g, Stir-fried bitter orange 15g, White peony root 21g, Red sage root 21g, Trichosanthes fruit 24g, Chuangxiong rhizome 12g, Safflower 10g, Stir-fried ground beetle 10g, Stir-fried corydalis tuber 10g, Licorice root 6g, for oral administration after being decocted in water, one dose a day.

Plus-minus: In case with restlessness and insomnia, plus stir-fried wild jujuba seed and capejasmine fruit; with abdominal distension and constipation, stir-fried radish seed and wine-fried rhubarb; with epigastric fullness and anorexia, magnolia bark and hawthorn fruit.

3. Acupoints: *Neiguan, Ganshu, Xingjian, Shanzhong* (all with reducing technique).

4. Ear acupuncture points: Heart, Liver, Sympathetic.

(Ⅵ) Stagnancy in the stomach

Key points of pathogenesis: Stomach damage due to overeating, food stagnancy in the stomach, obstruction of stomach collateral, acute pain over precordium.

Chief manifestations: Stabbing pain in the chest and stomach, epigastric fullness and abdominal distension. nausea and anorexia, palpitation with throbbing of the heart, constipation, plump tongue with teeth prints at its margins, tongue coat yellowish, thick and greasy, pulse taut, slippery and rapid.

1. Patent drugs: *Da Huang Pian* and *Fu Fang Dan Shen Pian* 4 tablets of each, t.i.d.

2. Decoction recipe: *Xiao Xian Xiong Tang* and *Dan Shen Yin* with modifications:

Trichosanthes fruit 30g, Red sage root 30g, Pinellia tuber 12g, Sandalwood 10g, Wine-fried rhubarb 6g, Amomum fruit 3g, for oral administration after being decocted in water, one dose a day.

Plus-minus: with abdominal distension and constipation, magnolia bark and radish seed are added; to treat remarkble epigastric stuffiness and anorexia, hawthorn fruit, germinated barley and stir-fried radish seed; to treat stabbing pain in the chest, cyperus tuber, stir-fried ground beetle, zedoary, chicken's gizzard-membrane and notoginseng powder.

3. Acupoints: *Zhongwan, Neiting, Neiguan, Shanzhong, Xinshu* (all with reducing technique).

4. Ear acupuncture points: Spleen, Stomach, Heart, Sympathetic, *Shenmen*.

II. Case report:

Case 1: Mr. Cui, 71 years old, worker, admitted into

hospital on Sept. 17, 1982, with complaint of paroxysmal chest pain for more than three years, aggravated for two days. On Dec. 1980, he was admitted into our hospital owing to anterior myocardial infarction. Having been treated with both traditional Chinese and western medicine for more than 80 days, he was discharged from the hospital. Two days ago, following vexation, the patient had such symptoms as violent chest pain, oppressed feeling in the chest with dyspnea, perspiration, aversion to cold, frequent hiccough, loss of appetite, constipation, listleesness, pinkish colour of the tongue with ecchymosis, tongue coat thin whitish and dry, pulse taut thready on the left side and thready weak on the right side. Examination: blood pressure 100/80 mmHg, ECG shows: 1. acute inferior myocardial infarction; 2. old anterior myocardial infarction; 3. chronic coronary insufficiency.

TCM syndrome differentiation and treatment: Blood stasis due to deficient *qi*, true cardiac pain caused by obstruction of stomach collateral. The treatment ought to be directed at replenishing *qi* and promoting blood circulation, removing obstruction in the channels to arrest pain.

Recipe: Astragalus root 30g, Red sage root 30g, Ginseng 10g, Cinnamon twig 10g, Sandalwood 12g, Chuanxiong rhizome 10g, Licorice root 6g, to be decocted in water for oral dose. one dose a day.

Therapeutic effect: After 4 doses of medication, Ginseng was replaced by *Dangshen* 30g. Another 10 doses of medication. ECG turned into subacute inferior myocardial infarction. 29 doses of medication in all. Thereafter, almost all the symptoms subsided. Tongue and pulse normal. ECG indicated old anterior myocardial infarction.

Case 2: Mr. Han, 36 years old, cadre, hospitalization on Dec. 30, 1982.

The patient had severe pain in the chest for a day. He had been staut in constitution. Over the recent three days, as his father was suddenly on critical condition (due to traffic accident), the patient was oversad and angry. Yesterday morning, he had sudden colicky pain in the chest, radiated to the left shoulder and back, oppressed sensation in the chest with dyspnea, dizziness, blurred vision, cold limbs, profuse sweating, general debility and fatigue. He melted three tablets of nitroglycerin in mouth without effect, and then he took *Guan Xin Su He Wan* and amyl nitrite, when his condition was a little bit better, he was hospitalized. The present symptoms: stuffiness and pain in the chest, distension and fullness in both hypochondria, dizziness, blurred vision, restlessness, insomnia, dark red colour of the tongue proper with thin yellowish coating, taut and slippery pulse. Examination: blood pressure 120/70mmHg, moist rales were heard from the inferior lobe of the left lung. ECG indicated acute anterior myocardial infarction.

Syndrome differentiation and treatment: Impairment of liver due to depression and anger, adversive flow of the vital energy, true heart colic caused by contracture of heart collateral. It is suitable to treat by soothing the liver and regulating the flow of *qi*, promoting blood circulation to stop pain.

Recipe: Bupleurum root 15g, White peony root 12g, stir-fried immature bitter orange 10g, Chuanxiong rhizome 10g, Cyperus tuber 10g, Curcuma root 10g, Safflower 10g, Moutan bark 10g, Red sage root 30g, Pueraria root 30g, Trichosanthes fruit 30g, to be decocted in water for oral dose. One dose a day.

Therapeutic effect: After three doses of medication, most symptoms subsided. Continuous intake of above modified recipe. 46 doses in succession. Infarction Q waves disappeared, ECG restored normal.

II. Personal experience

As far as the first case is concerned, combined treatment with traditional and western medicines was carried out during his first time's hospitalization. Finally, despite 80 days' stay in hospital, he was discharged from hospital still with subacute myocardial infarction. Three years after his discharge, again, myocardial infarction was found in different regions. Only with syndrome differentiation and treatment of traditional Chinese medicine, just 29 doses of medication of traditional Chinese drugs are enough. Even Q waves disappeared. Therefore, so long as the differentiation is right, prescription is proper, Chinese medicine can not only treat acute myocardial infarction but also be capable of attaining wonderful effect, which can also be proved in the second case. Both cases confirm that traditional Chinese medicine can work well as the drug for promoting the collateral circulation of the heart.

Variant angina pectoris

Variant angina pectoris differs widely from typical angina pectoris in clinical and EKG manifestations, and in some aspects even towards opposite or reverse direction thus also called reverse angina pectoris. Its clinical characteristic is that the seizure has no relation with physical effort or mental stress, the pain is more intense and it lasts of longer duration than the typical angina. The time of seizure is periodic, often at a certain time of a day or night, exactly the same hour. The more severe seizure is usually accompanied by electro-cardiographic changes such as elevated S-T segment in a certain leads, and depression of S-T segment in its corresponding opposite leads, but without abnormal Q wave. Arhythmia, especially of ventricular type is commonly met. The symptoms are severe and persist longer time, and the more occurrence of acute myocardial infarction, and high ratio of sudden death. This disease pertains to 'xiong bi (chest pain)', 'zhen xin tong (the real heart pain)', 'jue xin tong (the heart pain with syncope)' in TCM.

I. TCM syndrome differentiation and treatment

Pathogenesis in brief: The stagnation of liver *qi*, the maladjustment of *qi* mechanism, the *qi* stagnation and blood stasis. The impeded passage induces pain, and the fluent passage of *qi* and blood will arrest the pain.

Chief manifestations: Chest pain in paroxysmal attack, at a definite time, pain rather severe, referred to back and shoulder. The pain usually occurs during rest, diminish or disappear at motion. Accompanied by chest oppression, mental depression, in scanty hours of sleep interfered with plenty dreams, epigastric fullness and impaired appetite. Tongue proper red, with thin white slimmy coating. Pulse taut or hesitant pulse.

Therapeutic principle: To disperse the liver and regulate the *qi*, to activate the blood circulation and arrest the pain.

1. Patent drug:

(1) *Guan Xin Su He Wan*, one bolus t.i.d.

(2) *Hong Hua* injection, 2 ml I.M. t.i.d.

(3) *Kuan Xiong Wan*, one bolus b.i.d. half an hour prior to the episode.

(4) *Fu Fang Dan Shen Pian*, 4 tablets t.i.d. and *Shu Gan He Wei Wan* 10g t.i.d. regular intake even without seizure.

(5) *Chuan Dan* injection 20~30 ml in 5% glucose 250~500 ml intravenous drip, twice a day.

2. Decoction recipe: *Xue Fu Zhu Yu Tang* with modi-

fications: Bupleurum root 12g, Curcuma root 12g, Chinese angelica root 12g, Red sage root 15g, Peach kernel 15g, Safflower 10g, Stir-fried bitter orange 10g, Sandal wood 10g, Chuanxiong rhizome 12g, Stir-fried corydalis tuber 10g, Licorice root 3g, for oral administration after being decocted in water, one dose a day.

Plus-minus: In case chest pain severe, add musk 1g (in silk envelope, put in after other drugs), grass-leaved sweetflag rhizome 12g, decocted in 500 c.c. yellow rice wine; for constipation cases, add radish seed, wine treated rhubarb; dysphoria with inclination to anger, add rose, moutan bark, capejasmine fruit; sleepless and plenty dreams add fleeceflower vine, albizia flower.

3. Acupoints: *Xinshu, Jueyinshu, Neiguan, Jianshi, Ximen, Shanzhong, Sanyinjiao, Yinlingquan, Taichong* (reducing method during episode, at remissions moderate reinforcing and reducing).

4. Ear acupuncture points: Heart region, *Shenmen*, Endocrine, Subcortex. A pill of *Liu Shen Wan* put on the point and fixed with adhesive plaster, press it during seizure to relieve pain.

5. Digital acupoint pressing method: During acute episode select *Xinshu* or *Ganshu* (left), *Shanzhong, Sanyinjiao*, with thumb pinching and pressing with force, sometimes with immediate relief of pain.

II. Case report

Mr. Zhang, 56 years old, cadre, admitted to the hospital on March 2, 1984, with the chief complaint of severe chest pain for 4 months. Since November 9, 1983 sudden acute chest pain like twisting, associated with sweating, numbness of hands without palpitation and dyspnea. The pain lasted 2 minutes and spontaneously subsided without treatment. Another seizure of pain the very dawn. The electrocardiogram gave a picture of chronic coronary insufficiency and he was treated with sorbide nitrate (carvasin), persantin adalat, segontin, low molecular weight dextran, energy mixture, polarized liquid, Yi Xin Pian and other drugs for more than one month without effect, on the contrary the seizure became more frequent, $2\sim 13$ times a day, each seizure lasted $2\sim 16$ minutes, the severity of pain increased, pain referred to shoulder and back accompanied with profuse sweating. The seizures usually occurred in the morning, $2\sim 6$ A.M., having no relation with intake of food, emotional and weather change. In case no seizure for $1\sim 2$ day, then it is certain to be followed by a sudden and severe attack within $1\sim 2$ day. On physical examination B.P. 170/70 mmHg, heart rate 86/min, rhythm regular. no pathological murmur. Lungs breating sound normal. Tongue slender and lean, tongue proper red with ecchymosis, the hypoglossal veins crooked and engorged, dark purple in color, tongue coat yellow, thick and slimmy. Pulse taut and slippery. The electrocardiogram during severe episode revealed: ① acute subendocardial infarction; ② hypertrophy of left ventricle; ③ coronary artery insufficiency. $S_{V_1} + R_{V_5} = 4.5$ mv, ST segment: V_2 slightly elevated, V_{4-6} slightly lowered. T wave: I, AVL, V_{2-6} deeply inverted 4-16mm. During remission, the electrocardio-rheogram showed $HT = C/A - C = 7$, SV (systole volume) = 44ml/beat, SVI (systole volume index) = 24, CO(cardiac output) = 2.816 liter/min, CI (cardiac index) = 1.57 liter/min/m², IPR (intravascular peripheral resistance) = 2840 dyne.sec.cm^{-5}, apical cardio-gram: A/E-O: 14.2%, wave form: late systolic high plateau. Function of left ventricle: PEP/LVET = 41%. Blood lipids, blood sugar within normal limit. Liver function transaminase 7.

Diagnosis: TCM cardiac pain.

Chronic coronary artery insufficiency. Variant angina pectoris in modern medicine.

Therapy: He was treated with adalat 20mg, carvasin 10mg, aminophylline 0.1mg, valium 2.5mg, pentanitrol 10mg, all above the dose of each time, given three times a day for more than twenty days without effect, and with further addition of papaverine 90 mg in low molecular weight dextran 500ml intravenuous drip daily for seven days, the pain not relieved. TCM drugs used in accordance with the principle to replenish *qi* and activate blood circulation, to remove the obstruction in *yang qi* for 7 days, the principle to replenish *qi* and nourish *yin*, to remove stagnation and arrest pain for half month still no effect. With the therapeutic principle of dispersal of liver *qi*, and activation of blood, resolving stagnation and arresting pain for 25 days with some alleviation of symptoms.

And at last with dispersal of the depressed liver *qi* and removal of stagnation and purgation of bowel, to promote *qi* flow and arrest the pain.

Recipe: Bupleurum root 12g, Curcuma root 12g, Red peony root 12g, Stir-fried bitter orange 12g, Capejasmine fruit 10g, Stir-fried corydalis tuber 10g, Moutan bark 10g, Oriental wormwood 30g, Red sage root 30g, Peach kernel 10g, Chuanxiong rhizome 6g, Rhubarb 6g, Sandal wood 6g, Bamboo shaving 6g, to be decocted in water, one recipe dose daily.

After 31 recipe doses, the condition became gradually better, till the essential disappearance of chest pain. The food ingestion and sleep returned to normal, he could take a walk downstair. Tongue proper red, tongue coat thin and yellow. Pulse slightly taut. B.P. 130/80 mmHg, EKG changes gradually better, with chronic coronary insufficiency left only. T wave V_{4-5} slightly inverted, V_6 low and flat, liver function normal, other examinations all returned to normal. On discharge, he was advised to take *Fu Fang Dan Shen Pian* 4 tablets, *Guan Xin Su He Wan* one bolus, *Shu Gan He Wei Wan* 6g, three times a day, to fortify the therapeutic effect.

Follow-up 6 months later, no seizure.

III. Personal experience

According to TCM, varient angina pectoris pertains to chest pain due to stagnation of liver *qi*, the stagnation of *qi* and blood stasis. The therapeutic principle should aim at the dispersion of depressed liver *qi* mainly, and aided by activating the blood and arresting the pain. This disease pertains to exess syndrome in most cases, and it differs from the common '*xiongbi* (cardiac pain)' in pathogenesis which pertains to deficiency in fundamental and excess in incidental.

It is important advising the patient to eliminate worry and fear, cultivating optimistic spirit to conquer the disease.

Acute myocardial infarction

Acute myocardial infarction (AMI) is one of the most common type of manifestations of coronary artery disease. It is due to acute blockage of coronary artery with severe and persistent ischaemia and the occurrence of necrosis. Clinically with acute and persistent retrosternal pain, fever, leucocytosis, and increased erythrocyte sedimentation rate, increase of serum trans-aminase and other ferments, progressive electrocardiographic changes and others. This disease pertains to the category of 'true heart colic', 'heart colic with cold limbs', 'syncope syndrome', 'collapse syndrome' and others.

I. TCM syndrome differentiation and treatment

Pathogenesis in brief:

Longstanding heart disease, the gradual decline of heart *qi*, the obstruction of collateral with phlegm and stagnation, the body of heart damaged, the asthenia of the fundamental, the sthenia of the incidental.

(I) The impending collapse of heart *yang*

Key points of pathogenesis: The constitution of *yang* insufficiency, the loss of warmth of the heart collateral, the sudden damage of heart body, and the further exhaustion of heart *yang*.

Chief manifestations: Sudden faint and collapse with sweating and cold limbs, facial pallor. After the recovery of consciousness, oppressive chest pain, listlessness. Tongue proper pale, pulse thready and indistinct, knotted orintermittent.

Therapeutic principle: To recuperate the depleted *yang* and treat the cold limbs, to astringe the *yin* fluid, and rescue collapse.

1. Patent drug:

(1) *Shen Mai Zhen*, 20ml add to 50% glucose solution 40ml intravenous drip.

(2) *Sheng Mai Zhen*, the same as (1) or alternate use with (1).

(3) *Yi Xin Kou Fu Ye*, 20ml t.i.d.

2. Decoction recipe: *Shen Fu Tang* and *Sheng Mai San* with modifications:

Prepared aconite root 15g, Ginseng 24g, Red sage root 24g, Ophiopogon root 24g, Schisandra fruit 12g, Honey fried licorice root 10g, Cinnamon twig 6g, for oral administration after being decocted in water, one dose a day.

Plus-minus: Aversion to cold, cold limbs, nocturia, indicate insufficiency of kidney *yang*, add epimedium, bighead atractylodes; dyspnea and restlessness, cough with white sputum, awakened in night due to suffocation indicate up burst of evil fluid to heart and lung, add lepidium seed, acorus rhizome, peucedanum; puffiness of face, epigastric distension, belonging to *yang* deficiency of heart and spleen, minus honeyfried licorice, schisandra fruit, plus bighead atractylodes, poria, areca peel.

3. Acupoints: *Guanyuan, Qihai, Xinshu, Zusanli* (all with moxibustion), *Neiguan, Jianshi, Shanzhong, Tongli* (moderate reinforcing and reducing technique).

4. Pill pressing over ear acupoints: Heart, *Shenmen*, Sympathetic, Subcortex, *Liu Shen Wan* the pill used.

(II) Phlegm-stagnation obstruction

Key points of pathogenesis: Constitution of *yang* asthenia type, the endogenous formation of phlegm and its impediment of heart *qi* and obstruction of heart collateral.

Chief manifestations: Colicky pain of heart and chest, pain of definite site, referred to left shoulder, with oppressive sensation of chest, palpitation and dyspnea, dizziness, cough with plenty sputum. Tongue proper dark purple, with ecchymosis. Tongue coat white and slimmy. Pulse taut and slippery.

Therapeutic principle: To activate *yang* and eliminate phlegm, to resolve stagnation and arrest pain.

1. Patent drug: *Fu Zi* No. 1 injection (racemic demethyl aconitin), 5mg add to 10% glucose 250ml intravenous drip two or three times a day.

2. Decoction recipe: *Gua Lou Xie Bai Ban Xia Tang* and *Shi Xiao San* with modifications:

Trichosanthes fruit 15g, Macrostem onion 10g, Cattail pollen 10g, Trogopterus dung 10g, Corydalis tuber 10g Musk 1g (wrapped with silk), for oral administration after being decocted with water, one dose a day. *Su He Xiang Wan* half a bolus (taken seperately with fluid).

Plus-minus: Chilliness and cold limb, pulse deep and slow, plus cinnamon twig, aconite root, asarum herb; severe chest pain, add red peony root, safflower, chuanxiong, notoginseng powder.

3. Acupoints: *Xinshu, Yanglinquan, Neiguan* (all reinforcing), *Jueyinshu, Jianshi, Shanzhong, Fenglong* (all reducing).

4. Ear acupoints: Heart, *Shenmen*, Sympathetic, Subcortex.

(Ⅲ) Sudden collapse of heart *yang*

Key points of pathogenesis: Sudden collapse of heart *yang*, the loss of warmth of the channels and the obstruction of the blood vessels, spirit departure from the heart, loss of consciousness results.

Chief manifestations: Cloudiness of mind, cold limbs, profuse sweating, purpura of the skin, cyanosis of lips and finger nails, dull pain and oppressive sensation in the chest, respirations irregular, pulse faintly felt with impending stoppage.

Therapeutic principle: To rescue the *yang* from dropping and treat the collapse. To resolve stagnation and stimulate the sensitive orifices.

1. Patent drug: *Shen Fu* injection and *Sheng Mai Zhen*, 40ml each add into 50% glucose solution 50ml intravenous injection, in alternation at half an hour interval, till the rise of blood pressure, nearly to its original level, then change into *Sheng Mai Zhen* 60ml add into 10% glucose solution 250ml intravenous drip.

2. Decoction recipe: *Shen Fu Tang* with modification: Ginseng 15g, Astragalus 30g, Prepared aconite root 10g, Honey-fried licorice root 15g, Dogwood fruit 15g, Ophiopogon root 12g, Red peony root 10g, Chuanxiong rhizome 10g, Safflower 6g, Cinnamon twig 6g, Musk 1g (wrapped with dense silk), for oral administration after being decocted in water, one dose a day.

Plus-minus: Cloudiness of mind prominent add grass leaved sweetflag rhizome, curcuma root, polygala root.

3. Acupoints: *Baihui, Qihai, Guanyuan* (all moxibustion), *Xinshu, Zusanli* (both reinforcing technique of acupuncture), *Shanzhong, Jianshi, Neiguan* (all reducing tech-

nique).

II. Case report

Mr. Liu, 66 years old, cadre, was admitted to hospital on Sept. 30, 1985.

Chest pain, suffocation with impending death for 8 hours, pain referred to the two shoulders, continuous sweating, four limbs not warm, facial pallor, spiritless and malaise, shortness of breath, disinclination to talk. Tongue proper light red, with thin white and wet coating. Pulse thready and weak. B.P. 140/90mmHg. EKG showed acute inferior myocardial infarction.

Diagnosis: TCM *zhen xin tong* (real heart pain). Insufficiency of *qi* and blood, stagnation of heart collaterals.

Western medicine: Acute inferior mural myocardial infarction.

Therapeutic principle: To replenish *qi* and nourish *yin*, to resolve stagnation and make the collaterals patent.

Recipe: *Yi Xin Kou Fu Ye* 15ml t.i.d.

October 5, after medication all the symptoms gradually alleviated, he came out of bed to pass urine, and suddenly felt suffocation with impending death, profuse sweat, cold limbs, shortness of breath, reluctant to speak, tongue proper light red, tongue coat thin and white, pulse thready faintly palpable and intermittent, cardiac rhythm totally irregular, heart sound not uniform with strong and weak beats. Heart rate 65 times a minute. Small bubbling rales at the two bases of lungs. EKG showed: 1.

acute inferior mural myocardial infarction; 2. auricular fibrillation; 3. I° A-V block. In TCM this belonged to expenditure of *qi* on account of motion, the decline and fall of premordial *qi*, the impending collapse of heart *yang* and the impending exhaustion of heart *yin*. The therapeutic principle should be to warm up the *yang* and re plenish the *qi*, to nourish the *yin* and resume circulation.

Recipe: American ginseng 30g, Ophiopogon root 60g, Honey-fried licorice 20g, Cinnamon twig 6g, Flavescent sophora root 6g, Hawthorn fruit 30g, for oral administration after being decocted in water, one dose a day.

Therapeutic effect: 5 hours after the first recipe dose, auricular fibrillation, I° A-V block disappeared. After 6 doses, removed American ginseng, with astragalus and other drugs added. Medication till Oct. 25 all symptoms disappeared. EKG showed subacute inferior mural myocardial infarction, and discharged from hospital.

II. Personal experience

(I) About the classification of typees of acute myocardial infarction in accordance with the TCM syndrome differentiation and treatment: Strictly speaking, there are variations of clinical manifestations of a disease, unable to be entirely included in the types, no matter how many the types may be. So on the basis of type classification it is necessary to be aided by addition or diminution of ingredients with the changes of symptoms. This is beneficial towards the scheme planation and routinization of

TCM therapy.

(Ⅰ) About the therapeutic effect of TCM treatment of acute myocardial infarction (AMI): The prominent effect of TCM in treating AMI is by means of TCM syndrome differentiation and treatment, such as to rescue the fall of *yang* and treat the collapse; to keep the equilibrium balance of *yin* and *yang*, to regulate the activity of *qi* and blood, thus to attain the purpose of eliminating symptoms and curing the disease.

(Ⅱ) The treatment of severe cases of AMI, the TCM syndrome differentiation and treatment should be in accordance with the principle described under this section. In cases not severe or illness already become steady, the treatment may follow the descriptions under the topic of coronary atherosclerotic heart disease or coronary arterial disease (CAD).

Shock

Shock is an acute circulatory dysfunctional syndrome characterized by insufficient blood drainage of organs essential to maintain life. Its main clinical manifestations are drop of blood pressure, acceleration of heart rate, feeble pulse. general malaise, skin cold and wet, facial pallor, cyanosis of lips, oligouria, dysphoria, sluggish reactions, cloudiness of mind, even coma. This pertains to '*jue* syndrom', '*tuo* syndrome', (prostration), '*shen hun*', in

TCM.

I. TCM syndrome differentiation and treatment

Pathogenesis in brief: Extreme deficiency, with exhaustion of *yin* and *yang*, exhaustion of *yin* and exhaustion of *yang* have different manifestations.

(I) Exhaustion of *yang*

Key points of pathogenesis: Exhaustion of *yang qi*, and loss of astringent activity, *yin* fluid excretion from the exterior, and impaired mentality.

Chief manifestations: Cold limbs, profuse cold sweating, feeble respirations, listlessness, even coma. Thirsty, inclination to hot drink, chilliness and lie down curled up with folding of legs. Tongue proper light colored and wet, pulse barely palpable with impending stoppage.

Therapeutic principle: To replenish the *yang* and rescue the collapse.

1. patent drug:

(1) *Shen Fu* injection, 10~20ml added to 50% glucose solution 30~40ml intravenous injection 1~2 times, then 40~80ml, added to 10% glucose solution 250~500ml intravenous drip.

(2) *Fu Zi* No. 1 injection (racemic demethyl aconitin), 5mg add to 10% glucose solution 250ml intravenous drip once or twice daily.

2. Decoction recipe: *Shen Fu Tang* with additional ingredients:

Ginseng 30g, Prepared aconite root 30g, Dogwood

fruit 20g, Schisandra fruit 15g, Red sage root 30g, Licorice 6g, for oral administration after being decocted in water, frequent sip.

Plus-minus: In cases with palpitation or colicky pain in chest, use *Fu Shou Cao Zong Dai* each time 0.6~0.8mg, add to 50% glucose solution 20ml, intravenous slow push, once daily, with the removal of dogwood, and the addition of arborvitae seed, polygala root, grass-leaved sweetflag rhizome, ophiopogon root in the decoction. In cases with chronic cough, dyspnea, and shock, lepidium seed, ginger treated pinellia tuber, mulberry bark, gecko powder should be added.

3. Acupoints: *Baihui, Shenque, Guanyuan* (all moxibustion), *Zusanli, Hegu* (all acupuncture). For coma patient, add acupuncture *Yongquan*.

(Ⅱ) Exhaustion of *yin*

Key points of pathogenesis: The depletion of *yin* fluid unable to astringe the *yang*, and the escape of the asthenic *yang* leading to collapse.

Chief manifestations: Malar flush, dysphoria, mouth dry, thirsty, like to drink, palpitation, sweat a lot, fever, delirium, cold limbs, urine dark and stool constipated. Tongue proper deep red, tongue cost yellow and dry, pulse thready rapid or deep and indistinct, barely palpable.

Therapeutic principle: To rescue *yin* and treat collapse.

1. Patent drug: *Shen Mai Zhen*, 20~30ml add to equal amount of 50% glucose solution, intravenous injection,

repeat at 10~20 minutes interval, till the rise of blood pressure, then changed to intravenous drip.

2. Decoction recipe: *Sheng Mai San* with additional ingredients:

American ginseng 30g, Siberian solomonseal rhizome 24g, Ophiopogon root 30g, Schisandra fruit 15g, Dog wood fruit 20g, Honey-fried licorice root 10g, for oral administration after being decocted in water, one dose a day.

Plus-minus: In cases depletion of *yin* due to high fever, plus *Zi Xue San* 3g swallow with fluid and add scutellaria root, honeysuckle flower, forsythia fruit, capejasmine fruit, isatis leaf; in cases depletion of *yin* due to infectious dysentery, withdrawl of schisandra fruit, dogwood fruit, and addition of phellodendron bark, pulsatilla root, pueraria root, bupleurum root, white peony root; high fever with constipation and impaired consciousness, add rhubarb, scrophularia root, mirabilite; high fever with purpura, add red sage root, moutan bark, red peony root.

3. Acupoints: *Renzhong, Hegu, Shixuan* (all with reducing technique), *Yongquan, Zusanli* (all with reinforcing technique).

(Ⅲ) Exhaustion of *yin* and *yang*

Key points of pathogenesis: *Yang* can not hold the *yin*, the *yin* can not astringe the *yang*, *yin* and *yang* both exhausted, the life will be endangered very soon.

Chief manifestations: Comatous, eyes sluggish in motion, mouth open, pupils dilated, the sweat sticky as oil, rattling in the throat, shortness of breath, respirations rapid, curling of tongue and contraction of testicle coldness of the whole body, purpura, cyanosis of the lips or face and terminals of the limbs. In continence of the urine and stool. Pulse indistinct with impending stop.

Therapeutic principle: To rescue back the *yin* and *yang*, to treat the collapse and awaken the mind.

1. Patent drug: *Sheng Mai Zhen*, 40~60ml with equal amount of 50% glucose intravenous injection in alternation with *Fu Zi* No.1 injection (racemic demethylaconitin) 5mg add to 10% glucose solution 250ml intravenous drip.

2. Decoction recipe: *Sheng Mai San* and *Shen Fu Tang* with additional ingredients:

Red ginseng 30g, Ophiopogon root 45g, Schisandra fruit 15g, Red sage root 30g, Prepared aconite root 24g, Dried ginger 12g, Cinnamon bark 10g, for oral administration after being decocted in water, with the fluid by nasal feed or rectal drip.

Plus-minus: For deep coma plus musk, grass leaved sweetflag rhizome, curcuma root. For rattling in throat add red tangerine peel, bile treated arisaema tuber, grass leaved sweetflag rhizome. For purpura, cyanosis of lips add moutan bark, red peony root, safflower.

3. Acupoints: *Baihui, Shenque, Guanyuan, Qihai, Zusanli* (all moxibustion), *Neiguan, Hegu, Suliao, Yongquan, Renzhong, Shixuan* (all acupuncture, moderate reinforcing and reducing technique).

I. Case report

Mrs. Ni Ma, female, 23 years old, peasant, was admitted in emergency on Nov. 16, 1978 on account of menopause 6 months, coma for three days.

Patient had dragging pain in the lower abdomen with progressive exaggeration 3 days ago. Twelve hours after onset, the pain became very severe lacerating in character. and then spontaneous lysis, but nausea, vomiting, a feeling to defecate, dizziness, and then loss of consciousness. She received symptomatic treatment in a hospital. On account of the gradual downhill of the illness, with stoppage of breathing three times, B.P. 20/0 mmHg, no urine for 2 days, with a tentative diagnosis of rupture of uterus she was tranfered to our hospital.

In 1975, patient had obstructed vaginal passage and uterine rupture during delivery because of cicatrization of vagina, with stillbirth and hemorrhagic shock received emergency treatment in our hospital. After operation on account of fistula of urinary bladder and vagina, fistula of vagina and the rectum, with secondary septicaemia, the operation was to make artificial anus, the recto-vaginal fistula waiting for secondary stage operation.

On examination: Temperature no rise in thermometer, pulse indistinct. respiration 50 times/min, B.P. 40/20mmHg, skin cyanotic, comatous, eyes gazing upward, with the disappearance of ciliary reflex, pupils of equal size, loss of light reflex.Lips cyanotic dry and with fissures, rough breathing sound in both sides of lungs, heart sound low and feeble, heart rate 130 beats/min, abdomen bulging, board like rigidity, palpation not satisfactory, coldness of limbs, the scar formation in lower one third of vagina, only finger tip allowed to get into, and blocked by the softened fetal head. Pushing up the fetal head, from the vagina black putrefecation fluid of foul odor flowed out accompanied with gas bubble.

Continuous oxygen inhalation, after infusion of 5% sodium bicarbonate solution 400ml, heart rate 130 beats/min, respiration 40 times/min, B.P.60/50mmHg. Continued the infusion, and antibiotics, hormones and other emergent measures adopted for hours, B.P. 90/60mmHg, respiration 32/min. Scanty urine leaked out, still comatous. Under local anaesthesia exploration operation done. From the incision opening purple blue bloody fluid flowed out, a black necrotic fetus of the months pregnancy and placenta removed with very foul black fluid about 2000ml flowed out. The length of rupture of uterus 12cm long, endometrium of posterior wall edematous, necrotic. During operation, the blood pressure dropped to 20/0 mmHg, respirations irregular, abdominal cavity closed, abdominal wall and vagina open drainage, operation lasted 30 minutes. After operation continued oxygen inhalation, blood transfusion 400ml, and infusion of 5% sodium bicarbonate solution 200ml. Emergency call of traditional chinese medical doctor for consultation.

Patient comatous, with coldness of four limbs,

cyanosis of lips and the whole body, cold sweat. Pulse feeble, indistinct with impending stoppage. Laboratory examination: CO_2 combining power 19.76 milliequivalent/liter, WBC 2100, neutrophil 89% lymphocyte 11% B.P. 48/30 mmHg.

TCM syndrome differentiation and treatment: From the abdomen the removal of putrefied dead fetus with severe damage of guinuine *qi*, collapse of heart *yang*, the stagnation of blood vessels, the noxious evil not eliminated. The therapeutic principle was to rescue the *yang* and treat the collapse, to stimulate the sensitive orifice and activate the circulation, accompanied by clearing the heat and detoxification.

Recipe: Ginseng 30g, Astragalus 45g, Cinnamon twig 10g, Prepared aconite root 10g, Dogwood fruit 30g, Glehnia root 30g, Dendrobuim 20g, Ophiopogon root 20g, Honeysuckle flower 30g, Forsythia fruit 15g, Red peony root 10g, Polygala 10g, Honey fried licorice root 10g, Musk 1g (wrapped with silk), for oral administration after being decocted in water, one dose a day.

On Nov. 18, 1978, after one dose, the mentality became gradually clear, four limbs became warm, lips and skin color of the body resumed normal. Tongue proper red with little coating. Pulse feeble and weak, B.P. 90/60 mmHg.

Recipe: The above recipe with removal of musk, and the addition of Chinese yam 30g.

On Nov. 24, after four recipe doses, the illness gradually better, she could drink buttered tea, milk and broth. Blood count normal, she could come down from bed and walk. Tongue proper light red, tongue coat thin and white.

Continued the above recipe with the removal of ginseng and the addition of 15g pseudostellaria root. One recipe daily. After removal of the necrotic tissue by gynecologist and the whole layer stitching of the uterus, open drainage from the vagina and abdominal wall. 3 days later the wound healed and discharged from the hospital.

III. Personal experience

Clinically *Jue* or *Tuo* syndrome is an emergent syndrome, the ultimate thing is to adopt prompt treatment, with the acupuncture of digital acupoint pressing first. and medication given by intravenous or rectal route, and decoction should also be ready, and the integrated use of traditional Chinese and western medicine is necessary.

The differentiation of *yang* exhaustion, *yin* exhaustion, or *yin* and *yang* exhaustion is important in TCM. Shock due to infection, bleeding, cardiogenic shock or allergy shock may be treated according to the above mentioned.

Jue syndrome and *Tuo* syndrome can be transferred from each other. Usually *Jue* syndrome is the predromal omen of *Tuo* syndrome (collapse). So the addition of astringent drug even at *Jue* stage is necessary in order to prevent the further progress to *Tuo* syndrome.

Congestive myocardiosis

Congestive myocardiosis is a type of primary myocardiosis, most frequently met in clinic, with the chief manifestation of heart failure. Among the symptoms of which shortness of breath, edema, general malaise, and palpitation are essential. Its etiology still not well known, and the treatment of western medicine can only be symptomatic. This disease pertains to 'palpitation', 'edema', 'dyspnea syndrome'and others in TCM.

I. TCM syndrome differentiation and treatment

Pathogenesis in brief: *Qi* insufficiency of spleen and lung, the stagnation of cardiac blood, not relieved for long time. The damage from *yang* shifts to *yin*, resulting in the insufficiency of *qi* and *yin*, with the stagnacy of *yin* (such as phlegm or body fluid) formed in the interior.

Chief manifestations: Palpitation, chest oppression, shortness of breath, malaise, edema, anorexia, dysphoria and less sleep, even dyspnea, cough with sputum and saliva, restlessness, all the above symptoms aggravated after fatigue. Tongue proper dark red, with ecchymosis. Tongue coat white and slimmy. Pulse deep fine, unsmooth, knotty or intermittent.

Therapeutic principle: To replenish *qi* and nourish

the *yin*; to activate the pulse and sedate the mind.

1. Patent drug: *Shen Mai Zhen*, 40ml add to 10% glucose solution 250ml intravenous drip, once daily.

2. Decoction recipe: *Bao Yuan Tang* and *Sheng Mai San* with modifications:

Astragalus root 30g, Dangshen 15g, Ophiopogon root 30g, Schisandra fruit 6g, Cinnamon twig 10g, Red sage root 30g, Honey-fried licorice root 6g, Peach kernel 10g, Sandal wood 6g, Amomum fruit 6g, one dose daily, add water 500ml, with small fire decoct to 250ml, in two divisions, oral intake seperately.

Plus-minus: In-clination to deficiency of kidney *yang*, with generalized edema, plus prepared aconite root, poria, lepidium seed, alismatis rhizome, peucedanum root. In-clination to *yin* deficiency of heart and kidney with soreness and weakness of loin and knee, vexation and sleepless, remove cinnamon twig, honey-fried licorice, add prepared fleece-flower root, white peony root, lotus plumule, stirfried wild jujuba seed. In-clined to *yang* deficiency and perversion of fluid, with symptoms of epigastric fullness and distention, nausea and vomiting, oppression in chest and palpitation, remove schisandra fruit, honey fried licorice, add ginger treated pinellia tuber, red tangerine peel, poria. For stagnation of heart blood with symptoms of paroxysms of chest pain, tongue proper dark purple, or with ecchymosis, pulse unsmooth, remove schisantra fruit, add red peony root, moutan bark, peach kernal, amber powder (to be swallowed with fluid).

Course: 2 months for one course of treatment, generally 1~3 courses are needed.

3. Acupoints: *Guanyuan, Shenshu, Xinshu, Mingmen, Shenmen* (all moxibustion), *Zhongwan, Shuifen, Fenglong, Xuehai* (all reducing technique).

II. Case report

Mr. Yang 46 years old, peasant, came to clinic on Nov. 5, 1984, with the chief complaint of palpitation, shortness of breath and fatigue for 6 months. 3 years ago, after cold drinks he had dull epigastric pain, aggravated at night, relieved with press, anorexia. In recent 6 months he had palpitation with motion, shortness of breath, fatigue, associated with dryness of mouth and bitter taste in mouth, liquid stool, bad sleep. In the past, no other illness. Tongue proper light red, thin and white coat, pulse slow and weak. On examination: B.P. 140/90 mmHg. EKG showed nodal rhythm, ventricle rate 37 beats each minute, dynamic electrocardiogram calculator scanning: 1. Occasional auricular extrasystole, 2. Sinus bradycardia, 3. I° AVB, 4. Sinus asystole, 5. Nodal escape rhythm, X-ray fluoros-copy: heart enlarged to the left. Echocardiogram showed left and right ventricle cavity enlarged. Mitral valve double peak, inverted. An impression of congestive myocardosis of the expanding type made.

TCM syndrome differentiation: Insufficiency of *qi* and *yin*, with malnutrition of heart vessels.

Western medicine diagnosis: Primary congestive

myocardosis, expansion type.

Therapeutic principle: To replenish *qi* and nourish the *yin*, to activate the pulse and sedate the mind.

Recipe: Astragalus root 15g, Dangshen 15g, Cinnamon twig 12g, Red sage root 24g, Ophiopogon root 15g, White peony root 24g, Chinese angelica root 15g, White atractylodes rhizome 12g, Poria 15g, Peach kernel 10g, Pueraria root 30g, Amomum fruit 3g, Honey-fried licorice 6g, for oral administration after being decocted in water, one dose a day.

According to the above recipe with some modifications 15 doses taken, all the symptoms disappeared. After 185 doses, he could attain heavy physical labor work without any discomfort, just like before this illness. Tongue proper light red, with thin and white coating. Pulse was moderate. EKG showed sinus brady cardia. Echocardiogram revealed slight enlargement of left ventricle cavity, right ventricle cavity resumed normal. X-ray fluoroscopy: Heart and lung normal.

II. Personal experience

To treat this disease it is difficult to get prompt therapeutic effect. After medication, if there is no aggravation of symptoms, no need to alter the prescription till 10 recipe doses were taken. The drugs were capable to activate the blood and remove stagnation, such as peach kernel, ground beetle and others should be used from the beginning to the end, but it is no use to give overdosage, this is in accordance with the principle to stop while a bigger half of the illness removed, the rest left to the recovery on behalf of his own ability, including rest and proper diet.

During treatment the author had the impression that it is comparatively easy to attain the disappearance of symptoms, and is more difficult to get electrocardiographic improvement, and the most difficult of all is the echocardiogram improvement.

Gall bladder–heart syndrome

Gall bladder-heart syndrome is a myocardial metabolic disorder due to intoxication from the biliary tract infection and toxin absorption. Biliary hypertension can reflex ively induce precordial pain and arrhythmia. The chief clinical manifestations are precordial pain and arrhythmia. This disease pertains to the category of 'hypochondriac pain', *'xiong bi'* (*qi* obstruction in the chest) and 'palpitation'.

I. TCM syndrome differentiation and treatment

Pathogenesis in brief: Stagnation of biliary tract, the dysfunction of stomach, the stasis of gastric collateral and the impeded function of heart.

Chief manifestations: Paroxysmal attack of chest pain, referred to the hypochondria, distending pain of the right hypochondrium, with pain referred to the shoulder and back, palpitation and restlessness, accompanied by chest oppression and epigastric fulness, impaired appetite, bitter taste of mouth, dryness of throat, all symptoms aggravated by anger, slightly relieved after belching of gas. Tongue proper red, tongue coat white and slimmy. Pulse taut.

Therapeutic principle: To disperse the liver and biliary tract; to regulate stomach function and relieve the pain.

1. Patent drug: *Shu Gan He Wei Wan*, 10g t.i.d.

2. Decoction recipe: *Chai Hu Shu Gan San* with modifications:

Bupleurum root 12g, Curcuma root 12g, Stir-fried bitter orange 10g, Spikenard 12g, Sichuan chinaberry 12g, White peony root 15g, Stir-fried corydalis tuber 12g, Sandal wood 10g, Cyperus tuber 10g, Licorice 3g, for oral administration after being decocted in water, one dose a day.

Plus-minus: With fever and jaundice plus capejasmine fruit, Chinese gentian, dandelion herb; *Fu* in excess and constipated, add mirabilite, stir-fried radish seed; stone formation due to damp heat accumulation, add lysimachia, chicken's gizzard membrane.

3. Acupoints: *Ganshu, Danshu, Zhangmen, Qimen, Zhongwan, Taichong, Neiguan, Yanglingquan, Jianli* (all with reducing technique).

II. Case report

Ms. Xu, 42 years old, cadre, came to clinic on June 25, 1988, with the chief complaints of paroxysmal chest pain and palpitation for 25 days, she was examined in a certain hospital, with electrocardiogram showing myocardial *lao lei* (strain), auricular presystole, after treatment with nitroglycerine, sorbide nitrate, valium, amiodaronum and others, the chest pain not relieved, still had palpitation, thus came to our hospital. The present symptoms consisted of paroxysmal chest pain, palpitation and chest oppression, epigastric fulness and dull aching pain, referred to the right hypochondrium, bitter taste of mouth, throat dryness, nausea and retching, disgust to oily food, urination dark colored, stool constipated. Tongue proper red, with light yellowish and slimmy coating. Pulse taut, slippery and rapid. Ultrasonic B of liver and biliary tract suggested chronic cholecystitis. EKG showed myocardiac strain and frequent auricular extrasystole.

A diagnosis was made by western medicine of biliary heart syndrome.

TCM syndrome differentiation and treatment: Accumulated heat and dampness, disharmony between liver and stomach, *qi* stagnation, and blood stasis of heart collaterals. The reasonable treatment should be to disperse the *qi* of liver and biliary tract. To clear off heat and resolve stagnation.

Recipe: Bupleurum root 15g, Curcuma root 12g,

Capejasmine fruit 12g, Stir-fried immature bitter orange 12g, Rhubarb 6g, Oriental wormwood 30g, Flavescent sophora root 12g, Ginger treated bamboo shaving 10g, Stir-fried corydalis tuber 10g, Coptis root 6g, to be decocted in water one recipe dose daily.

The second visit on July 2. After 5 doses, the chest pain and palpitation disappeared, and the other symptoms alleviated too. Loose stool two times a day. Tongue proper light red, with thin, yellow coat. Pulse taut and slippery.

From the above recipe rhubarb and coptis root removed, and pinellia tuber 10g, poria 12g, barley sprout 15g, added, decocted in water, for oral take, one recipe dose daily.

The third visit on July 9. Another seven doses taken, nearly all the symptoms disappeared, still some anorexia and malaise. Tongue proper light red, tongue coat white and slimmy. Pulse moderate. She was given a prescription of *Xiao Yao Wan* 6g t.i.d. continued for another month in order to fortify the therapeutic effects.

III. Personal experience

In the clinic while encountering cases with paroxysmal attack of chest pain and cardiac arrhythmia not effective with medicines capable to dilate the coronary artery, and treat the cardiac arrhythmia, we have to keep this disease (the gallbladder-heart syndrome) in mind. Digital pressing and pinching the acupoints of *Ganshu*, or

Danshu, frequently with immediate relief of pain. Besides, complicated with cardiac arrhythmia, further addition of *Neiguan* point is helpful.

Viral myocarditis

Viral myocarditis refers to the myocarditis caused by varieties of viruses. The inflammatory lesions of the disease may be localized or diffuse, acute, subacute or chronic. The inflammation may invade the myocardial mesenchyme and the myocardial fiber showing various degrees of dys-tropic changes scattered between the regions of necrosis and fibrosis. In the recent years the research of the disease has been going on enthusiastically. Myocarditis may be induced by many pathogneic organisms and diseases such as Coxsackie virus, ECHO virus as well as viruses of poliomyelitis, measles, chicken-pox, parotitis, influenza, epidemic hemorrhagic fever and others, of which the disease caused by enterovirus is the most important and most common. The myocarditis which, in the past, was considered to be due to influenza virus is in fact induced by Coxsackie virus and ECHO virus. In TCM, this disease is categorized as 'epidemic febrile disease', 'palpitation', 'chest pain', etc.

I. **TCM syndrome differentiation and treatment**

Pathogenesis in brief: Invasion of virus into the

viscera, consumption of *yin* and impairment of *qi*, resulting in mal-nourishment of the heart.

(I) Blazing evil heat in both the *qi* and *ying* systems

Key points of pathogenesis: Virulence in both *ying* and blood systems, giving rise to extreme excess of *qi* and extreme heat of blood, persistant existence of evil-heat that threatens the internal organs.

Chief manifestations: High fever. flushed face, swelling and pain in the throat, dry mouth and tongue, thirst without wish to drink more, purple skin eruption, or hematemesis, hematuria, palpitation, irritability, even mania, delirium, deep red colour of tongue proper with thin yellowish coating, strong and rapid pulse.

Therapeutic principle: To clear off heat from *ying* system; to protect *yin* by detoxicating.

1. Patent drug:
(1) *Xi Ling Jie Du Pian*, 24 tablets, t.i.d.
(2) *Yin Huang* injection, 4ml t.i.d. i.m.

2. Decoction recipe: *Qing Wen Bai Du San* with modifications:

Honeysuckle flower 45g, Forsythia fruit 18g, Arctium fruit 10g, Peppermint 10g, Platycodon root 12g, Dried rehmannia root 30g, Ophiopogon root 30g, Moutan bark 15g, Isatis leaf 30g, Gypsum 45g, Common reed 45g, Licorice root 6g, for oral administration after being decocted in water, one dose a day.

Plus-minus: Anemarrhena rhizome, scrophularia root

ought to be added to the recipe for the case marked by remarkable high fever and thirst; additional administration of *Zi Xue San* for the case with loss of consciousness and constipation; cogongrass rhizome, capejasmine fruit and madder root for the case with epistaxis.

3. Acupoints: *Dazhui, Quchi, Shaoshang, Hegu, Laogong, Taichong* (all with reducing technique), *Houxi, Xinshu* (both with reinforcing technique).

(II) Deficiency of both *qi* and *yin*

Key points of pathgenesis: Prolonged invasion of noxious heat, consumption of *qi* and *yin*, obstruction in the heart collateral, disturbance in the blood transportation.

Chief manifestations: Severe palpitation, insomnia, dreamfulness, lassitude, vague pain in chest, restlessness, all aggravated during motion, pink colour of tongue proper, thready and weak pulse.

Therapeutic principle: To replenish *qi* and nourish *yin*; to remove obstruction in the channels and allay excitement.

1. Patent drug: *Ren Shen Jian Pi Wan* and *Bai Zi Yang Xin Wan*, 1 bolus of each t.i.d.

2. Decoction recipe: *Zhi Gan Cao Tang* with modifications:

Honey-fried licorice root 12g, Ginseng 10g, Astragalus root 45g, Ophiopogon root 30g, Dried rehmannia root 24g, Donkey-hide gelatin 10g (melted), Cinnamon twig 10g, Red sage root 15g, Arborvitae seed 12g, Stir-fried wild jujuba seed 18g, Tangerine peel 6g, for oral administration after being decocted in water, one dose a day.

Plus-minus: In case exhibiting more sign of *yang* deficiency of *qi*, palpitation and edema, plus 6 grams of poria, white atractylodes rhizome and sepium periploca bark; in case exhibiting more sign of insufficiency of yin-blood, tidal fever and irritability, plus scrophularia root, and capejasmine fruit; with obvious lassitude and anorexia, plus white actractylodes rhizome, poria and amomum fruit. If the illness is chronic and persistent, peach kernal, safflower, luffa, and sweet gum fruit are to be added.

3. Acupoints: *Guanyuan, Xinshu, Ganshu, Shenmen* (with reinforcing technique).

4. Ear acupoints: Heart, Kedney, Sympathetic.

I. Case report

Case 1: Mr. Wang, 38 years old, cadre, came to seek medical advice for the first time in 1979.

The patient suffered from one day's aversion to cold and high fever accompanied by discomfort in throat, continous violent palpitation and restlessness, pantalgia, some stiffness of neck, thirst with predilection of more drinking, epistaxis, deep-coloured urination, constipation, bright red colour of tongue proper with thin yellowish coating, full, rapid and running pulse. Examination: body temperature 39.5°C, WBC 6800, heart rate 115 beats/min, arrhythmia, ECG: ① sinus tachycardia; ② muscular strain of inferior mura of heart; ③ occasional premature beat. Diagnosis of western medicine: ① influenza; ② virus myocarditis.

TCM syndrome differentiation and treatment: Invasion of epidemic toxins, blazing of evil-heat in both the *qi* and *ying* systems. It is advisable to direct the treatment at clearing away heat and toxic material, reducing the heat in *ying* system and promoting blood circulation.

Recipe: Honey suckle flower 45g, Frosythia fruit 15g, Isatic leaf 30g, Pueraria root 15g, Gypsum 45g, Anemarrhena rhizome 12g, Dried rehmannia root 30g, Red peony root 15g, Moutan bark 12g, Red sage root 20g, Capejasmine fruit 10g, Common reed 45g, Licorice root 6g, for oral administration after being decocted in water, one dose a day.

Therapeutic effect: After 5 doses of medication, body temperature 37.5°C, all the symptoms were relieved. Continuous administration of above recipe with exclusion of gypsum, anemarrhena rhizome, red peony root, moutan bark and isatic leaf, and with addition of opiopogon root, pseudostellaria root, glehnia root, coix seed, white atractylodes rhizome, poria, and hawthorn fruit. After another 21 doses of medication, all the symptoms disappeared, body temperature normal, ECG normal.

Case 2: Mr.Yang, 43 years old, hospitalized for treatment on April 9, 1979.

The patient has had palpitation, shortness of breath,

and chest pain for three months. Three months ago, after exposure to cold he had high fever palpitation and stuffy sensation in chest . Having been treated with western medicine, his high fever subsided, but palpitation and stuffiness in chest were not relieved. From western medicine, his disease was diagnosed as virus myocarditis, arrhythmia. While treated with a variety of drugs such as lidocaine, segontin, dilantin, sorbid nitrate, prednisone, creatinine, and decoction of honeyfried licorice root, the effect was poor. The following symptoms still present: severe palpitation, shortness of breath, weakness, stuffiness in chest with dyspnea, dizziness, irritability, insomnia, anorexia, pink colour of tongue proper with whitish coating, thready weak pulse which was also uneven or intermittent. ECG: ventricular premature beat presenting trigeminal pulse, left anterior branch block.

TCM syndrome differentiation and treatment: The disease was ascribed to the deficiency of both *qi* and *yin*, lack of nourishment of the heart and the mind. It was advisable to aim the treatment at replenishing *qi* and tonifying *yin*, removing obstruction in the channels and tranquilizing the mind.

Recipe: Honey-fried licorice root 30g, Astragalus root 30g, Dangshen 30g, Cinnamon twig 30g, Schisandra fruit 18g, Red sage root 21g, Curcuma root 9g, Spatholobus stem 30g, Stir-fried ground beetle 12g, Ophiopogon root 15g, Stir-fried wild jujuba seed 20g, Tangerine peel 10g, for oral administration after being decocted in water, one dose a day.

Therapeutic effect: With 12 doses of medication, all the symptoms basically disappeared. ECG restored normal.

II. Personal experience

In the clinical treatment of viral myocarditis, what counts is the early treatment of primary disease, to prevent noxious pathogen from invading the heart. Hence, at the beginning, antipyretics and detoxicants should be large in dosage to dominate the treatment in order to attack evils with drastic action. In the course of treatment, to nourish *yin* and replenish *qi* should be focused all the time to nourish heart and restore its function. Prolonged disease will invade collateral, for this reason, it is necessary to supplement drugs for activating *qi* and promoting blood circulation in the late stage of the disease.

Sick sinus syndrome

Sick sinus syndrome is the consequence of the disorders of automatic pacing function or transmission due to ischemia or inflammation of sinus node and its surrounding tissue, thus resulting in bradycardia and a series of symptoms including general symptoms, nerve and heart symptoms and others, to constitute a syndrome entity. In severe cases, there might occur Adams-stokes syndrome or sudden death. In TCM, the disease pertains to the category of 'vertigo', 'palpitation', 'cold limbs', 'prostration syndrome', and others. At present time, the treatment with western medicine can manage to reduce and prevent the attack of Adam-stokes syndrome, but the therapeutic effect is not stable, especially in the later period. Although to install an artificial pacemaker is a new therapeutic method, it is limited by many conditions, and therefore, not readily accepted by patients. To treat with traditional Chinese medicine has clinically proved to be quite effective, and quite a few patients have recovered from the illness. This illustrates that the pathologic change of sick sinus is not irreversible.

I. TCM syndrome diffierentiation and treatment

Pathogenesis in brief: Prolonged illness impairing *yang*, insufficiency of the heart-*yang*, the phlegm obstruction of the collaterals and the stagnation of blood vessels.

(I) Insufficiency of the heart-*qi*

Key points in pathogenesis: Long-standing illness injuring *qi*, and the *qi* loses its ability to lead blood as a guide, thus blood circulation slowed and even complicated with blood stasis.

Chief manifestations: General debility, fatigue, shortness of breath with disinclination to talk, palpitation, spontaneous perspiration, plump tongue with whitish coating, deep slow and weak pulse. In case with stagnation, often with stabbing pain in the chest, dark red color of the tongue proper or with ecchymosis, pulse deep slow and hesitant.

Therapeutic principle: To replenish *qi* and warm the *yang*, so as to promote blood circulation.

1. Patent drug: *Ren Shen Jian Pi Wan*, 1 bolus each time, t.i.d. Concurrently, *Fu Fang Dan Shen Pian* 4 tablets each time, t.i.d.

2. Decoction recipe: *Bao Yuan Tang* and *Dan Shen Yin* with modifications:

Astragalus root 30g, Ginseng 10g, Cinnamon twig 10g, Honey-fried licorice root 6g, Sandal wood 10g, Amomum fruit 10g, for oral administration after being decocted in water, one dose a day.

Plus-minus: In case with remarkble chest pain, plus rose, peach kernel and chuanxiong rhizome; with remarkble spontaneous perspiration, plus white atrctylodes rhizome and ledebouriella root.

3. Acupoints: *Qihai*, *Mingmen*, *Xinshu* (all with moxibustion technique), *Zusanli*, *Shanzhong*, *Shenmen* (all with reinforcing technique), *Xuehai* (with reducing technique).

(II) Insufficiency of heart-*yang*

Key points of pathogenesis: *Qi* deficiency involving *yang*, loss of warmth of heart channel, slow blood circulation, with production of a lot of cold manifestations.

Chief manifestations: Dizziness, aversion to cold, palpitation, shortness of breath, urine clear, urination long even sudden fall with unconsciousness, cold limbs, and recover consciousness soon after, pale tongue proper with thin whitish coating, deep and slow pulse.

Therapeutic principle: To warm and invigorate the heart-*yang*, to disperse coldness, to activate collateral.

1. Patent drug:

(1) *Guan Xin Su He Wan*, 1 pill each time, t.i.d.

(2) *Fu Fang Dang Gui* injection, 2 ml each time, i.m. once a day.

2. Decoction recipe: *Ma Huang Fu Zi Xi Xin Tang* with modifications:

Honey-fried Ephedra 12g, Prepared aconite root 10g, Asarum herb 6g, Cinnamon twig 10g, Honey-fried licorice root 10g, Chinese ange-lica root 12g, Epimedium 12g, for oral administration after being decocted in water, one dose a day.

Plus-minus: Psoralea fruit, antler, and morinda root are to be employed for the case with cold pain in loin and knees exhibiting more signs of the deficiency of kidney-*yang*; Poria, white atractylodes rhizome and sepium periploca bark for the case with flooding of body fluid due to *yang* deficiency.

3. Acupoints: *Guanyuan, Qihai, Shenshu, Xinshu, Mingmen* (all with moxibustion technique), *Shuifen, Fenglong* (both with reducing technique).

(III) Insufficiency of *yin*-blood

Key points in pathogenesis: Prolonged and persistant illness, impairment of *yang* affecting *yin*, disability of *yin* to astringe *yang*, disability of blood to nourish the heart.

Chief manifestations: Severe palpitation, insomnia, dreamfulness, dry mouth and throat, irritability, night sweat, red colour of tongue proper with little coationg, fine and slow pulse, or sometimes slow, sometimes rapid.

Therapeutic principle: To replenish yin and nourish blood, to remove obstruction in the channels and tranquilize the mind.

1. Patent drug: *Yi Xin Kou Fu Ye*, 10ml each time. t.i.d.

2. Decoction recipe: *Sheng Mai San* with additional ingredients:

American ginseng 10g, Ophiopogon root 30g, Siberian solomonseal rhizome 15g, Schisandra fruit 8g, Red peony root 12g, Fleece flower stem 30g, Licorice root 3g, for oral administration after being decocted in water, one dose a day.

Plus-minus: In case complicated with blood stasis, notoginseng powder (taken after mixing with water), moutan bark are employed; if complicated with yang deficiency, epimedium and cinnamon twig employed; for those with exuberance of fire of deficient type, anemarrhena rhizome, phellodendron bark and cinnamon bark added.

3. Acupoints: *Taixi, Shenshu, Xinshu, Sanyinjiao, Xuehai* (all with reinforcing technique), *Taichong, Laogong Xinjian* (all with reducing technique).

II. Case report

Mr. zhang, 60 years old, came to see medical advice on April 6, 1984. Hospitalization No. 33995. Stuffy pain in the chest for years and aggravated for half month.

On April 5 last year, after exposure to cold, the patient abruptly produced such symptoms as dizziness, fatigue, chest pain, cold limbs, palpitation, shortness of breath, and he went to a doctor without delay. ECG suggested chronic coronary insufficiency, sinus bradycardia, heart rate 45 beats per minute, incomplete right bundle branch block. After intake of sorbide nitrate, and persantine and melting nitroglycerin, his symptoms were relieved. From then on, whenever he was run down, or emotional excited or overeating, the above symptoms appeared. However, ECG sometimes indicated tachycardia, heart rate 105~120 beats per minute. 15 days ago, all the symptoms were aggravated owing to fatigue.

Present symptoms: Stuffy pain in the chest, fatigue and weakness, vertigo, blurred vision, cold limbs, poor appetite, palpitation, shortness of breath, abdominal distension, liquid or loose stool, dark colored tongue proper with thin whitish coating, pulse deep, slow and weak. Blood pressure: 120/80 mmHg. Heart sounds low and blunt, heart rate regular, 46 beats per minute. ECG: chronic insufficiency of blood supply of coronary artery, sinus bradycardia, heart rate: 43 beats per minute, incomplete right bundle branch block.

Diagnosis of western medicine: 1. chronic insufficiency of blood supply of coronary artery. 2. sick sinus syndrome.

TCM syndrome differentiation and treatment: This disease is caused by deficiency of heart-*yang*, and obstruction of heart collateral. It is advisable to treat by replenishing *qi* and warming *yang*, promoting blood circulation to remove obstruction in the channels.

Recipe: Astragalus root 30g, Dangshen 15g, Cinnamon twig 12g, Honey-fried licorice 10g, Red sage root 24g, Chuanxiong rhizome 12g, Rose 10g, Sandal wood 10g, Amomum fruit 6g, Stir-fried radish seed 12g, for oral administration after being decocted in water, one dose a day.

Acupoints: *Guanyuan, Qihai, Xinshu, Mingmen* (all with moxibustion), *Zusanli, Shanzhong* (all with reinforcing technique), *Xuehai* (with reducing technique), once a day.

Therapeutic effect: With 41 doses of medication and 41 times of acupuncture, almost all the symptoms disappeared, pink tongue proper with thin whitish coating, pulse moderate and forceful. ECG indicated: chronic insufficiency of blood supply of coronary artery, (better than the previous ECG). Heart rate: 62 beats per minute.

III. Personal experience

In regard to pathogenesis and treatment: This syndrome is clinically differentiated into three type, these three are related and annexed to one another, so they can not be completedly seperated. For example, prolonged deficiency of *qi* would develop into deficiency of *yang*, consequently, deficienty of *yang* must be complicated with deficiency of *qi*, therefore, to warm *yang* and to replenish *qi* are usually employed simultaneously. The existence of *yin* is the prerequisite of the existence of *yang*. The impairment of *yang* would impede the generation of *yin* and in turn impairment of *yin* would impede the generation of *yang*, giving rise to the deficiency of both *yin* and *yang*, so the treatment principle is to employ both nourishing *yin* and warming *yang*, both replenishing *qi* and nourishing *yin*. The relationship between *qi* and blood is particularly close, deficiency of *qi* leads to its disability to take the guiding role of blood, and this results in blocked blood flow, while deficiency of blood leads to its disability to carry *qi*, resulting in exhaustion of *qi*. Hence, replenishment of *qi* is usually combined with the promotion of blood circulation, and the replenishment of *qi* and replenishment of blood usually applied together.

The pathogenesis of the disease: It begins with deficiency of *qi*, gradually invades *yang*, and results in deficiency of both *yin* and *yang*, *qi* and blood. Analyzing and differentiating pathological conditions in accordance with the eight principal syndromes, deficiency is considered to be fundamental and among the deficiencies the deficiency of *yang* is essential. As internal organs concerned, the fundamental is the kidney and the incidental is the heart.

As for stagnation of phlegm, blood stasis and accumulated cold, they are merely the pathological results of deficiency of *qi* and *yang* and in turn acting as causes for some symptoms.

Cardiac arrhythmia

Cardiac arrhythmia is the complication or sequale of many kinds of heart disease. Cardiac arrhythmia may also exist as an isolated entity, and commonly met in clinics. In severe cases, it may aggravate the diseased condition, even endanger life. It belongs to the category of *'xin ji','zheng chong'* (palpitation with or without external stimuli).

I. TCM syndrome differentiation and treatment

Pathogenesis in brief: The prosperity or decline of *yin* and *yang*, the waxing and waning of *qi* and blood, either belonging to cold or heat, being of excess or sthenia, of deficiency or asthenia, all capable to retard the circulation and induce arrhythmia with the appearance of irregular pulses the knotty, the intermittent and the runing pulses.

(I) Sthenic cold syndrome

Key Points of pathogenesis: Cold evil has the property to make things contract, thus the contraction of blood vessels resulting in blood stasis. The pulse is usually slow.

Chief manifestations: Palpitation and shortness of breath, chest oppression and pain, alleviated while warm, exaggerated after exposure to cold. All symptoms slightly attenuated during motion. Urine clear and amount not scanty. Tongue proper light red, with white and wet coating, pulse slow and forceful.

Therapeutic principle: To warm up the channel and expel the cold, to activate the collaterals and attain recovery of pulse.

1. Patent drug: *Fu Zi Li Zhong Wan*, one bolus t.i.d. swallow the bolus with decocted fluid of fresh ginger.

2. Decoction recipe: *Ma Huang Fu Zi Xi Xin Tang* with additional ingredients:

Honey-fried ephedra 12g, Prepared aconite root 10g, Asarum herb 3g, Chinese angelica root 12g, Cinnamon twig 12g, Honey fried licorice 15g, Fresh ginger 10g, for oral administration after being decocted in water, one dose a day.

Plus-minus: Associated with phlegm stagnation plus pinellia tuber, macrostem onion; with *qi*-stagnation plus cyperus tuber, curcuma root; with blood stasis, plus chuanxiong rhizome, safflower.

3. Acupoints: *Fengchi, Dazhi, Waiguan*(indirect moxibustion with ginger in between), *Xinshu, Pishu, Feishu* (all acupuncture with reinforcing technique).

(II) Asthenic cold syndrome

Key points of pathogenesis: Asthenia of *yang qi* with

exuberance of cold in the interior the loss of warmth and activation of blood vessels.

Chief manifestations: Palpitation and restlessness, chest oppression and shortness of breath, feeling of vacancy, dizziness and malaise, with aggravation after physical strain. Aversion to cold, cold limbs. Tongue proper light colored, coat thin and white. Pulse deep, slow and without strength.

Therapeutic principle: To warm up the *yang* and dispel the cold, to replenish the *qi* and restore the pulse.

1. Patent drug: *Jin Gui Shen Qi Wan* and *Bu Zhong yi Qi Wan*, one bolus t.i.d. with white wine 15g as guiding drug.

2. Decoction recipe: *Er Xian Tang* with modifications: Curculigo rhizome 12g, Epimedium 12g, Indian mulberry root 10g, Chinese angelica root 12g, Psoralea fruit 12g, Prepared aconite root 10g, Cinnamon twig 10g, Sepium periploca bark 6g, Honey fried licorice 10g, Astragalus root 15g, for oral administration after being decocted in water, one dose a day.

Plus-minus: Complicated with phlegm, plus macrostem onion, pinellia tuber, asarum; with blood stasis, add chuanxiong rhizome, safflower.

3. Acupoints: *Qihai, Guanyuan, Xinshu, Pishu, Shenshu* (all moxibustion), *Shenmen, Zusanli, Neiguan* (all acupuncture with reinforcing technique).

(III) Sthenic heat syndrome

Key points of pathogenesis: Exuberance of heat, with

strong propelling force and accelerated blood circulation, the pulse in most cases rapid.

Chief manifestations: Palpitation, fever, thirsty with preferance to cold drink, vexation, dreamfulness, urine dark colored and constipation. Tongue proper red with yellow coating. Pulse slippery, rapid and forceful.

Therapeutic principle: To clear off heat and purge the fire. To cool the blood and sedate the mind.

1. Patent drug:

(1) *Niu Huang Qing Xin Wan* one bolus t.i.d.

(2) *Ba Li Ma* injection, 1mg, i.m. once a day.

2. Decoction recipe: *Qing Xin Tang* with modifications:

Rehmannia root 30g, Ophiopogon root 24g, Coptis root 10g, Capejasmine fruit 10g, Flavescent sophora root 10g, Lotus plumule 10g, Licorice 3g, for oral administration after being decocted in water, one dose a day.

Plus-minus: With phlegm in addition, plus trichosanthes fruit, thunberg fritillary bulb, anemarrhena rhizome. High fever, sore throat, further add subprostrate sophora root, platy-codon root, isatidis root, gypsum, scrofularia root, rhinoceros horn powder, dry stool, add scrofularia, rhubarb. In cases with food stagnancy add radish seed, hawthorn fruit, forsythia fruit. For blood stasis add red sage root, moutan bark, red peony root.

3. Acupoints: *Hegu, Neiguan, Zusanli, Fenglong, Laogong, Yongquan, Xinshu* (all with reducing technique).

(IV) Asthenia fever syndrome

Key points of pathogenesis: Insufficiency of *yin* and blood, no filling of blood vessel, asthenic fever agitation, pulse fine and rapid.

Chief manifestations: Palpitation, easily frightened, scanty sleep, forget-fulness, tidal fever, sweat while asleep, feverishness over palms, soles and in the chest. Body of tongue thin, tongue proper red with little coating. Pulse fine rapid and weak.

Therapeutic principle: To nourish the *yin* and reinforce the *qi*, to clear the heat and sedate the mind.

1. Patent drug:

(1) *Bu Xin Dan*, 10g t.i.d.

(2) *Zhu Sha An Shen Wan*, 10g t.i.d.

2. Decoction recipe: *Sheng Mai San* with modifications:

Pseudostellaria root 30g, Rehmannia root 30g, Schisandra fruit 10g, Ophiopogon root 24g, Lotus seed 6g, Licorice root 3g, for oral administration after being decocted in water, one dose a day.

Plus-minus: Sweat while sleep, add dragon's bone, oyster shell, floating wheat; dysphoria with little sleep, add capejasmine fruit, stir-fried wild jujuba seed.

3. Acupoints: *Xinshu*, *Shenshu*, *Houxi*, *Shenmen* (all with reinforcing technigue), *Neiguan*, *Hegu* (all with reducing technique).

(V) Deficiency of *yin* and *yang*

Key points of pathogenesis: Both deficiency of *yin* and *yang*, no filling of blood vessels, pulse weak, knotty pulse and intermittent pulse.

Chief manifestations: Palpitation, dizziness, chest oppression, shortness of breath, chilliness and cold limbs, soreness and weakness of loin and knees. Tongue proper light colored, tongue coat white, pulse weak and knotty and intermittent.

Therapeutic principle: To reinforce the *qi* and activate *yang*, to nourish blood and recovery of pulse.

1. Patent drug:

(1) *Jin Gui Shen Qi Wan*, one bolus t.i.d.

(2) *Wan Nian Qing* injection, each time 2~4 ml. with 50% glucose solution 20 ml, diluted and slow push, three times a day, or i.m., each time 4 ml q.i.d.

2. Decoction recipe: *Zhi Gan Cao Tang* with modifications:

Honey fried licorice 12g, Dangshen 15g, Cinnamon twig 10g, Rehmannia root 30g, Ophiopogon root 30g, Donkey-hide gelatin 12g (melted with heat), Stir-fried wild jujuba seed 30g, Arborvitae seed 12g, Fresh ginger 6g, Chinese date 5 pieces, for oral administation after being decocted in water, one dose a day.

Plus-minus: Vexation and less sleep, plus lotus plumule, flavescent sophora root; for chest pain add cat-tail pollen, peach kernel; oppressive ache over chest and epigastrium, minus rehmannia root, Donkey-hide gelatin, plus red sage root, sandal wood, amomum fruit; chest oppression with plenty sputum, remove rehmannia root, donkey-hide gelatin, add trichosanthes fruit, peucedanum root;

dizziness and malaise add astragalus root, pueraria root. With *yin* deficiency prominent, vexation and hotness over palms, soles and in the chest, remove cinnamon twig, and add anemarrhena rhizome, phellodendron bark, lotus plumule, cinnamon bark; *yang* deficiency with aversion to coldness, cold limb, minus rehmannia root, plus epimedium.

3. Acupoints: *Shenshu, Xinshu, Houxi, Neiguan, Zusanli, Sanyinjiao* (all with reinforcing technique). Vexation and less sleep, add *Shenmen* (reinforcing); chest pain add *Shanzhong, Xuehai* (both with reducing technique), chest oppression and much sputum, add *zhongwan* (reinforcing), *Fenglong, Shanzhong* (both reducing).

II. Case report

No. 1: Mr. Yang, 43 years old, came to attain the clinic on Mar. 28, 1980, with the complaint of palpitation and chest oppression for 3 months. Three months ago after a severe attack of common cold with high fever, and then the appearance of palpitation and chest oppression. In another hospital the EKG revealed frequent ventricular extrasystole of bigeminal rhythm, and was given a diagnosis of viral myocarditis, with the use of lidocaine, segontin and others without much effect.

The present symptoms consisted of palpitation with or without external stimuli, chest oppression and shortness of breath, aggravated after fatigue, and more prominent in the afternoon and at night, accompanied with dizziness, insomnia, dysphoria, anorexia, stool constipated, tongue proper light red, with thin white, slimmy coating. Pulse reluctant weak and intermittent. This belonged to the deficiency of both *yin* and *yang*. The therapeutic principle of replenishing *qi* and warming up the *yang* and nourishing the *yin* and arresting the palpitation adopted.

Recipe: Honey-fried licorice 30g, Cinnamon twig 15g, Dangsen 30g, Rehmannia root 30g, Ophiopogon root 30g, Schisandra fruit 15g, Red sage root 24g, Spatholobus stem 30g, Curcuma root 12g, Flavescent sophora root 12g, Arborvitae seed 12g, decoct in water, one recipe dose daily by mouth.

After 14 doses, the effect not prominent, still with chest pain at times, the dosage of cinnamon twig increased to 30g, with further addition of ground beetle 12g, clematis root 15g, seven recipe doses taken with marked relief of all symptoms, EKG returned to normal, another forty some doses taken and all the symptoms disappeared. The above prescription was used continuously with one recipe every other day for consecutive two months in order to fortify the therapeutic effect. Follow up half a year later, he remained healthy.

No. 2 : Ms. Liu, 50 years old, came to attain the clinic on Jan.21, 1980, with the chief complaint of chest oppression and palpitation for more than one year, exacerbated in recent 20 days.

One year ago in a night, she had syncope, each time lasting half an hour, consecutively for two times, after the seizure of syncope she felt chest oppression, palpitation and malaise aggravated. EKG examination revealed I° A-V block, II° one type A-V block, chronic coronary insufficiency, and then received medical treatment consisting of atropine, dibazole, sorbide nitrate, aminophylline, composite red sage root injection and others without much improvement. 20 days ago after a cold, the symptoms further aggravated, EKG showed III° A-V block, chronic coronary insufficiency.

The symptoms at time of clinic consisted of chest oppression, palpitation, shortness of breath, puffiness of face, general malaise, coldness of limbs, dreamful sleep, facial pallor, tongue proper light red, tongue coat thin and white, pulse deep and deficient (sun mai). Blowing systolic murmur of third grade over the apex of heart. B.P. 170/90 mmHg, heart rate 34 beats/min., EKG showed AVB III°, imcomplete right bundle block, chronic coronary insufficiency.

From TCM syndrome differentiation this case was due to the decline of *yang* and the excess of *yin*, no inspiration of heart *yang*, the delayed blood circulation. The principle of treatment should be to warm up the channel and activate the *yang*, to make the collateral patent and the restoration of pulse. The prescription recipe Decoction of ephedra, aconite root, asarum with additional ingredients.

Recipe: Honey fried ephedra 12g, Prepared aconite root 30g, Asarum 3g, Psoralea fruit 21g, Honey fried locorice 15g, Chinese angelica root 15g, decoct in water, one recipe dose daily.

After 10 recipe doses, most of the symptoms disappeared, only slight palpitation after motion. Tongue proper light red, tongue coat thin and white, pulse moderate. B.P. 190/70 mmHg. Two EKG tracings both I° AVB, imcomplete right bundle block, chronic coronary insufficiency.

Discussion:

1. This was a case of coronary artery disease complicated with II° auriculo-ventricular block, pertaining to severe cardiac arrhythmia. A certain hospital decided to treat her with an artificial pacemaker, but the patient refused. In TCM the arhythmia is ordinarily classified into three groups: the slow pulse, rapid pulse and irregular pulses.

The author in clinic usually classed the arhythmia into two types, the rapid type and the slow type. The slow pulse is chiefly responsible for cold, the excess or deficiency in accordance with its force. Slow pulses with force indicate old and obstinate cold. Slow, forceless pulses indicate *yang* dificiency with the formation of cold. The rapid pulse is chiefly responsible for heat, and the determination of excess or deficiency in accordance with its force too. Rapid pulses with force indicate the exuberance of evil heat, while rapid pulses without force indicate *yin* deficiency with the formation of heat in the interior. This case gave deep and deficient pulse, *Sun Mai* (the deficient pulse) pertains to the category of slow pulse group. In a respiratory cycle of the doctor, there are only two pulse beats, the half of the normal pulse namely 32-40 beats in a minute. The appearance of deficient pulse was a sign of severe condition of the disease.

2. From the change of blood pressure, the decoction of ephedra, aconite and asarum lowered the blood pressure instead of the suspected elevation. This indicated that TCM syndrome differentiation and treatment is to regulate the *yin* and *yang*, to correct its deviation to excess or deficiency, and a new equilibrium condition established. With the disappearance of symptoms, the elevation of blood pressure lowered, and the lowered blood pressure elevated. The composite recipe had therapeutic effects different from the pharmaclogical effects of its components. In this case, among the six drugs used there are four drugs having hemopiesic action, while after medication the blood pressure rapidly lowered to normal. This phenomenon needs further research to find out the real explanation.

3. This case is an evident proof that chinese herb medicine is efficient in treating conduction block of myocardium, and render them recovering to normal state. The mechanism require further investigations.

III. Personal experience

Heart belonging to *yang* viscera is chiefly responsible for circulation, propelling the blood endlessly circulating in the vessel and thus the pulse moderate, even and with spirit. The florescence or decline of heart *qi*, the filling or vacancy of blood influenced by many exopathic or endogenic factors, especially by the cold evil or heat evil. The cold evil may render the pulse become slow. Slow and forceful pulse indicates the exuberance of cold in the interior and the cold in excess. As cold has the property to constrict, to astringe the *qi*, thus the constriction of vessel and the stasis of *qi* and blood, among this type of arhythmia a number of them belongs to functional. Slow and forceless pulse is a manifestation of asthenia syndrome which is a result of *yin* deficiency with cold formation. In this case the insufficiency of heart *qi* and the decline of heart *yang* with impaired propelling force, and thus the stasis of blood flow, the majority among this group belong to organic heart disease, with impeded heart function. Rapid pulse is usually due to heat pathogen. Pulse rapid and forceful pertains to heat in excess The agitation of evil heat makes the heart *qi* abundant, and the rapid filling of the vessels, the rapid blood flow results. Its pathophysiology may be related to the high metabolism and increase of susceptibility of myocardial excitation. Among this type most belongs to functional. Rapid and forceless pulse pertains to asthenic heat. As the *yin* deficiency due to lingering illness, with the endogenous asthenic heat or weakness of heart *yang* and weakness of propelling force thus the pulse without force. The pathophysiology is related to the diminished heart function or heart failure of organic heart disease, its diminished blood volume and the increased metabolic demand lead to the increase of cardiac pulsatile ability. No matter the exuberance of pathogen or the decline of propriel vital energy, the disharmong between *yin* and *yang*, the disorder of *qi* and blood, therefore the slow and rapid pulse frequently in combination with other pulses such as *cu* pulse (running pulse), *jie* pulse (knotted pulse), *dai* pulse (intermittent pulse).

The decoction of prepared licorice is one of the most frequently used recipe in treating cardiac arrhythmia with good therapeutic effects. A statistic of 70 cases of arhythmia, 39 cases used this recipe. This recipe puts the emphasis on reinforcing the heart *qi*, activating the heart *yang*, which are the key points in treating knotty pulse or intermittent pulse. Assisted with medicine to replenish blood and nourish the *yin*, to fill in and nourish the blood vessel, the *yang qi* capable to attach and adhere to the *yin* and blood, the reestablishment of *yin* and *yang* equilibrium, thus the knotty and intermittent pulse cured and the palpitation arrested.

Migraine

Migraine, or vascular hemicrania, is a kind of paroxysmal headache due to an impeded function of contraction and relaxation of cerebral blood vessels. There may be omen symptoms of visual hallucination, hemianopia and other transcient cerebral functional disturbances. During the episode, it is usually accompanied by nausea, vomiting and other manifestations of vegetative nerve functional disorders. Its etiology still not well known. This disease pertains to the category of 'pian tou feng (hemicrania)' and others.

I. TCM syndrome differentiation and treatment

Pathogenesis in brief: The stagnation of liver *qi* with the invasion of stomach, the tranference of stagnated *qi* to fire, and the production of wind from exuberance of fire. The perversive upward invasion of wind and fire, and the spasm of vessels and muscles.

Chief manifestations: Sudden episode of headache, rather severe, left or right, may refer to eye or tooth, sparkling of eyes before the episode, with frequent accompaniment of nausea, vomiting, and paroxysmal sweat. After the arrest of pain, the same as without illness. Tongue proper red, with thin and yellowish coating. Pulse taut fine and rapid.

Therapeutic principle: To sooth the liver and extinguish the wind, to clear the heat and arrest the pain.

1. Patent drug:

(1) *Long Dan Xie Gan Wan*, 6g t.i.d. and whole scorpion powder 5g t.i.d.

(2) *Qi Ju Di Huang Wan*, one bolus t.i.d. and *Long Dan Xie Gan Wan* 6g. t.i.d.

2. Decoction recipe: *Tian Ma Gou Teng Yin* with modifications:

Gastrodia tuber 12g, Uncaria stem with hooks 24g,

Sea-ear shell 30g, Scutellaria root 10g, Capejasmine fruit 10g, Gypsum 30g, Earthworm 12g, Bupleurum root 6g, Chrysanthemum flower 12g, Vitex fruit 12g, Licorice root 3g, Scorpion 12g, Centipede 3g, for oral administration after being decocted in water, one dose a day.

Plus-minus: In cases with exuberance of liver fire, vexation with anger inclination, plus gentian root, moutan bark, pinellia tuber; tangerine peel, bile treated arisaema tuber, white mustard seed in cases of wind-phlegm obstruction of collateral, and muscular contracture; acute pain followed by lingering pain add peach kernel, safflower, red peony root. During remission, add prepared fleece-flower root, white peony root, and glossy privet fruit.

3. Acupoints: *Ganshu, Danshu, Dadun, Xingjian, Taichong, Touwei, Fengchi, Qubin* (all with reducing technique); wind fire obstruction of collateral, plus *Fengfu, Waiguan, Qiuxu, Hanyan* (all with reducing technique); complicated with phlegm, add *Weishu, Zhongwan, Fenglong, Daling, Neiguan* (all with reducing technique); blood stasis, add *Ganshu, Xiehai, Sanyinjiao* (all reducing).

4. Ear acupoints: Liver, Gallbladder, Heart, Sympathetic, Endocrine.

II. **Case report**

Mr. Sun, 39 years old, worker, came to the clinic on May 5, 1978. Paroxysmal headache for 5 years. On account of anger and insomnia for a whole night, in the morning he had dazzle or sparkling of eyes followed by headache of left, lacerating or penetrating with an awl in character, associated with nausea, vomiting, vexation, muscular spasm over the pain site. Tongue proper red, with thin yellow coat, pulse taut and rapid. Each year he had 5~10 episodes like that described above. A diagnosis of migraine made. With the use of oryzanol, new preparations of ergot (methyl-butanyl ergine) without much effect. A diagnosis of upward invasion of wind-fire of liver channel made, and the principle of treatment was to allay the liver and extinguish the wind, to clear down the fire and arrest the pain.

The disposal consisted of firstly acupuncture *Dadun*, *Xingjian*, *Taichong*, *Hegu*, *Touwei*, *Qubin*, *Fengchi*, *Fengfu*, *Danshu* (all with reducing technique). After the gradual improvement of the symptom, the oral recipe given below prescribed:

Gastrodia tuber 12g, Uncaria stem with hook 30g, Gentian root 10g, Capejasmine fruit 12g, Sea-ear shell 30g, Gypsum 30g, Chuanxiong rhizome 12g, vitex fruit 12g, Earthworm 12g, Whole scorpion powder 6g (to be swallowed with fluid) Centipede 5g (to be swallowed with fluid), Curcuma root 12g, Fleece-flower stem 30g, Bupleurum root 6g, for oral administration after being decocted in water, one dose a day.

The third vist on May 9. After three doses of the above decoction, no headache and other symptoms gone too, except some discomfort of left side of head. Vexation and inclination to anger, insomnia and dreamfulness, bitter taste in mouth, urine deep colored, stool constipated. Tongue proper red with scanty coat, pulse taut, fine, and rapid. This indicated the insufficiency of *ganyin*, and the liver fire not cleared up yet.

Recipe: *Qi Ju Di Huang Wan*, one bolus t.i.d. and *Long Dan Xie Gan Wan*, 5g t.i.d. The continuous use of the above bolus and pill for two months, in order to fortify the therapeutic effects.

One year later, no episode of pain.

III. Personal experience

Migraine is a stubborn disease, yet with precise syndrome differentiation, proper well selected medication, the therapeutic effect is satisfactory. This is due to wind fire of the liver channel, and the flare up of wind fire along the channels to the head, frequently complicated with wind cold, phlegm and blood stagnation. In cases complicated with wind cold, ligusticum root, ephedra asarum herb should be prescribed. Complicated with phlegm stagnancy pinellia tuber, bile treated arisaema tuber, white mustard seed should be given. Complicated with stagnated blood, peach kernel, safflower, ground beetle and others should be added.

During the episode, the emergent uses of acupuncture, ear acupuncture, or digital acupoint pressure to relieve the pain as an incidental therapy. After the relief of pain, the principle of treatment should direct to the foundamentals, the method of increasing water and fluid and irrigating the wood, nourishing the liver to relieve pain should be adopted.

Hyperlipoidemia

The elevation of several or all the blood-lipid components in the plasma is named hyperlipoidemia which is the major factor leading to atheroslerosis. The treatment of this disease is of important significance in preventing and treating the disorders caused by atheroslerosis such as cerebrovascular accident, insufficiency of blood supply, myocardiac infarction, etc. In view of the main symptoms occuring in the disease: vertigo, palpitation, oppressed sensation in chest, shortness of breath, numbness of limbs, lassitude, etc., it is in TCM attributable to the category of 'phlegm-dampness', 'obstruction of turbid *qi*', 'obstruction of *qi* in the chest',etc.

I. **TCM syndrome differentiation and treatment**

Pathogenesis in brief: Deficiency of the liver-*yin* and kidney-*yin*, the abnormality of the transporting function of the spleen, the upward flaming of fire and phlegm obstruction, stasis in the blood vessels, mal-nourishment of the channels.

(I) Deficiency of liver-*yin* and kidney-*yin*

key points in pathogenesis: Deficiency of liver-*yin*

and kidney-*yin,* stagnation of asthenic fire in the interior, phlegm formation caused by burning fluid, obstruction of phlegm, blood stasis.

Chief manifestations: Dizziness, headache, hemianesthesia, palpitation, restlessness and irritability, loss of appetite, sleep disturbed with dreams, chest stuffiness and pain, dry stool, red colour of the tongue proper with ecchymosis, pulse taut slippery or taut hesitant.

Therapeutic principle: To replenish the kidney and sooth the liver, to resolve phlegm and promote blood circulation.

1. Patent drug:
   (1) *Liu Wei Di Huang Wan,* 1 bolus t.i.d.
   (2) *Xin Xue Ning Pian,* 5 tab. t.i.d.
   (3) *Zhi Bai Di Huang Wan,* 1 bolus, t.i.d.

2. Decoction recipe: *Jiang Zhi Tong Mai Yin* with additional ingredients:

   Fleece-flower root 30g, Eclipta 24g, Bupleurum root 10g, Curcuma root 12g, Oriental wormwood 24g, Alismatis rhizome 24g, Cassia seed 24g, Rhubarb 6g, Hawthorn fruit 20g, for oral administration after being decocted in water, one dose a day.

3. Acupoints: *Shenshu, Ganshu, Houxi* (all with reinforcing technique), *Xingjian, Fenglong, Xuehai, Sanyinjiao* (all with reducing technique).

(II) In sufficiency of the spleen with overabundance of dampness

Key points of pathogenesis: Excessive dampness due

to deficient spleen, accumulation of excessive fluid in the interior to be coagulated into phlegm which blocks channels.

Chief manifestations: Dizziness, a feeling of distension in the head, lassitude and weakness, wish to sleep after meal, epigastric distress, abdominal distension puffy face and eyelids, numbness of limbs, even stiffness of the tongue and difficulty in speaking, involuntary drooling, plump tongue with teeth-prints at its borders, tongue coat thin, white and wet, pulse deficient and slow.

Therapeutic principle: To invigorate the spleen and clear off dampness, to resolve phlegm and remove obstruction in the channels.

1. Patent drug:

(1) *Ren Shen Jian Pi Wan*, 1 bolus each time, t.i.d.

(2) *Mai An Chong Ji*, 10g each time to be taken after being infused with boiling water, t.i.d.

2. Decoction recipe: *Er Chen Tang* with modifications: Lotus leaf 15g, Atractylodes rhizome 12g, Poria 15g, Pinellia tuber 12g, Bile-treated-arisaema tuber 10g, Tangerine peel 10g, Alismatis rhizome 24g, Earthworm 12g, Batryticated silkworm 12g, White mustard seed 10g, for oral administration after being decocted in water, one dose a day.

Plus-minus: Grassleaved sweetflag rhizome, curcuma root and prepared polygala root should be added to the recipe for cases with stiffness of the tongue and difficulty in speaking; scorpion and centipede for those with facial hemiparalysis; radish seed and magnolia bark for treating abdominal distension; agastache, eupatorium and red bean for evil-dampness.

3. Acupoints: *Pishu, Weishu, Zusanli* (all with reinforcing technique), *Yinlingquan, Fenglong, Xuehai, Sanyinjiao* (all with reducing technique).

II. Case report:

Mr. wang, 55 years old, came to seek medical advice on Dec. 16,1987.

The patient suffered from chest stuffiness and chest pain for more than a year, and aggravated for half a month. Fifteen days ago, his overwork in mentality and body gave rise to paroxysmal chest stuffiness and pain accompanied by palpitation, shortness of breath, dizziness and fidgets which were aggravated by movements. ECG indicated ventricular bundle block in the left anterior branch, frequent ventricular premature beats (mostly interpolated extrasystole). Blood lipid: Tch 210 mg%, TG 311 mg%, HDL-ch 55mg%, LDL-ch 928mg%, VL DL-ch 62.2 mg%; apolipoprotein APoA-I 173.1 mg%, APoA-II 39.6 mg%, $APoB_{100}$ 151.6 mg%. Red colour of tongue proper with whitish greasy coating, pulse taut thready and intermittent uneven. Blood pressure 120/80 mmHg. He usually suffered from hyperlipemia and took atromid-S and elastase for five months, 2 tab. of each t.i.d. From the view point of western medicine, his disease was diagnosed as hyperlipemia and cardiac arrhythmia. From the syndrome differentiation and treatment, it was diagnosed as chest pain, palpitation caused by *yin* deficiency of the liver and kidney, stasis of blood in heart collateral. The therapeutic principle was to treat by tonifying the liver and kidney, removing blood stasis and obstruction in the channels. *Jiang Zhi Tong Mai Yin* (drink for lowering blood-lipid and promoting blood circulation) was prescribed, one dose a day (at the meantime the intake of western medicine should be stopped). With two month's medication various symptoms disappeared, tongue and pulse normal, ECG normal. Blood-lipid Tch 138 mg%, TG 136 mg% HDL-ch 58mg%, LDL-ch 53 mg%, VLDL-ch 27 mg%; Apolipoprotein: APo A-I 170 mg%, APo A-II 38 mg%, $APoB_{100}$ 121 mg%. Blood pressure 120/80 mmHg.

III. Personal experience

In the treatment of hyperlipoidemia with TCM, special attention should be paid not only to exopathic factors manifested as improper diet and wind-cold invasion into the body but also to endopathic factors marked by both deficiency of the spleen and kidney which is considered as the fundamental and dominant factor; in relation to the fundamental is the incidental which refers to the stagnation of *qi* and blood stasis or dominant phlegm-dampness. In general, treating both the incidental and the fundamental aspects of a disease (its symptoms and cause) at the same time is the therapeutic principle to be adopted namely; on one hand to nourish the liver and kidney or to remove dampness by invigorating dampness, on the other hand, equally and simultaneously to regulate the flow of *qi* and promote blood circulation or to resolve phlegm and remove obstruction in the channels. In this way, to gain tonifying action while eliminating greasy and astringent components, otherwise tonification would be followed by more extreme obstruction of *qi* and blood stasis, and more severe domination of phlegm-dampness.

In the course of treatment, there might be a transient elevation of blood-lipids. This is one form of the manifestations indicating that the drug works, because, through pharmacological action of the drug, evil phlegm of atheromatous plaques attaching to the blood wall is dissolved in the blood, when the dissolving rate faster than the excretion rate, blood lipid would be increased. When these lipids excreted out of the body, blood-lipid would gradually come down and subjective symptoms would subside correspondingly.

For patients with hyperlipoidemia, it is better to alternate work with rest and recreation and to keep on diet. Rest is not important for patients who do not undertake hard physical labour. If the patient is a mental worker, physical training should be encouraged. At ordinary times, it is proper to eat more vegetable food, less oily and greasy food, so as to avoid damage of the spleen and stomach.

Respiratory and cardiac failure of pulmonary encephalopathy

This syndrome is a developmental stage of pulmonary heart disease (cor pulmonale) which is resulted from chronic bronchitis, pulmonary emphysema and finally pulmonary heart disease. When reaching this stage, the condition is dangerous, critical and sometimes fatal, so it is really the final or terminal stage. In spite of the adoption of numerous emergency measure of western medicine, the mortality rate is still very high. With the simultaneous use of the syndrome differentiation and treatment of TCM, not only the mortality rate lowered, but also the course of treatment shortened. This syndrome pertains to the category of 'coma', 'edema', 'asthma', 'syncope' and others.

I. TCM syndrome differentiation and treatment

Pathogenesis in brief: The deficiencies of lung, heart, kidney, with accumulation of fluid and phlegm, the upward invasion of heart and lung. The stasis of heart blood, the impeded pulmonary function of dispersion and descending, the impaired kidney function of astringency and inspiration. Many dangerous phenomena break out.

(I) The retention of water due to *yang* deficiency

Key points of pathogenesis: The retention of water due to *yang* deficiency, the upward invasion of heart and lung, the stasis of heart blood, and the failure of pulmonary dispersing and descending function.

Chief manifestations: Cough and dyspnea, palpitation without external stimulation, generalized edema, especially in the lower limb. Cough with clear diluted frothy sputum. Face, lips, finger nails cyanotic, listless, or coma, sweating and cold limbs. Scanty and short urination. Tongue proper purplish blue. Tongue coat white and wet. Pulse deep, fine and weak.

Therapeutic principle: To warm up the kidney and circulate the water; to clear off the lung and resolve stagnation.

1. Patent drug: *Jin Gui Shen Qi Wan*, one bolus, t.i.d. *Ren Shen Ge Jie San*, 5g t.i.d. Tablet of composite red sage root 4 tablets t.i.d.

2. Decoction recipe: *Zhen Wu Tang* and *Dan Shen Yin* with modifications:

Prepared aconite root 12g, Cinnamon twig 12g, Poria 30g, Ginseng 12g, White atractylodes rhizome 12g, Red sage root 24g, Sandal wood 8g, Peach kernel 10g, Sepium periploca bark 12g, Lepidium seed 15g, Peucedanum root 12g, for oral administration after being decocted in water one dose a day.

Plus-minus: In cases cough with much sputum, dyspnea indicating phlegm stagnation in lungs add perilla fruit, ginger treated pinellia, eagle wood; epigastric oppression, abdominal distention, anorexia, slimmy tongue coat indicating spleen deficiency add amomum fruit, stir-fried radish seed, haw-thorn fruit. In case the heart orifices blocked with phlegm, at times mentality clear, at times cloudy, addition of borax pill; the occurrence of coma further addition of grassleaved sweetflag rhizome, curcuma root.

3. Acupoints: *Shenshu, Guanyuan, Qihai, Zusanli* (all with reinforcing technique), *Pishu, Shuifen, Fenglong* (all moxibustion).

(II) The impending exhaustion of *qi* and *yin*

Key points of pathogenesis: The impending exhaustion of real *yin* which can not astringe the *yang*, and the *qi* losing its astringint and inspirating power, the upward climbing of the solitary *yang* resulting in the excess of the upper, and deficiency of the lower with impending collapse of real *yang*.

Chief manifestations: Severe dyspnea with mouth open, and elevation of shoulder, nares flaring, swaying of the body, and evident movement of abdomen during respirations, sweating of head, cold feet, palpitation, face and lips cyanotic, absentminded, dysphoria and restless ness, eyes gazing forward, incontinence of urine and stool. Tongue proper red and dry, with yellow black dry coating. Pulse superficial, large rootless, or thready in-distinct, knotty or intermittent.

Therapeutic principle: To astringent the *yin* and enhance the inspiration. To support the *yang* and treat the collapse.

1. Patent drug: *Sheng Mai Zhen*, 20 ml added into 50% glucose 40 ml intravenous push, two or three times a day.

2. Decoction recipe: *Shen Fu Tang* with modifications:

American ginseng 30g, Prepared aconite root 20g, Schisandra fruit 15g, Dogwood fruit 20g, for oral administration after being decocted in water, one dose a day. *Hei Xi Dan* 2.5g to be taken with decoction fluid, b.i.d.

Plus-minus: High fever, dysphoria and listless, removal of prepared aconite root, add *An Gong Niu Huang Wan* one bolus two or three times a day; in case coma with phlegm rattling in the throat, add grass-leaved sweetflag rhizome, curcuma root, bile treated arisaema tuber, prepared polygala root, bamboo juice.

3. Acupoints: *Shenshu, Guanyuan, Qihai, Gaohuang, Zusanli* (all with reinforcing technique). Much sputum coma, add *Fenglong, Pishu, Xinshu, Shenmen* (moderate reinforcing and reducing technique).

II. Case report

Mr. Li, 64 years old, a worker, came to clinic on Feb. 24, 1982, with history of cough for more than twenty years. In last 5 years the repeated recurrence and gradual aggravation of cough, sputum, fever, chest oppression, palpitation, edema. The occurrence of seizure was in winter, with remissions in summer. Recently he had fever up to 39 °C, clear mind at one time, drowsy at another, cough, dyspnea, respirations rapid, face purple dark in color, lips and the whole body cyanotic. Tongue proper purple and dark, yellow slimmy coatings. Pulse fine weak rapid and intermittent. Heart sounds low and blunt, heart rate 128 beats/min, cardiac rhythm irregular. Moist rales in both sides of lungs, respiration 28 times/min. Liver enlarged. Blood gas analysis pH 13.1, $PaCO_2$ 80 mmHg, PaO_2 45 mmHg, HCO_2 350 mmHg, BE 41 mmHg, a diagnosis of pulmonary encephalopathy, respiratory and heart failure, respiratory acidosis, and metabolic alkalosis. Emergent disposal consisting of antibiotics, oxygen inhalation, diuretics, cardiac stimulants, respiratory stimulants for 2 days, the disease condition became worse with development of coma, fever still, facial color black, spitting foam, sputum rattling in throat like pulling a saw to and fro, chest full and respirations rapid, severe dyspnea with body swaying and pronounced abdominal respirations, sweating and cold limbs, convulsion, incontinence of urine and stool, pulse deep indistinct with impending stoppage, This indicated the impending exhaustion of *qi* and *yin*, the block of phlegm-heat in the interior. The therapeutic principle was to replenish *yin* and reinforce *yang*, to clear up heat and arouse the mind (other emergency disposals of western medicine continued).

1. Patent drug: *An Gong Niu Huang Wan*, one bolus each time, two or three times a day, dissolved in fluid and nasal feed.

2. Decoction recipe: American ginseng 30g, Schisandra fruit 12g, Ophiopogon root 45g, Cinnamon twig 10g, Grass leaved sweetflag rhizome 12g, Curcuma root 12g, for oral administration after being decocted in water one recipe dose daily.

3. Acupoints: *Qihai*, *Guanyuan*, twice a day moxibustion.

After medication, the gradual recovery of clear mentality, 3 days afterwards he could talk and protrude the tongue. High fever subsided. Body temperature 37.6°C. He could take liquid diet after removal of the nasal tube, but listless, cold wet limbs, rattling in the throat. Tongue proper bluish purple with scanty saliva, greyish black dry coat. Pulse fine rapid and weak. *An Gong Niu Huang Wan* one bolus daily. Decoction recipe American ginseng reduced to 12g, with further addition of glehnia root, pueraria root 12g, sepium periploca bark 6g, licorice root 3g, with removal of grass leaved sweetflag rhizome. 15 days after patient's symptoms markedly improved, blood gas analysis within normal limit. He was advised to continue the intake of *qi* replenishing and *yin* nourishing drugs in order to fortify the therapeutic effects.

III. **Personal experience**

This disease is a knotty problem in medical science.

With the only use of western medicine in emergency cases, some without much effect. In combination with treatment of traditional Chinese medicine, not a few dying cases can be brought back to life. In comatous patient unable to take medicine by mouth, other paths can be used, nasal tube or rectal tube may be inserted, and slow dripping recommended.

In critical condition, the number of herb drugs should be few and the quantities used large, such as American ginseng 30g is used. This single drug has eminent therapeutic effect and can snatch a patient from the jaws of death. when the critical condition is tided over, the recipe may include more kinds of medicines, each kind of suitable dosage, namely the commonly used quantity, with the consideration of all aspects, *yin* and *yang*, *qi* and blood, gradual regulation and avoid acting with undue haste, as haste makes waste and the aim can not be attained.

Heart failure of chronic pulmonary heart disease

Chronic pulmonary heart disease (cor pulmonale) is mostly derived from chronic bronchitis, pulmonary emphysema. The increased resistance of pulmonary circulation leads to hypertrophy of right ventricle, and finally heart failure. In TCM this disease pertains to *tan yin* (phlegm-liquids), *shuigi* (edema), cough and dyspnea and others.

I. **TCM syndrome differentiation and treatment**

Pathogenesis in brief: Long standing cough and dyspnea develope pulmonary emphysema which in turn leads to the obstruction of the pulmonary collaterals and the impeded circulation.

(I) Pulmonary stagnation with phlegm-heat

Key points of pathogenesis: Sick of cough and dyspnea for long time, with further invasion of wind-heat, phlegm and heat block of the lung, the impaired dispersion of the lung *qi*.

Chief manifestations: Cough with yellow thick sticky sputum, suffocation and shortness of breath, dyspnea and dysphoria, unable to lie flat, fever, thirsty, urine dark colored, stool dry. Tongue proper red, tongue coat yellow and slimmy. Pulse slippery and rapid.

Therapeutic principle: To clear up the heat and resolve the sputum; to moisten the lung and allay the dyspnea.

1. Patent drug:

(1) *She Dan Chuan Bei Me*, 1~2 tube t.i.d.

(2) *She Dan Chuan Bei Ye* and *Da Qing Ye He Ji*, one tube each, t.i.d.

(3) *Kang Yan injection*, each time one ampoule i.m. t.i.d.

2. Decoction recipe: *Sang Xing Tang* and *Xie Bai San* with modifications:

Mulberry leaf 12g, Bitter apricot seed 12g, Adenophora

root 24g, Thunberg fritillaria bulb 12g, Pear peel 15g, Houttuynia 30g, Trichosanthes peel 20g, Ophiopogon root 15g, Reed stem 30g, Mulberry bark 10g, Wolfberry bark 12g, Platycodon root 12g, Licorice root 6g, for oral administration after being decocted in water, one dose a day.

Plus-minus: Severe cough and dyspnea, plus stemona root, coltsfoot flower, belamcanda rhizome; severe heat, plus honeysuckle flower, dande-lion herb; much sputum, add pumice, lepidium seed, pyrrosia leaf; fullness and oppressed feeling in chest and diaphragm, add immature bitter orange, magnolia bark, eagle wood.

3. Acupoints: *Feishu, Lieque, Waiguan, Tiantu, Fenglong, Shanzhong* (all with reducing technique).

(II) Attack of the heart by retained fluid

Key points of pathogenesis: On account of the *yang* deficiency of spleen and kidney. The accumulation and flooding of water dampness, the involvement of heart and lung, with *yin* in excess, and *yang* in decline.

Chief manifestations: Edema, palpitation with or without external stimuli, shortness of breath, malaise, unable to lie flat, dyspnea and restlessness at motion, scanty and short urination, epigastric fullness, oppression and anorexia. Lips cyanotic, tongue plump with imprint at margins. Tongue thin white and slimmy, pulse weak rapid or knotty, or intermittent.

Therapeutic principle: To warm up the *yang* and remove body fluids with diuretics; to resolve stagnation and sedate the mind.

1. Patent drug: *Fu Shou Cao Zong Dai* injection, each time 0.25~0.50 mg, added to 50% glucose solution 20 ml intravenous, slow push, once a day, and take Tablet of composite red sage root each time 4 tablets, three times a day.

2. Decoction recipe: *Zhen Wu Tang* and *Ling Gui Zhu Gan Tang* with modifications:

Prepared aconite root 10g, Cinnamon twig 10g, Poria 30g, Big head atractylodes rhizome 24g, Umbellate pore fungus 15g, Red sage root 24g, Bugleweed 15g, Sepium periploca bark 10g, Lepidium seed 18g, Platycodon root 6g, for oral administration after being decocted in water, one dose a day.

Plus-minus: Prominent palpitation, add magnetite, amber powder; nausea, anorexia, add ginger treated pinellia tuber, magnolia bark, fresh ginger.

3. Acupoints: *Neiguan, Zusanli, Sanyinjiao* (all with reinforcing technique), *Fuliu, Shuifen* (both with reducing technique).

(III) Mental confusion due to phlegm

Key points of pathogenesis: weakened body resistance, pathogens in excess. Heart confused by phlegm.

Chief manifestations: Cloudiness of mind, phlegm rattling in throat, respirations rapid, feverish and restless, even becoming comatous. Tongue proper purple dark. Tongue coat thick and slimmy. Pulse slippery and rapid.

Therapeutic principle: To clear up heat and remove the

phlegm, to stimulate the sensitive orifices and arouse the spirit.

1. Patent drug: *Zi Xue San*, 3g t.i.d. and drink bamboo juice 30g, two or three times a day.

2. Decoction recipe: *Di Tan Tang* with modifications: Pinellia tuber 12g, Red tangerine peel 12g, Prepared arisaema tuber 10g, Ginseng 10g, Poria 15g, Immature bitter orange 12g, Bamboo shaving 10g, Scutellaria root 12g, Lotus plumule 6g, Curcuma root 12g, Prepared polygala root 10g, Grass-leaved sweetflag rhizome 10g, for oral administration after being decocted in water, one dose a day.

Plus-minus: Dampness in excess with edema, add atractylodes rhizome, *Su He Xiang Wan*; abdominal fullness with scanty urine, add eagle wood, amber; fever, with yellow thick sticky sputum, add scutellaria root, trichosanthes fruit, bamboo juice with further addition of *An Gong Niu Huang Wan* or *Zhi Bao Dan*.

3. Acupoints: *Renzhong, Yongquan, Taichong* (all with reducing technique).

4. Ear acupoints: Heart, brain, subcortex, sympathetic.

II. **Case report**

Ms. Wang, 54 years old, peasant, came to the clinic on Jan. 15,1988, with a history of cough and dyspnea for 15 years exaggerated in the last 5 days. 5 days ago on account of fatigue, generalized edema, especially in the lower limbs, palpitation, dyspnea aggravated with motions, unable to lie flat, cough, foamy sticky sputum, epigastric fullness, nausea, anorexia, short urination and scanty in amount, cyanotic lips. Tongue proper plump with tooth imprint over margin. Tongue coat thin white and slimmy. Pulse rapid and without force, jugular vein engorged, liver enlarged, the upper margin at 4th i.c.s, the lower margin 4 cm below the costal margin, 7 cm below the xiphoid process. Liver tough, tender on palpation; edema of the lower limbs. P_2 accentuated over tricuspid region Ⅱ° systolic murmur, lungs breathing sound low, moist rales over the two bases. X-ray flouroscopy of chest right anterior oblique position the right ventricle enlarged. EKG right axis deviation. Pulmonary P wave, V1 $R/S>1$, V5 $R/S<1$, QRS low voltage.

western medicine diagnosis: Pulmonary heart disease, heart failure.

TCM syndrome differentiation *yang* deficiency of spleen and kidney, water retention with invasion of heart and lung. The therapeutic principle of warming up the *yang*, and remove water with diuretics, to resolve stagnation and sedate the mind.

Recipe: Prepared aconite root 10g, Cinnamon twig 10g, Poria 30g, White atractylodes rhizome 15g, Red sage root 21g, Pyrrosia leaf 20g, Sepium periploca bark 10g, Bugleweed 12g, Peach kernel 10g, Lipidium seed 18g, Ginger treated pinellia tuber 12g, Magnolia bark 10g, Stir fried radish seed 15g, for oral adinistration after being decocted in water, one dose a day.

After 10 recipe doses, edema disappeared, appetite increased, she could walk but felt palpitation and shortness of breath if rapid. The above recipe, with the removal of aconite root, and lipidium seed, add dangsen 15g, amomom fruit 10g, licorice root 3g, one recipe dose every other day to fortify the therapeutic effects.

III. Personal experience

This disease is difficult to be radically cured, only with symptomatic relief and easy recurrence especially in winter. The above is only incidental treatment which is commonly used during the seizure. When the heart failure corrected, the continuous treatment is still neccessary, this is what we called "diseases occur in winter, the treatment should start from summer". The methods commonly adopted are of two kinds, one is "to strengthen the lung (metal) by way of reinforcing the spleen (earth)". The second is "to tonify the kidney and improve inspiration". By mean of the above two principles, in majority of cases the disease will have less seizure and once the occurrence of seizure, the attack less severe. The commonly used recipe is: Astragalus root 15g, Dangsen 12g, White atractylodes 10g, Siberian solomonseal rhizome 15g, Schisandra fruit 6g, Poria 12g, Chinese angelica root 12g, Peach kernel 12g, Tangerine peel 10g, Sichuan fritillary bulb 10g, Fermented leaven 12g, for oral administration after being decocted in water, one dose a day.

Lung abscess

Lung abscess is an infection of the lung caused by a variety of pyogenic organisms, at early stage being purulent inflammation and later abscess formation. Clinically, the main manifestations are high fever, cough, and the expectoration of a large amount of purulent and foul phlegm. The disease, in TCM, is categorized as *'fei yong'*

I. TCM syndrome differentiation and treatment

Pathogenesis in brief: Stagnation of the lung by noxious heat, hectic fever due to accumulation of heat, heat stagnation, and blood stasis, putrefaction of flesh and blood.

(I) Wind-heat attacking the lung

Key points of pathogenesis: Wind-heat attacking the exterior, excessive heat in the lung, weakness of *wei* (the defense principle) *qi*, the lung losing its clearing and descending function.

Chief manifestations: Chill and fever, cough with scanty sputum, chest pain aggravated while coughing, dry mouth and nose, difficulty in breathing, tongue coat thin and yellowish, pulse floating and rapid.

Therapeutic principle: To disperse wind-heat, and remove pulmonary heat and resolve phlegm.

1. Patent drug: *Yin Qiao Jie Du Pian*, 24 tab. t.i.d., to be taken after being ground into powder and mixed with boiled water.

2. Decoction recipe: *Yin Qiao San* with modifications: Honeysuckle flower 30 g, Forsythia fruit 15 g, Schizonepeta 10 g, Reed rhizome 45 g, Peppermint 10 g, Platycodon root 12 g, Houttuynia 30 g, Lophatherum 10 g, Scutellaria root 12 g, Licorice root 6 g; for oral administration after being decocted in water, one dose a day.

Plus-minus: In case with headache, plus mulberry leaf, chrysanthemum flower, and chastetree fruit; with severe cough and profuse phlegm, plus trichosanthes seed, Zhejiang fritillary bulb and bitter apricot kernel; with severe chest pain, plus trichosanthes fruit, curcuma root, and peach kernel.

3. Acupoints: *Quchi, Waiguan, Hegu, Chize, Dazhui, Xiangu* (all with reducing technique).

(Ⅱ) Accumulation of noxious heat in the lung

Key points in pathogenesis: Accumulation of noxious heat in the lung, giving rise to blood stasis, putrefaction of flesh and blood, rupture of abscess to interior.

Chief manifestations: High fever, chill, profuse sweat, chest pain, dysphoria in breathing, expectoration of fishy and stinky, purulent and bloody sputum, fidget, thirst with likeness of drinks, bright red colour of tongue proper with yellowish and thick coating, slippery and rapid pulse.

Therapeutic principle: To clear away heat and toxic material from the lung, to promote pus discharge and remove obstruction in the channels.

1. Patent drug:

(1) *Jin Lian Hua* injection, 1 amp. each time, i.m. t.i.d.

(2) *Xi Ling Jie Du Pian* 24 tab. each time, taken after being ground into powder and mixed with boiled water, t.i.d.

2. Decoction recipe: *Qian Jin wei Jing Tang* with additional ingredients:

Coix seed 45 g, Waxgourd seed 30 g, Peach kernel 15 g, Honeysuckle flower 30 g, Forsythia 15 g, Houttuynia 30 g, Isatis leaf 30 g, Platycodon root 12 g, Licorice root 6 g, Reed stem 15 g; for oral administration after being decocted in water, one dose a day.

Plus-minus: Gypsum, anemarrhena rhizome and scutellaria root are supplemented to treat extreme heat; *Xi Huang Wan* is selected for treating cases with unbearable foul sputum; trichosanthes fruit, rhubarb, and immature bitter orange added to treat constipation; glehnia root, ophiopogon root and anemarrhena rhizome to those with dry mouth and throat; cogongrass rhizome, moutan bark, node of lotus rhizome and rehmannia root to those with hemoptysis.

3. Acupoints: *Feishu, Yuji, Chize, Fuliu, Fenglong*

(all with reducing technique).

(Ⅲ) Deficiency of both *qi* and *yin*

Key points of pathogenesis: Gradual subsidence of noxious heat with impairment of both *qi* and *yin*.

Chief manifestations: Expectoration with a small amount of purulent blood, tidal fever, irritability, dry mouth and throat, spontaneous perspiration, night sweat, emaciation, shortness of breath, bright red colour of tongue proper, deficient and rapid pulse.

Therapeutic principle: To replenish *qi* and tonify *yin*; to moisten the lung and resolve phlegm.

1. Patent drug: *Zhi Ke Qing Guo Wan*, two pills, t.i.d.

2. Decoction recipe: *Qing Zao Jiu Fei Tang* with modifications:

Root of American ginseng 10 g, Glehnia root 24 g, Zhejiang fritillary bulb 12 g, Loquat leaf 12 g, Honey-fried lily bulb 24 g, Ophiopogon root 30 g, Moutan bark 12 g, Wolfberry bark 15 g, Platycodon root 12 g, Apricot kernel 12 g, Licorice root 3 g, for oral administration after being decocted in water, one dose a day.

Plus-minus: In case with anorexia, plus coix seed, white atractylodes rhizome, and germinated barley; with persistant feverishness, plus stellaria root, sweet wormwood, and dried rehmannia root; with profuse sputum, plus trichosanthes fruit, stir-fried radish seed and anemarrhena rhizome.

3. Acupoints: *Feishu, Pishu, Zusanli* (all with reinforcing technique), *Fenglong, Yinlingquan* (both with reducing technique).

II. Case report:

Mr. Guo, 54 years old, worker, came to clinic on April 24, 1986.

With three days high fever and chill, at the beginning, the patient was diagnosed to have a cold and so was prescribed *Xi Ling Jie Du Pian*, medemycin, PPC and so on, but the therapeutic effect was not remarkble. In recent days his symptoms were aggravated gradually, with manifestions of chill, and high fever, which could not be relieved by sweating, spells of coughing, stuffy sensation in the chest with pain aggravated by cough, expectoration of yellow and thick sputum which smelled stenchy and occasionally mixed with purulent blood, dry mouth and throat, scanty dark urine, constipation, bright red colour of tongue proper with its coating yellowish, thick and greasy, slippery and rapid pulse. Examination: body temperature 39.5°C, WBC 19500. Differential count: Neutrophile 84%, lymphocyte 16%. X-ray fluoroscopy: lung abscess of the left upper lobe. Diagnosis of western medicine: Lung abscess.

Syndrome differentiation of TCM: Invasion of the lung by noxious heat, decomposition of the blood and putrefaction of flesh. It is advisable to treat by clearing away heat and removing the poisonous substances, promoting pus discharge and resolving phlegm.

Recipe: Coix seed 45 g, Waxgourd seed 30 g, Peach kernel 12 g, Honeysuckle flower 30 g, Forsythia fruit 15 g, Houttuynia 30 g, Isatis leaf 30 g, Scutellaria root 15 g, Platycodon root 12 g, Licorice root 6 g, for oral administration after being decocted in water, one dose a day.

Therapeutic effect: After the medication of 15 doses, all the symptoms were relieved, body temperature: 37.5℃; WBC 8600, tongue proper red, tongue coating whitish, pulse thready and weak. Continuous medication of the above recipe with exclusion of scutellaria root, isatis leaf, houttuynia and with addition of pseudostellaria root, ophiopogon root, glehnia root, germinated barley. Another 15 doses of medication, all the symptoms disappeared. X-ray fluoroscopy of chest: Abscess on the upper lobe of left lung absorbed, linear stripe shadow being the only finding.

III. Personal experience

The three syndromes classified above refer to the three stages of pulmonary abscess, namely, the primary, the middle and the last. Proper medication at primary stage would make a quick recovery. Therefore, the treatment at primary stage is most important, especially the application of antipyretics and detoxicants, such as honey suckle flower, forsythia fruit, houttuynia, isatis leaf, patrinia, dayflower, etc. The dosage of drugs should be large. Be sure to eliminate the disease after medication. Since the lung and large intestine are interior-exteriorly related, the propelling of large intestine is helpful in the purification and descendance of pulmonic *qi*, care should be taken all the time of the free movement of the bowels, frequently used drugs are trichosanthes fruit, rhubarb, peach kernel and others.

Tuberculous pleuritis with effusion

Tuberculous pleuritis with effusion is the further development of dry pleuritis. Generally speaking, the onset is sudden, accompanied by prominent chest pain, aversion to cold, spontaneous perspiration, general discomfort, cough, fever, even complicated with critical symptoms like shortness of breath, dyspnea, and cyanosis. In TCM the disease pertains to the category of 'pain in chest and hypochondrium', '*xuan yin*', '*shaoyang* syndrome', 'accumulation of pathogens in chest', and others.

I. TCM syndrome differentiation and treatment

Pathogenesis in brief: Phlegm, heat accumulated in *Shaoyang*, disharmony of channels and collaterals, impairment of *yin* due to prolonged illness.

(I) Stagnancy of evil in *shaoyang*

Key points in pathogenesis: Accumulation of phlegm-heat in the lung invading *shaoyang*, giving rise to disturbances of *shaoyang* acting as pivots, and obstructions in blood vessels.

Chief manifestations: Alternate spells of fever and chills, fever not relieved by sweating, cough with little sputum, stabbing pain of the chest and hypochondrium, aggravated by breathing and turn on one's side, bitter taste, dry throat, lumpy feeling of epigastrium, thin and yellowish coating of the tongue, taut and rapid pulse.

Therapeutic principle: To clear away heat and resolve phlegm; to mediate *shaoyang*.

1. Patent drug: *Shu Gan He Wei Wan* and *Long Dan Xie Gan Wan*, 5 g of each, t.i.d.

2. Decoction recipe: *Xiao Xian Xiong Tang* and *Xiao Chai Hu Tang* with modifications:

Bupleurum root 15 g, Pinellia tuber 12 g, Scutellaria root 12 g, Coptis rhizome 10 g, Trichosanthes fruit 24 g, Stir-fried bitter orange 12 g, Safflower 10 g, Red peony root 12 g, Platycodon root 10 g, for oral administration after being decocted in water, one dose a day.

Plus-minus: Plus mulberry bark, white mustard seed and wolfberry bark for cases with obstruction of the lung by phlegm retention; plus coptis rhizome, Zhejiang fritillary bulb and stemona root for cases with remarkble accumulation of phlegm-heat.

3. Acupoints: *Feishu, Ganshu, Xinjian, Qimen, Fenglong, Zhangmen* (all with reducing technique).

(Ⅱ) Phlegm retention in the chest and hypochondrium

Key points of pathogenesis: Stagnancy of the lung *qi* failing to resolve body fluid, giving rise to retention of phlegm and fluid in the chest and hypochondrium.

Chief manifestations: Gradually relieved pain with cough, and gradually aggravated dyspnea, distension and fullness in the affected side of the chest and hypochondrium, thoracic bulging, unable to lie flat, low-grade fever, palpitation, thin and whitish coating of the tongue, deep and slippery pulse.

Therapeutic principle: To soothe the liver and facilitate the flow of the lung-*qi*, to expel water and phlegm retention.

1. Patent drug:

(1) *Kong Xian Dan* 5 g, to be taken at one draught on empty stomach, 5 days' administration in succession. In the duration, the dosage can be increased bit by bit in accordance with the reaction to the drugs.

(2) Capsules made of ground drugs of kansui root, knoxia root, and genkwa, 2~3 g each time, to be taken on an empty stomach in the morning with decoction of ten Chinese-date, one time every 1~2 days, 5~6 times in succession. After medication, there may appear slight borborygmi, abdominal pain, vomiting, diarrhea. If these symptoms are severe, medication should be stopped.

2. Decoction recipe: *Jiao Mu Gua Lou Tang* with

modifications:

Lepidium seed 15 g, Mulberry bark 15 g, Bupleurum root 12 g, Peach kernel 10 g, Trichosanthes fruit 15g, Perilla seed 12 g, Pinellia tuber 12 g, Pepper seed 12 g, Poria 21 g, Fresh ginger peel 10 g, for oral administration after being decocted in water, one dose a day.

Plus-minus: In case with excessive turbid phlegm, fullness in chest, and greasy coating of the tongue, onion bulb and apricot kernel are included in the recipe; with cases marked by persistant retention of fluid, weak constitution and want of appetite, cinnamon twig, white atractylodes rhizome licorice root and luffa supplemented; as for those with continuous stabbing pain in the chest and hypochondrium, attributable to the stagnancy of excessive fluid, the dosage of both lepidium seed and mulberry bark are reduced to 10 grams, meanwhile, add to the recipe the following ingredients: red peony root, sweetgum, cyperus tuber, safflower, waxgourd peel, etc.

3. Acupoints: *Zhangmen, Qimen, Ganshu, Xingjian, Taichong, Zhongwan, Fenglong, Sanyinjiao* (all with reducing technique).

(II) Interior heat due to deficiency of *yang*

Key points of pathogenesis: Prolonged obstruction with phlegm retention, transmission into heat impairing *yin*, lung dryness due to deficiency of *yin*, obstruction of collaterals.

Chief manifestations: Frequent choking cough, expectoration with little amount of mucous sputum, dry mouth and throat, accompanied by tidal fever, red cheeks, dysphoria with feverish sensation in chest, palms and soles, hypochondriac pain with stuffiness, emaciation, red coloured tongue proper with little coating, fine and rapid pulse.

Therapeutic principle: To nourish *yin* and clear off heat, to remove stasis and promote collateral circulation.

1. Patent drug: *Yang Yin Qing Fei Wan*, 1 bolus t.i.d. along with *Fu Fang Dan Shen Pian* 4 tablets, t.i.d.

2. Decoction recipe: *Sha Shen Mai Dong Tang* with modifications:

Glehnia root 20 g, Ophiopogon root 20 g, Fragrant solomonseal rhizome 24 g, Trichosanthes root 15 g, Mulberry bark 12 g, Wolfberry bark 12 g, Stemona root 12 g, Red peony root 10 g, White peony root 10 g, Red sage root 15 g, Licorice root 3 g, for oral administration after being decocted in water, one dose a day.

Plus-minus: Bupleurum root and fresh-water turtle shell are supplemented to treat cases with evident tidal fever; trichosanthes bark, curcuma root, bitter orange and luffa to treat distinct stuffy pain in the chest and hypochondrium; oyster shell, lepidium seed and alismatis rhizome to treat prolonged retention of fluid. When the case is complicated with deficiency of *qi*, mental fatigue, spontaneous sweating, and shortness of breath, pseudostellaria root, astragalus root and so on are to be employed.

3. Acupoints: *Shenshu, Taixi, Feishu, Xinshu, Sanyinjiao* (all with reinforcing technique), *Ganshu, Xingjian, Fenglong, Qimen* (all with reducing technique).

II. Case report

Ms. Jiang, 45 years old, worker, came to seek medical advice on June 27, 1986.

The patient had pulmonary tuberculosis for more than 10 years. And her condition of disease has been no better or worse. 10 days ago, she was ill with chills and fever. The intake of drugs didn't work well, for with the exception of vanishment of headache and pantalgia, she was still troubled with such symptoms as alternate attacks of chills and fever, obvious feverish body in the afternoon, cough, expectoration with thick yellowish sputum, stabbing pain in the left chest and hypochondrium, aggravated with cough and turning, bitter taste, dry throat, lumpy and stuffy feeling in the chest and stomach, anorexia, disturbance in bowel movement, insomnia, red coloured tongue proper with yellowish coating, pulse taut fine and rapid. Physical examination: body temperature (T) 38.1℃, fullness and dullness on percussion in the right-sided chest and hypochondrium, no breathing sound heard, a little rhonchi could be heard over the rest part, heart rate was regular, 96 beats per minute. Chest X-ray fluoroscopy excessive fluid in the right thoracic cavity, lung-markings increased, scattered calcified lesion over the upper lobe of right lung. Blood WBC: 12000. DC (differential count): neutrophil 84%, lymphocyte 16%; E.S.R. 86mm per hour. A diagnosis of tuberculous pleuritis with effusion made in western medicine. Diagnosis of TCM: 'hypochondrial pain', 'pleural effusion'.

TCM syndrome differentiation and treatment: stagnancy of the lung with phlegm-heat, dysfunction of *Shaoyang*, failure of facilitating the flow of the lung-*qi*, breaking out of various syndromes. The treatment should be directed at promoting the dispersing function of the lung, clearing up heat and resolving phlegm.

Therapeutic means:

1. Acupuncture: Acupoints *Feishu, Ganshu, Xingjian, Qimen, Zhangmen, Fenglong, Taichong* (all with reducing technique). Once a day.

2. Recipe: Bupleurum root 15 g, Coptis rhizome 10g, Scutellaria root 10 g, Trichosanthes fruit 24 g, Pinellia tuber 12 g, Stir-fried bitter orange 10 g, Platycodon root 12 g, Red peony root 12 g, Gypsum 30 g, White mustard seed 10 g, Stir-fried apricot kernel 12 g, Stemona root 12 g, Licorice root 6 g, for oral administration after being decocted in water, one dose a day.

The second visit on July 13. With 14 doses of medication and 14 days' acupuncture, all the symptoms vanished gradually except for slight cough, dry mouth without thirst, vague pain in the right hypochondrium on deep breathing, red coloured tongue proper with little coating, fine pulse. E.S.R. normal. WBC normal, T: 36.9℃. Chest X-rayed: thickened crura of diaphragm of the right hypochondrium. What is above showed that phlegm heat had been removed, vital-*qi* had not yet been restored, and the stagnancy in collaterals had not been completely removed. It is advisable to deal with the above by nourishing *yin*, regulating *qi* and promoting collateral circulation.

Recipe: Trichosanthes fruit 24 g, Glehnia root 20 g, Red sage root 24 g, Peach kernel 12 g, Pinellia tuber 10g, Red peony root 12 g, Bupleurum root 10 g, Zhejiang fritillary bulb 10 g, Licorice root 3 g, for oral administration after being decocted in water, one dose a day.

The third visit on July 29. With still another 15 doses of medication, all the symptoms faded away. Diet and sleep became normal. Advice was given to take *Xiao Yao Wan*, half a bag, t.i.d. Continuous administration for one month, in order to consolidate therapeutic effects.

Ⅲ. Personal experience

Thoracic excessive fluid is the chief pathological result of the disease. Hence, to eliminate water and phlegm retention is the basic treating principle for the disease. As hydrugogues and drugs for expelling fluid retention are drastic in action and would damage the stomach function, so, when given, they should be firstly, assisted by stomach protecting drugs and secondly, increased in dosage bit by bit. And the reaction to medication should be under observation.

At the time the method of eliminating water and expelling phlegm retention is utilized, the drugs for regulating *qi* and removing obstruction in collaterals ought to be administered simultaneously to support the action of medicine, in order that the promoted flow of *qi* is matched with the elimination of water, and the activated blood is matched with removal of obstruction in collaterals.

In case the prolonged illness is still marked with depleted vital energy and persistent water retention. Differentiation of symptom-complexes should be involved in the application of warming and removing obstruction in collaterals and removing excessive fluid, or nourishing *yin*, promoting blood circulation and removing dampness through diuresis.

For cases complicated with symptoms associated with oppression of the heart and lung such as excessive fluid in chest marked by dyspnea and tachypnea, shortness of breath, and cyanosis, aspiration of pleural effusion can work as the means to deal with the emergency case.

Carcinoma of lung

The statistical data of quite a few countries illustrate that case-fatality rate of pulmonary cancer is the first among the list of all cancers. The clinical manifestation of the disease is characterized by long-standing cough, with blood-stained sputum or hemoptysis, chest stuffiness and pain, dyspnea and tachypnea and shortness of breath. The disease, in TCM pertains to the category of 'cough', 'dyspnea syndrome', 'hypochondrial pain', 'blood syndrome', etc. By applying the theories, methods, recipes and chinese medicinal herbs of TCM to plan treatment for cancer of lung according to diagnosis, better curative effect is usually produced.

I. TCM syndrome differentiation and treatment

Pathogenesis in brief: Phlegm, heat, stasis, and asthenia prolonged retention of noxious-heat and stagnation leading to excess of the incidental and deficiency of the fundamental.

(I) Deficiency of *yin* with phlegm heat

Key points of pathogenesis: Lung damage due to prolonged cough, stagnancy of phlegm heat damaging the lung collaterals, resulting in the loss of the lung function to clear and descend.

Chief manifestations: Cough with dyspnea, expectoration of purulent sputum with stinking smell as of rotten fish, often stained with blood, stuffy feeling in the chest with dyspnea, sometimes accompanied by fever, dry mouth and throat, red coloured tongue proper with yellowish greasy coating, fine, slippery and rapid pulse.

Therapeutic principle: To nourish *yin* and resolve phlegm; to clear up heat and remove toxic material.

1. Patent drugs: *Yang Yin Qing Fei Wan*, 2 bolus t.i.d. together with the administration of *Xi Huang Wan*, 1 bolus, b.i.d. in the morning and evening.

2. Decoction recipe: *Sha Shen Mai Dong Tang* and *Xie Bai San* with modifications:

Glehnia root 15 g, Ophiopogon root 15 g, Trichosanthes root 12 g, Chonglou rhizome 12 g, Mulberry bark 12 g, Wolfberry bark 12 g, Trichosanthes fruit 20 g, Coix seed 30 g, Stemona root 10 g, White hyaciath bean 30 g, Licorice root 3 g, Common reed 30 g, for oral administration after being decocted in water, one dose a day.

Plus-minus: In case with fever, plus houttuynia and forsythia fruit; with blood stained sputum, plus node of lotus, capejasmine fruit and powder of pseudoginseng root.

3. Acupoints: *Feishu, Shenshu, Taixi, Fuliu* (all with reinforcing technique), *Tuiyuan, Lieque, Fenglong, Chize, Xingjian* (all with reducing technique).

(Ⅱ) Blood stasis due to impairment of collaterals

Key points of pathogenesis: Prolonged accumulation of noxious heat, giving rise to damage of lung-collaterals, bleeding in the interior forming blood stasis and obstruction in the interior.

Chief manifestations: Chest stuffiness with violent pain, a large amount of hemoptysis with purple dark colour, or intermingled fresh red and purple, expectoration of yellowish sputum, dyspnea and shortness of breath, dark purple colour of lips and finger nails, dark purple tongue proper with thin yellowish coating, taut rapid or hesitant pulse.

Therapeutic principle: To promote blood circulation and remove blood stasis; to clear away heat and remove toxic material.

1. Patent drug:

(1) *Yun Nan Bai Yao* 1.5 g each time, to be taken with decoction of node of lotus 30 g, t.i.d.

(2) *San Qi Fen* 2 g, t.i.d.

(3) *Zhi Zi Yan Qin Gao Pian* 5 tablets, t.i.d.

2. Decoction recipe: *Zhi Xue Hua Yu Tang* with modifications:

Inula flower 12 g (wrapped), Paris rhizome 15 g, Trichosanthes fruit 24 g, Chinese angelica root 12 g, Red sage root 12 g, Node of lotus 30 g (taken with fluid), for oral administration after being decocted in water, one dose a day.

Plus-minus: Corydalis tuber, cat-tail pollen, and

trogopterus dung are added for cases with severe chest pain; houttuynia, edible tulip bulb, belamcanda rhizome, stemona root and sun-plant, or along with *Xi Huang Wan* for cases with fever and foul yellowish sputum.

3. Acupoints: *Feishu, Lieque, Shaoshang, Fenglong, Xuehai, Sanyinjiao* (all with reducing technique).

(Ⅲ) Deficiency of both *qi* and *yin*

Key points of pathogenesis: Noxious heat impairing the lung, leading to consumption of *qi* and *yin*, disturbance of lung function to clear and to descend.

Chief manifestations: Dry cough with scanty sputum, dry throat and mouth, mental fatigue and weakness, low and husky voice, spontaneous sweating and shortness of breath, emaciation, anorexia, red coloured tongue proper with little coating, deep fine and weak pulse.

Therapeutic principle: To replenish *qi* and nourish *yin*, to remove stasis and toxic material.

1. Patent drug:

(1) *Shi Quan Da Bu Wan* 1 bolus each time, t.i.d. along with the intake of *Xi Huang Wan*, 1 bolus, b.i.d. in the morning and evening.

(2) *Ren Shen Jian Pi Wan* and *Xi Huang Wan* the method of administration same as above.

2. Decoction recipe: *Sheng Mai San* with additional ingredients:

Root of American ginseng 10 g, Ophiopogon root 18 g, Schisandra fruit 6 g, Astragalus root 15 g,

Glehnia root 15 g, Honey-fried lily bulb 15 g, Poria 15 g, White atractylodes rhizome 10 g, Atractylodes rhizome 10 g, Long-noded pit viper 12 g, Arnebia or Lithosperm root 12 g, Rice sprout 15 g, Barley sprout 15 g, Licorice root 13 g, for oral administration after being decocted in water, one dose a day.

Plus-minus: In case with low-graded fever, freshwater turtle shell, starwoot root, and chonglou rhizome are employed; with nonproductive cough, trichosanthes fruit and Zhejiang fritillary bulb supplemented; with anorexia, hawthorn fruit, tangerine peel and medicated leaven added.

3. Acupoints: *Feishu, Pishu, Shenshu, Sanyinjiao, Houxi* (all with reinforcing technique), *Qihai, Zusanli* (both with moxibustion).

II. Case report

Case 1: Mr. Wang, 56 years old. In October 1983, since one month ago he had symptoms of fever, cough and bloody sputum. In November, an exploratory operation of chest done a big carcinoma on the inferior lobe of left lung with adhesion to surrounding tissue found and 5~6 metastatic lymph nodes 2 × 3 (cm) size over the hilus of lung and mediastinum. Pathological report was poorly differentiated squamous epithelial carcinoma. The chest was closed without resection of carcinoma because of wide spread metastasis. During the three weeks of post operation, the patient was haunted by persistent existence of high fever which did not respond to antibioties, expectoration of red-yellowish bloody sputum, chest pain, insomnia, poor appetite, shortness of breath, scanty urine, constipation, irritable, feverish sensation in the chest. X-ray film revealed the further extension of lesions. The manifestations of red lips, flushed face, high fever, fidget, red coloured tongue without coating, taut and rapid pulse were ascribed to the syndrome of deficiency of both *yin* and *qi*, accumulation of noxious heat in the lung. In accordance with the principle of treating the incidental for emergency, large dosage of nourishing *yin*, and fluid-producing drugs, as well as detoxicating and heat clearing drugs given, such as dried rehmannia root, scrophularia root, ophiopogon root, red sage root, white peony root, wasp's nest, node of lotus, honey suckle flower, scutellaria root, dendrobium, winetreated rhubarb, black nightshade, buffalo horn and others prescribed. Baby's urine used as it is effective in clearing away noxious heat. Seven doses of medication stopped the bloody sputum, and ten doses complete subsidence of fever and all the symptoms relieved. Having been treated according to doctor's order for more than one month, the lesions were somewhat lessened. In view of the large range of lesions, radiotherapy was suggested to coordinate the treatment (7000 rad on the chest over the lesion, 6900 rad between the hilus of lung and mediastinum), as a result, lesions were further reduced to some extent, and the patient's constitution was recovering day by day. After radiotherapy, he learned to do traditional Chinese breathing exercise and at the same time, took decoction recipe of Chinese medicinal herbs. Up to now two years and four months have passed. Follow-up no recurrence except for reactional pericarditis as a sequele after radiotherapy (abstract of characteristic experiences of famous doctors Yu Rencun's medical records).

II. Personal experience:

To treat carcinoma of the lung with TCM, the key is to strengthen vital *qi* for the sake of strengthening the patient's resistance against diseases. Hence, it is dominant therapeutic principle to invigorate the spleen and tonify the lung, and to replenish *qi* and nourish *yin*. Some drugs share the action of treating the fundamental such as astragalus root, Dangshen, ginseng, American ginseng, pseudostellaria root, glehnia root, lily bulb, dried rehmannia root, scrophularia root, and so on. Phlegm heat, noxious heat, stagnancy are the factors inducing incidental syndrome, the following drugs with the action of treating the incidentals are recommended: trichosanthes fruit, paris rhizome, longnoded pit viper, honey suckle flower, forsythia fruit, sun-plant, *quan shen* (rhizome bistortae), poria, prunella spike, scutellaria root, stemona root, patrinia, houttuynia, wasp's nest, red peony root, red sage root, notoginseng, peach kernel, ect. In the course of treatment, it is frequently preferable to treat both the incidental and the fundamental. It is strictly forbidden to list drugs bitter in flavour and cold in nature with the action of removing toxins, which are thought to be "anti-cancer agents", to form a prescription for patients. So doing not only runs against the principle of syndrome differentiation, owing to bitter and cold nature of the drugs, the stomach will be damaged and the material basis of acquired constitution will be impaired. Thus the disease will become worse and even to critical condition.

Xi Huang Wan possesses a certain curatove effect to carcinoma of the lung and can be administered simultaneously with the decoction recipe.

Esophageal carcinoma and gastric carcinoma

Esophageal carcinoma and gastric carcinoma are clinically characterized by progressive dysphagia, blockage of the swallowed food in its passage from mouth to stomach and vomiting after eating. In TCM, it belongs to the category of *'ye ge'* (dysphagia), *'fan wei'* (regurgitation of food from stomach), 'vomiting' and others.

I. TCM syndrome differentiation and treatment

Pathogenesis in brief: Intermingled obstruction of phlegm and *qi*, accumulation of blood stasis in the interior giving rise to blockage of stomach-*qi* and consumption of stomach-*yin*, the impairment of *yin* affecting *yang*, invading the spleen and kidney.

(I) Intermingled obstruction of phlegm and *qi*

Key points of pathogenesis: Stagnancy of *qi*, dysfunction of fluid distribution. Condensation and accumulation into phlegm, mutual obstruction of phlegm and *qi*, failure of the stomach *qi* to propel downwards

Chief manifestations: Dysphagia, felling of fullness and stuffiness in chest, epigastric distension with vague pain, belching, salivation, dry mouth and throat, emaciation. Red coloured tongue proper with thin greasy coating. Taut and fine pulse.

Therapeutic principle: To regulate the flow of *qi* to alleviate mental depression, to resolve phlegm and moisten dryness.

1. Patent drug: *Mu Xiang Shun Qi Wan*, 6 g each time, t.i.d.

2. Decoction recipe: *Qi Ge San* with modifications: Curcuma root 12 g, Amomum fruit 10 g, Sandal wood 10 g, Glehnia root 15 g, Sichuan fritillary bulb 12 g, Poria 12 g, Garden balsam seed 10 g, Trichosanthes fruit 15 g, for oral administration after being decocted in water, one dose a day.

Plus-minus: In case with depressed *qi* turning into fire, amomum fruit is to be with-drawn while coptis root, India trumpet flower and red peony root are supplemented; in case with constipation due to the impairment of body fluid, scrophularia root, rhubarb and radish seed added; for cases with marked phlegm obstruction, pinellia tuber, tangerine peel and inula flower included.

3. Acupoints: *Shanzhong, Juque, Ganshu, Geshu, Weishu, Geguan* (all with reducing technique).

(II) Phlegm accumulated in the interior

Key points of pathogenesis: Prolonged stagnancy of *qi* responsible for accumulation of phlegm in the interior, as a blockage in the esophagus resulting in difficulty of swallowing.

Chief manifestations: Pain in chest, difficulty of swallowing food, vomiting immediately after swallowing, the material vomited just like red bean juice, stools as hard as faeces of sheep, emaciation, withered skin. Cyanosis of tongue proper. Weak and hesitant pulse.

1. Patent drug: *Xi Huang Wan*, 1 bolus, t.i.d. together with *Liu Shen Wan*, 5 pills, t.i.d.

2. Decoction recipe: *Tong You Tang* with modifications:

Dried rehmannia root 15 g, Chinese angelica root 12 g, Peach kernel 12 g, Red sage root 20 g, Trogopterus dung 10 g, Sichuang fritillary bulb 10 g, Notoginseng powder 3 g (swallow with boiled fluid),

Dung bettle 10 g, Curcuma root 10 g, Trichosanthes fruit 20 g, Licorice root 3 g, for oral administration after being decocted in water, one dose a day.

Plus-minus: Burreed tuber, zedoary, and vinegar-fried pangolin are employed for cases of marked stagnancy of phlegm; pinellia tuber and powder of clam shell for cases with extreme stagnancy of phlegm. If vomiting occurs immediately after administration, it's better to take *Yu Shu Dan* before hand.

3. Acupoints: *Shanzhong, Juque, Geshu, Neiguan, Xinshu, Geguan* (all with reducing technique).

(Ⅲ) Consumption of body fluid leading to heat accumulation

Key points of pathogenesis: Exhaustion of *yin*-fluid, impaired moistening of esophagus, fire of deficient type flaming upward, consumption of the source of nutrients for growth and development.

Chief manifestations: Blockage of swallowed food, unsmooth swallowing with pain, even difficulty to swallow water; distress in the stomach with burning heat; pain in the chest and hypochondria; sensation of heat felt in the chest, palms and soles, constipation; dry mouth and throat; dry red coloured tongue proper; taut fine and rapid pulse.

Therapeutic principle: To nourish *yin* and blood, to moisten dryness and promote the production of fluid.

1. Patent drug: *Wu Zhi An Zhong Yin,* 10 ml each

time, 3~5 times a day.

2. Decoction recipe: *Sha Shen Mai Dong Tang* with modifications:

Glehnia root 20 g, Ophiopogon root 15 g, Dried rehmannia root 20 g, Dendrobium 15 g, Black plum 10 g, Reed rhizome 30 g, Peach kernel 10 g, White honey 15 g (mixed with the ready decoction), for oral administration after being decocted in water, one dose a day.

Plus-minus: In case with stagnated heat in the stomach, coptis root and capejasmine fruit are supplemented; with constipation, trichosanthes fruit and rhubarb added, while black plum withdrawn; in cases with impairment of *yin* affecting *yang* marked by puffy face and edema of limbs, American ginseng, poria, dried ginger and pinellia tuber added, while ophiopogon root and dried rehmannia root with-drawn.

3. Acupoints: *Pishu, Weishu, Zusanli, Sanyinjiao* (all with reinforcing technique), *Shanzhong, Geguan* (both with reducing technique). For cases with distinct *yang* deficiency, additional acupoints: *Qihai, Gongsun* (all with reinforcing technique); for cases with vomiting immediately after eating, additional acupoint: *Zhongkui* (with moxibustion).

II. Case report

Case 1: Mr. Zhao, 50 years old, worker, came to seek medical advice on Nov. 5, 1974.

The patient complained of abdominal distension and fullness with vague pain and vomiting for three months. Recently, he felt difficulty in swallowing food. In some hospital he was diagnosed as carcinoma of pylorus in advanced stage to which surgery seemed helpless. He was advised to go back to his local hospital for treatment. On the way, a thought to consult doctor of TCM in our hospital came upon to his mind.

The patient had withered and yellowish face, emaciated body, distension and fullness in the stomach and abdomen, swollen in right-upper abdomen which would cause pain when pressed, the swelling hard as stone. Withered and grey yellowish colour of skin, weak breath, dull look in the eyes, vomiting a small amount of liquid like red bean juice, red-coloured tongue proper with dry yellowish coating, fine and hesitant pulse. All the above manifestations were ascribable to the syndrome of "regurgitation (of food from stomach)". Arising from obstruction of phlegm-stagnancy, taking food became difficult, the source of growth and development was exhausted, as the result, various symptoms broke out and life was in a critical condition. The treatment for it ought to focus at invigorating the spleen, replenishing *qi*, resolving phlegm and eliminating stagnancy.

Recipe: American ginseng 20 g, Smilax glabra rhizome 30 g, Glehnia root 20 g, Pinellia tuber 10 g, Trichosanthes fruit 20 g, Burreed tuber 6 g, Zedoary 6 g, Peach kernel 6 g, White atractylodes rhizome 12 g,

Chicken's gizzard-membrane 10 g, Licorice root 3 g, to divide decocted liquid into 5~10 portions, one portion each time, one dose a day.

The second visit on Nov. 10. After 4 doses of medication the patient's symptoms took a turn for better. He was in the mood with tendency to get up and move about, tongue proper red with its coating thin, yellowish and dry, pulse fine and hesitant.

Recipe: Continuous administration of above recipe with addition of dendrobium 20 g and germinated barley 30 g.

The third visit on Nov. 13. Another 2 doses of above recipe. As he took a change for the better, he sat up to have his hair cut, but, suddenly, he began to vomit blood mixed with purple dark blood clots and material like mashed flesh, amounting to 500 ml or so. The patient was collapsed and then given blood transfusion in the hospital of the factory he worked in. The patient was listlessness and his swelling on the right upper abdomen disapperared and felt soft when pressed. The mass over right upper abdomen not palpable but the right upper abdomen still fuller than left side, and tender. His tongue proper red with scanty coating, and pulse weak and faint.

Recipe: Ginseng 30 g, Schisandra fruit 12 g, Ophiopogon root 30 g, Burreed tuber 6 g, Peach kernel 6 g, Notoginseng powder 5 g, Chicken's gizzard-membrane 12 g, Licorice root 3 g, to divide decocted liquid into 10 portions, one portion each time, one dose a day.

The fourth visit on Nov. 17. Still another three doses of above recipe. The patient was in high spirit, all his symptoms took a marked change for better. He could take liquid food without vomiting and no longer given blood transfusion. His tongue proper red with its coating thin, whitish and slightly greasy, his pulse fine and weak.

Recipe: Continuous administration of above recipe with its ginseng being added up to 15 g, and with some additional ingredients: White atractylodes rhizome 12 g, Poria 15 g, Germinated barley 30 g, Sichuan fritillary bulb 10 g, Trichosanthes fruit 20 g, for oral administration after being decocted in water, one dose a day.

The fifth visit on Dec. 25. After 32 doses of above recipe, the symptoms nearly disappeared. Tongue proper pink, tongue coating thin and white, and pulse moderate. Later, the patient went to that hospital where he was once diagnosed as carcinoma of pylorus of stomach for examination, and this time the given diagnosis was denied. He was ordered to take *Ren Shen Jian Pi Wan* 1 bolus each time, t.i.d. two months as a course for the purpose of strengthening curative effect.

Follow-up half a year later, and the patient was basically recovered from his illness except for leanness.

Case 2: Mr. Hou, 47 years old, first visit on Oct. 23, 1979.

The patient's complaints were disturbance in taking food and eructation of gas for two months, difficulty in swallowing for 20 days. He was given X-ray esophagoscopy first in the staff hospital of Yima Mining burean in Henan Province and in the first affiliated hospital of the Fourth Army Medical University. Their X-ray films all revealed an irregular filling defect, about 10 mm, rigidity of esophageal wall, interruption of esophageal mucosa. The physio-therapy department of the affiliated hospital discovered cancer cells from the smear got through a net put in through esophagoscope. The patient was hereby diagnosed to suffer from carcinoma of the middle and lower esophagus in advanced stage. Surgery being impossible, he was advised to go back home for non-surgical treatment.

On Oct. 23, 1979, the patient came to our department to consult doctor, with the symptoms and signs of emaciation, bluish and dark complexion, puffiness of eyelid, hiccup, phlegm rattling in the throat, deficient, taut and hesitant pulse. These are ascribable to *yeshi* (dysphagia), caused by long-standing stagnancy of phlegm and salvation, obstruction of *qi* and stasis of blood. It was preferred to resolve phlegm and remove stasis, to promote digestion by invigorating the stomach.

Recipe: Poria 13 g, Pinellia tuber 13 g, Tangerine peel 10 g, Stir-fried Hawthorn fruit 13 g, Stir-fried barley sprout 10 g, Chicken's gizzard mombrane 10 g (stir-baked to brown), Stir-baking pangolin scales 9 g,

Stir-fried calyx and receptacle of a persimmon 9 g, Garden balsam seed 15 g, Airpotato yam 15 g, Chinese sage 16 g, all the drugs are first mixed with water 1500ml, honey 120 ml, and then decocted to boiling, to be taken in four portions, at four times, one dose a day.

Subsequent visit on Dec. 5. After the medication with 40 doses of above recipe, swallowing became smooth, hiccup absent and phlegm eliminated, but the throat was still dry and unsmooth and stool dry. The principle drawn up for the treatment was to promote the production of body fluid, to moisten dryness, and to nourish *yin* and replenish the stomach, assisted by softening masses, removing stagnation, detoxicating and clearing up carcinoma.

Recipe: Adenophora root 24 g, Ophiopogon root 15 g, Sichuan fragrant solomonseal rhizome 24 g, Chinese yam 24 g, Airpotato yam 16 g, Garden balsam seed 16 g, Chinese sage 16 g, Cogongrass rhizome 60 g, Long-noded pit viper 120 g, all the drugs are first mixed with water 2500 ml, honey 120 ml, and then decocted to boiling point, to be taken in two portions at two times, one dose a day. Simultanuously with administration of carcinoma resolving powder (fresh leech 180 g, carbonized tail hair of white goose 30 g, bear gall 16 g all ground into powder) 7 g, to be taken in two portions with boiled water.

The third visit on Jun. 12, 1980. The patient's throat was dry and unsmooth, stool dry and appetite restored to normal. Esophagus X-ray film revealed: posterior border was unsmooth and irregular, local filling defect 1.5 mm, block indistinct while barium meal passing, the upper part not extended, mucoss more regular than the previous one. The patient's condition took a change for better. The above recipe was prescribed again with the dosage of adenophora root, sichuan fragrant sdomonseal rhozome and airpotato yam, reduced to 15 g, ophiopogon root reduced to 10 g, carcinoma-reducing powder added up to 9 g per day. The method of making decoction and administration were the same as mentioned above.

The fouth visit on Feb. 7. The patient felt well. X-ray film indicated: Smooth downward passing of barium meal in the esophagus, clear mucosa, smooth and regular, exhibition of extension softness and peristalsis. Still furthur, the patient was prescribed 15 doses of above recipe and 60 bags of carcinoma-reducing powder, and ordered to continue with the medication after discharge from hospital in order to strengthen the curative effect.

In April, 1980, the patient went to visit the Staff Hospital of Yima Mining bureau again. A X-ray film was taken for him and it revealed a normal esophagus. In December of the same year, he came to our hospital to have another X-ray film taken, which showed, smooth downward passing of barium meal in the middle and lower parts, non-existence of distinct narrowness and extension, clear mucosa, no interruption and damage. Esophageal net smear discovered no cancer cells [adapted from 《Medicine and pharmacology of Guangxi》 (2), 29,1982, 20 Issue. by Chen Bang hong].

Ⅲ. Personal experience

How to cure cancer is a difficult question in the medical field all over the world. TCM syndrome differentiation and treatment is an effective measure and in some cases can produce satisfactory and even curative effect. The main therapeutic principle is to strengthen the body resistance and restore normal functioning of the body to consolidate the constitution, to resolve phlegm and eliminate stagnancy. Sometimes detoxicants and cancerocidal agents are used as assistant drugs but do not play dominant role in the treatment because only when vital *qi* is replenished, resistance is strengthened, can the self-cancerocidal mechanism be aroused and strengthened, and cancer cells flinched naturally and died. If detoxicants and cancerocidal agents dominate the medication, cancer cells can not be destroyed, instead the vital *qi* will be depleted, immunity will be lowered. Consequently, cancer is not cured but the body deteriorated.

Atrophic gastritis

Atrophic gastritis is considered to be the premonitary disease of gastric carcinoma, as without punctuate and adequate treatment of the former, there is a great probability developing into the latter. The clinical manifestations of atrophic gastritis are epigastric fullness or pain, anorexia, nausea, vomiting, anemia and emaciation. This disease pertains to the category of 'gastric pain', 'fullness and stuffiness of epigastrium' and others.

I. **TCM syndrome differentiation and treatment**

Pathogenesis in brief: Long standing stagnation of gastric qi with the transference into fire which in turn induces exhaustion of qi and yin on account of the asthenic heat in the interior.

(I) Deficiency of qi and yin, damp heat obstruction in the interior.

Key points of pathogenesis: Prolonged stagnation of stomach with fire production, and exhaustion of qi and yin.

Chief manifestations: Oppression and fullness over the epigastrium, dull aching, abdominal distension immediately after meal mouth bitter taste and sticky, general malaise, anorexia, belching of gas. Tongue coat light yellow and slimmy. Pulse soft and slippery.

Therapeutic principle: To activate spleen and remove dampness, to clear the heat and remove stagnation.

1. Patent drug: *Xiang Sha Liu Jun Zi Wan*, 10 g t.i.d. and tablet berberine, *Fu Fang Dan Shen Pian* each 4 tablets t.i.d.

2. Decoction recipe: *Ban Xia Xie Xin Tang* with modifications:
Ginseng 10 g, Glehia root 12 g, Coptis root 10 g, Scutellaria root 6 g, Dried ginger 3 g, Stir-fried immature bitter orange 10 g, Atractylodes rhizome 12 g, Poria 12 g, Honey-fried licorice 8 g, for oral administration after being decocted in water, one dose a day.

Plus-minus: Severe *qi* deficiency, add astragalus root, epimedium; *yin* deficiency prominent, add fragrant solomonseal rhizome, dendrobium, black plum; associated with stagnation, add red sage root, peach kernel; extreme heat, add dandelion herb, forsythia fruit; severe dampness, add amomum fruit, agastache.

3. Acupoints: *Zhongwan, Qihai, Zusanli, Neiguan* (all with reinforcing technique), *Jiuwei, Tianshu* (both with reducing technique).

4. Ear acupoints: Stomach, Spleen, Sympathetic, Iiver, Endocrine.

(II) Insufficiency of gastric *yin*, disturbance of dry heat in the interior

Key points of pathogenesis: Stagnation of gastric

qi with transference to fire, the excess of fire leading to damage of *yin*, and resulting in the dryness and heat disturbance in the interior.

Chief manifestations: Burning pain over the epigastrium, causalgia and inclination to hunger, abdominal distension immediately after eating, emaciation and anorexia. Dryness of mouth and throat, and stool constipated. Tongue proper red with little coating. Pulse taut and fine.

Therapeutic principle: To nourish the *yin* and replenish the stomach; to clear heat and moisten the dryness.

1. Patent drug: *Xiang Sha Yang Wei Wan*, 6 g t.i.d.

2. Decoction recipe: *Sha Shen Mai Dong Tang* with modifications:

Pseudostellaria root 15 g, Ophiopogon root 12 g, Dendrobium 12 g, Dandelion herb 20 g, White peony root 12 g, Hawthorn fruit 15 g, Licorice root 3 g, Finger citron 6 g, for oral administration after being decocted in water, one dose a day.

Plus-minus: With prominent *yin* deficiency, and gastric acid deficiency plus black plum, schisandra fruit; *qi* stagnancy with dry heat, plus curcuma root, rose, capejasmine fruit; bleeding due to trauma of collaterals add reed, rehmannia root, notoginseng powder.

3. Acupoints: *Zhongwan, Zusanli, Sanyinjiao, Neiguan, Shenshu* (all with reinforcing technique), *Jiuwei, Ganshu* (both with reducing technique).

4. Ear acupoints: Kidney, Spleen, Stomach, Sympathetic, *Shenmen*.

I. Case report

Mr. Wang, 43 years old, worker, came to our clinic on June 25, 1987, with the chief complaint of history of epigastric pain for 5 years, aggravation in the last 10 days. Through Barium meal fluoroscopy of stomach and gastroscopy examination, a diagnosis of atrophic gastritis made. With medication of pepsin, 1% dilute hydrochloric acid, atropine, terramycin, prednisone, the therapeutic effect not evident. After getting angry, all symptoms exaggerated. The symptoms presenting was epigastric fullness, paroxysmal vague pain, abdominal distension after taking food, emaciated, fatigue, general malaise, loss of brilliance of facial color, anorexia, belching of gas. Tongue proper light red. Tongue coat thin white and slimmy. Pulse fine and weak. This pertained to dificiency of both *qi* and *yin*, stagnation obstruction. The therapeutic principle was to reinforce spleen *qi*, to disperse stagnation and resolve dampness.

Recipe: Dangshen 15 g, Atractylodes rhizome 10 g, Poria 12 g, Ginger-treated pinellia tuber 10 g, Coptis root 6 g, Dried ginger 3 g, Magnolia bark 10 g, Rose 12g, Barley sprout 20 g, Licorice 3 g, for oral administration after being decocted in water, one dose a day.

The second visit on July 15. After 19 doses, all symptoms alleviated except the prominent dryness of mouth and throat. Tongue proper light red, tongue coat white and dry. Pulse fine. In the above recipe the removal of dried ginger, with the addition of glehnia root 15 g, red sage root 12 g, continued the oral administration.

The third visit on Sept. 10, another 50 doses taken, all the symptoms disappeared, body weight increase 5 kg. Tongue proper light red, tongue coat thin and white. Pulse moderate. Barium meal fluoroscopy of stomach gave normal picture. He was advised to continue *Xiang Sha Liu Jun Zi Wan* 6 g, t.i.d. for another month. One year later, no relapse.

II. Personal experience

Chronic atrophic gastritis, clinically usually divided into two types as above. From the basic point of view, the fundamental is insufficinecy of spleen *qi* and stomach *yin*. The incidental is *qi* stagnation, blood stasis and phlegm retention in the interior, ascending and descending dysfunction of *qi*. This pertains to deficiency complicated with excess, intermingled *yin* and *yang*, cold and heat. The therapeutic principle should direct chiefly to the fundamental, and subsidiary to the incidental. Clinically, ginseng, danseng, pseudostellaria root to reinforce spleen, support the *qi* and promote the formation of body fluid. Red sage root, peach kernel, rose, hawthorn fruit to regulate *qi* and activate blood, to remove stagnation. The synchronus use of coptis root, dried ginger and pinellia tuber, with cold and hot properties for dispersion and for purgation, for regulating ascending and descending, thus to enhance the physiological function of stomach, to improve the cellular degeneration of tissue, to promote the recovery of microcirculation and absorption of inflammation to alleviation of the atrophy of glands till recovery.

Chronic nonspecific ulcerative colitis

This is a kind of chronic colitis of unknown origin, the pathological changes are mainly of ulcerative in character, and the site of pathology mostly at terminal colon or rectum. The chief clinical manifestations consist of diarrhea, abdominal pain and mucus, pus and blood in the stool. This disease belongs to 'dearrhea', 'abdominal pain', 'dysentery' or 'recurrent dysentery' in TCM.

I. **TCM syndrome differentiation and treatment**

Pathogenesis in brief: Accumulation of damp heat in the large intestine for long time with the damage of mucous membrane and collaterals, the dysfunction of transportation, the putrefaction of *qi* and blood, and the excretion of pus and blood.

(I) Accumulated damp heat in the intestine

Key points of pathogenesis: Stagnation of damp heat in the intestine with impeded function, putrefaction of *qi* and blood and resulting in formation of pus and blood.

Chief manifestations: Abdominal pain and diarrhea, with intermingled white (pus) and red (blood), tenesmus, urination short and dark in color, may be associated with high fever, palpitation, distending pain over abdomen or epigastrium. Tongue proper red, tongue coat yellow and slimmy. Pulse slippery rapid.

Therapeutic principle: To clear heat and attain detoxification; to regulate the mechanism of *qi* and resolve dampness.

1. Patent drug: *Xiang Lian Wan*, 10 g t.i.d.

2. Enema recipe: Pulsatilla root 30 g, Phello-dendron bark 15 g, Portulaca 30 g, Hawthorn fruit 30g, Coptis root 12 g, Aucklandia root 10 g The above decocted in water and concentrated to 100 ml for retention enema, once a day.

3. Decoction recipe: *Shao Yao Tang* with modifications:

White peony root 20 g, Honeysuckle flower 30 g, Pulsatilla root 30 g, Licorice root 10 g, Aucklandia root 10 g, Coptis root 10 g, Phellodendron bark 10g, Red bean 30 g, Poria 12 g, Hawthorn fruit 20 g, for oral administration after being decocted in water, one dose a day.

Plus-minus: Noxious heat in excess, high fever with impaired consciousness, plus antelope's horn, fresh rehmannia root, and simultanuous intake of *Zi Xue San* exopathogen still existing, plus puerarum root, scutellaria root.

4. Acupoints: *Tianshu, Dachangshu, Xiawan, Neiting, Hegu*(all with reducing technique).

(II) Body resistance weakened while pathogens still prevailing.

Key points of pathogenesis: Diarrhea for long duration, the vital energy already weakened, while the pathogens still prevailing, the intermingled cold and heat, disease lingering.

Chief manifestations: Diarrhea at times, impaired appetite, general malaise, inclination to lie down and to warm. Aversion to cold. During defecation abdominal pain and tenesmus. Stool intermingled with mucous or blood. Tongue proper light red, with white slimmy coating. Pulse weak and rapid.

Therapeutic principle: To warm up the mid-burner (digestive tract) and clear up the intestine to resolve stagnation and activate the blood.

1. Patent drug:

(1) *Fu Zi Li Zhong Wan*, one bolus t.i.d. and tablet berberine and *Fu Fang Dan Shen Pian* each 5 tablets, t.i.d.

(2) *Wu Mei Wan*, one bolus t.i.d.

2. Decoction recipe: *Lian Li Tang* with modifications:

Ginseng 12 g, White atractylodes root 12 g, Dried ginger 10 g, Coptis root 10 g, Aucklandia root 10 g, Smilax glabra rhizome 20 g, Cinnamon bark 3 g, Peach kernel 12 g, Forsythia fruit 15 g, Licorice root 3 g, for oral administration after being decocted in water, one dose a day.

Plus-minus: In cases due to weakness of spleen and stomach, upward perversion of gastric *qi*, vomiting immediately after meal, plus ginger treated pinellia tuber, ginger juice, amomom fruit, grass-leaved sweetflag rhizome; in case with *yang* deficiency of spleen and kidney, chilliness, cold limbs, plus prepared aconite root, honey-treated ephedra.

3. Acupoints: *Pishu, Zusanli, Shenshu* (all with reinforcing technique), *Guanyuan, Qihai, Baihui* (all moxibustion), *Tianshu* (with reducing technique).

II. Case report

Ms. Yang, 45 years old, came to our clinic on January 21, 1988, with a history of diarrhea passing blood and pus for 5 years, with aggravation in 6 days. She was hospitalized many times with a diagnosis of chronic ulcerative colitis, and was treated with sulfadiazine, prednisone, probanthine, the ill condition sometimes better, sometimes worse; recently the condition aggravated after over-indulgence in sea fishy foods and mutton preparations. The diarrhea, 4~6 times a day, abdominal pain, temporarily relieved after defecation, tenesmus. Stool intermingled with mucus and pus and blood, jellylike. Emaciated, general malaise, inclination to lie down and keep warm, aversion to cold. Tongue proper light red, tongue coating white and slimmy. Pulse weak and rapid. This pertained to *yang* deficiency of spleen and kidney, stagnation in the interior. The therapeutic principle should direct to warm up spleen and kidney, to resolve stagnation.

Recipe: Coptis root 10 g, Dried ginger 6 g, Prepared aconite root 10 g, Phellodendron bark 10 g, Aucklandia root 10 g, Atractylodes root 12 g, Smilax glabra rhizome 24 g, Red and white peony root each 12 g, Areca seed 10g, Hawthorn fruit 30 g, Pueraria root 24 g, for oral administration after being decocted in water, one dose a day.

The second visit on Mar. 10. After 36 doses, all the symptoms alleviated, stool once daily, appetite improved, the meal intake increased, abdominal pain disappeared. The stool semiliquid with mucus. Tongue proper light red, coat thin and white. Pulse fine and weak.

The above recipe with addition of astragalus root 30 g, dahurian angelica root 10 g, honeysuckle flower 30g, peach kernel 10 g, with removal of dried ginger, for oral administration after being decocted in water, one dose a day.

The third visit on May 5. 51 doses taken, all symptoms disappeared. Stool once daily, formed without mucus, pus or blood. Tongue proper light red, tongue coat thin and white. Pulse moderate. On sigmoidoscopey, the surface of ulcer healed. She was told to continue intake of *Xiang Sha Liu Jun Zi Wan* 10 g, b.i.d., for two months to fortify the therapeutic effects.

Ⅲ. Personal experience

This is a chronic lingering disease, as the retention of damp heat in the colon, with crosion of its membrane, collaterals damaged. The therapeutic principle is to clean up the damp heat, remove stagnation in the gastro-intestinal tract, to regulate *qi* and activate the blood.

To astringe too early or drastic purgation, diuresis should be avoided, this should be strictly followed.

Senile constipation

Senile constipation here indicates the constipation not the result of illness, but due to slowed intestinal peristalsis in aged people, and the prolonged stay of digested food in the intestine. This pertains to the category of *"xu bi"* (asthenic constipation) in TCM.

I. TCM syndrome differentiation and treatment

Pathogenesis in brief: Debility of the aged, whether insufficiency of *yin* blood or *yang qi*, or stagnation of *qi*. The dryness and impaired moistening of intestine leads to constipation.

(I) The impaired moistening of the intestine

Key points of pathogenesis: Insufficiency of *yin* and blood, deficiency of body fluids, and the impaired moistening of intestine with the result of constipation.

Chief manifestations: Constipation. Facial appearance without brilliance, dizziness, palpitation, lumbar soreness. Tongue proper light red. Pulse fine and sluggish.

Therapeutic principle: To nourish the *yin* and blood, to moisten intestine and promote defecation.

1. Patent drug: *Wu Ren Wan*, 10 g t.i.d.

2. Decoction recipe: *Zun Sheng Run Chang Wan* with modifications:

Rehmannia root 30 g, Chinese angelica root 15 g. Prepared fleece-flower root 24 g, Hemp seed 30 g. Peach kernel 15 g, Stir-fried bitter orange 10 g, Cassia seed 12 g, for oral administration after being decocted in water, one dose a day.

Plus-minus: In cases with *yin* deficiency and heat in the interior, plus scrofularia root, anemarrhena rhizome, fleece-flower root.

3. Acupoints: *Pishu, Weishu, Zusanli, Qihai* (all

with reinforcing technique).

(Ⅱ) Intestine cold

Key points of pathogenesis: The asthenia of kidney *yang*, with formation of internal cold which causes stagnation of *qi* and the weakness of transportation.

Chief manifestations: Difficulty in expelling the stool, urine clear and large in amount, pallor of face, soreness of loin and spinal column, thermophilia, aversion to cold, tongue proper light colored, with white coat, pulse deep and slow.

Therapeutic principle: To warm up and reinforce the kidney *yang*; to moisten the intestine and promote defecation.

1. Patent drug: *Ban Liu Wan*, 5 g t.i.d.

2. Decoction recipe: *Ji Chuan Jian* with modifications:

Desertliving cistanche 30g, Chinese angelica root 15g, Achyranthes root 15g, Cimicifuga rhizome 10g, Stir-fried bitter orange 10g, Cinnamon bark 6g, for oral administration after being decocted in water, one dose a day.

Plus-minus: In cases with *qi* deficiency, plus astragalus root, ginseng; with kidney *yin* deficiency, plus wolfberry fruit prepared rehmannia root.

3. Acupoints: *Guanyuan* (moxibustion), *Shenshu, Dachangshu, Zhigou, Zhaohai* (with reinforcing technique).

I. Case report

Mr. Lu, 60 years old, cadre, came to clinic on August 5, 1978. With the chief complaint of constipation for 3 years, Tab. phenolphthaleinum, senna leaf, Tab. including rhubarb and others used, after purgation, the constipation became more resistent. Bowel moved with difficulty, accompanied with facial pallor, loin aching, cold limbs, urination clear and large in amount, general malaise. Tongue proper light red, tongue coat white. Pulse deep and slow. This was considered to be deficiency of kidney *yang*, impeded moistening of the intestine. The principle of treatment should be to warm up *yang* and promote defecation.

Recipe: Desertliving cistanche 30g, Chinese angelica root 15g, Ginseng 10g, Cinnamon bark 6g, Achyranthes root 15g, Stir-fried bitter apricot seed 12g, Stir-fried bitter orange 10g, for oral administration after being decocted in water, one dose every other day.

After 10 doses, the defecation became normal, all symptoms disappeared. With 5 times the recipe doses, ground into fine powder, mixed with heated honey, each bolus 10g, t.i.d. to fortify the results.

II. Personal experience

In senile age, the depletion of blood and essence, the decline of kidney *yang*, during acutely ill stage, acupuncture and medication have to be employed. In common occasions, dietary therapy should be more suitable. The dietary therapy as follows.

1. Tyemella 15g, oral administration after being decocted in water and mixed with honey 15g, one dose daily, divided into two portions taken seperately.
2. Banana, pears, radish and others after meal.
3. Pig's blood, spinach, carrot and others.
4. Sesame, peanut, walnut, rice ground into fine powder suitable amount each time, twice a day.

Cirrhosis of liver with ascites

Cirrhosis of liver with ascites is due to hypertension of portal vein, usually associated with hepatosplenomegaly, varicose veins of abdominal wall, varicoses of esophagus and fundus of stomach with rupture and hemorrhage, hepatic coma and others. It pertains to the category of 'tympanitic distension','single abdominal distension','spider tympany' and others.

I. **TCM syndrome differentiation and treatment**

Pathogenesis in brief: The disease starting from liver, and later with involvement of spleen and kidney couses qi stagnation and blood stasis with obstruction of water passage. The mutual accumulation of liver, spleen and kidney pathology in the abdomen.

(I) Damp-heat stagnancy

Key points of pathogenesis: The excess of damp-heat with stagnancy in middle burner, the dysfunction of spleen, resulting in *qi* stagnation and water retension.

Chief manifestations: Abdomen big and full, distension resistant to palpation, dysphoria, bitter taste of mouth, nausea, anorexia, thirsty, with disinclination to drink, urination dark colored and unsmooth. There may be jaundice, or hematemesis, hematochezia. Tongue proper red, with yellow slimmy coat. Pulse taut and repid.

Therapeutic principle: To clear up heat and resolve dampness, to get rid of water retension by duiretics and remove distension.

1. Patent drug: *Long Dan Xie Gan Wan* 10g, t.i.d. and *Chen Xiang Hua Zhi Wan* 5g, t.i.d.

2. Decoction recipe: *Zhong Man Fen, Xiao Wan* and *Yin Chen Hao Tang* with modifications:

Oriental wormwood 24g, Capejasmine fruit 10g, Curcuma root 12g, Scutellaria root 12g, Magnolia bark 12g, stir-fried bitter orange 10g, Poria 18g, Alismatis rhizome 24g, Plantain seed 21g, Lysimachia 20g, Talc 12g, for oral administration after being decocted in water, one dose a day.

Plus-minus: Exuberance of noxious heat, constipated, plus rhubarb, anemarrhena rhizome, gypsum; accumulated heat in urinary bladder, urination dark colored and unsmooth, add mole cricket, cricket, eagle wood; bleeding due to heat, with hematochezia, epistaxia, add notogensing, hairy vein agrimony, cogongrass rhizome ,biota tops; high fever, impaired consciousness Qing Kai Ling injection 20ml added to glucoss 500ml intravenuous drip or oral intake of An Gong Niu Huang Wan.

3. Acupoints: *Pishu, Danshu, Shuigou, Yinlingquan, Sanyinjiao, Pangguangshu* (all with reducing technique).

(Ⅱ) Blood stasis of liver and spleen

Key points of pathogenesis: Blood stasis of liver and spleen, obstruction of blood vessels, water retension in the interior.

Chief manifestations: Fullness and rigidity of abdomen, abdominal masses bulging, veins engorged over abdomen, facial color dark, spider angioma, venules simulating crab's foot, red patches over palms, mouth dry, and disinclination to drink. Stool black. Tongue proper dark purple or with ecchymosis over the margins. Pulse deep taut and unsmooth.

Therapeutic principle: To activate the blood, and remove stagnation, and to activate the *qi* and remove fluids with diuretics.

1. Patent drug:

(1) *Fu Fang Dan Shen Pian* 4 tablets t.i.d., swallowed with Decoction fluid of motherwort 30g.

(2) *Zhou Che Wan*, 5g t.i.d.

(3) *Bie Jia Jian Wan*, 5g t.i.d.

2. Decoction recipe: *Tiao Ying Yin* with modifications:

Chinese angelica root 12g, Red peony root 12g, Red sage root 24g, Bupleurum root 10g, Burreed tuber 6g, Zedoary 10g, Corydalis tuber 12g, Rhubarb 6g, Chinese pink herb 15g, Lepidium seed 12g, Mulberry bark 12g, Areca seed 10g, for oral administration after being decocted in water, one dose a day.

Plus-minus: Black stool plus notoginseng powder, biota top; ascites prominent, plus alismatis rhizome, bugleweed, princesplume ladysthumb fruit.

3. Acupoints: *Xuehai, Geshu, Zhongji, Shuigou, Fuliu, Yinlingquan* (all with reducing technique), *Zhangmen, Qimen* (both moxibustion)

(Ⅱ) *Yang* deficiency of spleen and kidney

Key points of pathogenesis: Weakness of *yang qi*, water dampness not resolved, stagnation in abdomen, abdominal distension as frog.

Chief manifestations: Abdomen enlarged and distended, as a bag enveloping water, edema of lower limb. Face bluish yellow, malaise, aversion to cold, epigastric fullness, anorexia, urination short and scanty in amount. Tongue proper plump, light purple. Pulse deep taut and without force.

Therapeutic principle: To warm and tonify the spleen and kidney, to resolve dampness and remove water with diuretics.

1. Patent drug:

(1) *Fu Zi Li Zhong Wan*, one bolus t.i.d. and *Ji Sheng Shen Qi Wan*, one bolus t.i.d.

(2) *Yu Gong San*: morning glory seed 120g, Common fennel fruit 30g, both ground into fine powder 2g, t.i.d.

2. Decoction recipe: *Zhen Wu Tang* with modifications:

Prepared aconite root 12g, Cinnamon twig 10g, White atractylodes root 20g, Alismatis root 24g, Umbellate pore fungus 24g, Fresh ginger 10g, Cogongrass rhizome 30g, for oral administration after being decocted in water, one dose a day.

Plus-minus: Inclination to deficiency of spleen *yang*, plus dangshen, astragalus root; inclination to deficiency of kidney *yang*, add epimedium; after the clearance of edema, *Xiang Sha Liu Jun Zi Wan* in the morning, *Jin Gui Shen Qi Wan* at night.

3. Acupoints: *Shenshu, Pishu, Qihai, Shuifen* (all with reducing technique).

(Ⅳ) *Yin* deficiency of liver and kidney

Key points of pathogenesis: *Yin* deficiency of liver and kidney, impaired distribution of body fluid, water fluid retention in the middle burner, the blood stasis as the result.

Chief manifestations: Abdomen big and full, with prominence of veins over the surface, abdomen rather tense; four limbs thin, dark color of face, dryness of mouth and throat, dysphoria, insomnia, gum bleeding, epistaxis, urination short and scanty. Tongue proper red with little salivation. Pulse taut, fine and rapid.

Therapeutic principle: To nourish liver and kidney,

to resolve stagnation and remove fluids with diuretics.

1. Patent drug: *Liu Wei Di Huang Wan*, one bolus t.i.d., mole cricket and cricket equal amount, baked dry and ground to powder, 5g, t.i.d.

2. Decoction recipe: *Liu Wei Di Huang Tang* with modifications:

Pseudostellaria root 24g, Ophiopogon root 24g, Rehmannia root 24g, Dogwood fruit 10g, Chinese yam 15g, Red sage root 20g, Moutan bark 12g, Alismatis rhizome 30g, Bugleweed 12g, Cogongrass rhizome 30g, for oral administration after being decocted in water, one dose a day.

Plus-minus: For low grade fever, add swallowwort root, turtle shell, sweet worm-wood, wolf-berry bark; much bleeding, add hairy vein agrimony, stir-fried capejasmine fruit, small thistle and Japanese thistle, notoginseng powder; in cases complicated with damp-heat, add oriental wormwood, anemarrhena rhizome, phellodendron bark, pronounced abdominal distension, add radish seed, shell of areca nut.

3. Acupoints: *Ganshu, Pishu, Zhangmen, Qimen* (all with reinforcing technique), *Shuigou, Yinlingquan, Xuehai, Geshu* (all with reducing technique).

I. **Case report**

Mr. Li, 42 years old, cadre, came to clinic on Dec. 5, 1978, with abdominal fullness and distension for more than one year, with exacerbation one week. He was diagnosed cirrhosis of liver complicated with ascites, abdominal paracentesis for several times, and the recurrence of fluids soon after tapping. Ono week ago, sudden spell of chill and fever, body temperature 40°C, temperature gradually lowered, and still had aversion to cold, cold limbs, needling pain over chest and hypochondria, abdomen full and distended, abdominal circumference 103cm, mentally fatigued, anorexia, urination short and scanty, stool liquid or semiliquid, emaciated, facial color black yellow, several spider angioma over face and chest simulating the crab's feet called xie zhao wen luo. Tongue proper dark purple, tongue coat white and dry, with scanty salivation. Pulse deep, fine and unsmooth.

TCM syndrome differentiation and treatment: This pertained to *yang* deficiency of spleen and kidney, obstruction in interior with water dampness. *Qi* stagnation and blood stasis. The therapeutic principle adopted was to warm and tonify spleen and kidney, to resolve stagnation and remove dampness with diuretics.

Recipe: Prepared aconite root 10g, Dangshen 15g, White atractylodes root 12g, Chinese yam 15g, Dogwood fruit 10g, Poria 24g, Alismatis rhizome 24g, Shell of areca nut 15g, Amomum fruit 10g, Peach kernel 10g, Zedoary 12g, Indian mulberry root 10g, Chicken's gizzard membrane 10g, Bupleurum root 10g, for oral administration after being decocted in water, one dose a day.

The second visit on Dec, 14. After 8 recipes taken,

the aversion to cold and cold limb disappeared, urine increase in amount, abdominal distension alleviated, abdominal circumference 98cm. Still dull vague aching over right hypochondrium, liquid stool, anorexia. Tongue proper dark purple. Pulse deep fine and weak.

From the above recipe the removal of prepared aconite root, the addition of cinnamon twig 6g, ginseng 10g, stirfried haw-thorn fruit to black 15g, stir-fried radish seed 12g, oral decoction as before, one dose daily.

The third visit on Feb. 3, 1979. Another 45 doses taken, gradual increase of urine amount, appetite gradually turned better, abdominal distension alleviated and ascites entirely gone. Abdominal circumference 78cm. Sleep sound, stool normal. Tongue proper dark red, with thin white coating, pulse deep and fine.

Recipe:Took *Xiang Sha Liu Jun Zi Wan* 10g in the morning, *Jin Gui Shen Qi Wan*, one bolus at night, to fortify the therapeutic effects.

II. Personal experience

Cirrhosis of liver with ascites is a stubborn disease often resistent to treatment, often ineffective with simple use of diuretics. In TCM there is the hydragogue method, the suitable use of which may get instant results just like setting up a pole and see its shadow.

1. Iudication: The course comparatively short, the vital *qi* not declined, appetite still not bad, severe abdominal distension, urine scanty and stool constipated.

Pulse forceful.

2. The commonly used recipe: *Zhou Che Wan* or *Kong Xian Dan* and others.

3. Methods of administration:

(1) In the morning while the stomach is vacant, bolus swallowed with decoction of Chinese date, one course, consecutive intake for 3 days.

(2) "To attenuate the bigger half of a disease", to avoid damage of spleen and stomach, and exhaustion of vital energy which may lead to hemorrhage and coma.

(3) The alternate use of hydragogues and tonic drugs, such as American ginseng 12g, white atractylodes root 30g, or astragalus root 45g, Chinese angelica root 10g, using the water decoction fluid.

Besides, after the subsidence of ascites, still the enlargement of liver and spleen, the following recipe can be used for gradual resolution: Vinegar fried turtle shell 12g, Ground beetle 12g, Mole cricket 10g, Oyster shell 12g, Stir-fried pangolin scales 6g, Burreed tuber 6g, Zedoary 6g, Peach kernel 6g, Rhubarb 10g, Chicken's gizzard membrane 10g, Bupleurum root 5g, Curcuma root 10g, Tangerine peel 10g, America ginseng 10g, Hawthorn fruit 6g, Barley sprout 6g.

5 times the doses of the above recipe, ground into fine powder, with the addition of heated honey to make pills, each time 6g, two or three times a day.

Cholelithiasis

Cholelithiasis is mostly the result of intestinal helminthiasis and biliary tract infection. Its clinical manifestations are sudden acute pain over the epigastrium or right hypochondrium. The pain is so severe as to make patient doubled up, rolling in the bed, restless and cry, often referred to the right shoulder or right back below the right shoulder girdle. During the episode of attack, the patient may be found with his fist pressing over the abdomen, wet with profuse sweat, facial pallor, nausea and vomiting. This disease pertains to the category of hypochondriac pain, abdominal pain, epigastric pain, jaundice in TCM.

I. TCM syndrome differentiation and treatment

Pathogenesis in brief: The stagnation of liver *qi*, with damp heat accumulation in the interior, the decoction and cooking of the body fluid with stone formation.

(I) Stagnation of liver *qi*

Key points of pathogenesis: Liver damage due to *qi* stagnation and anger, the dysfunction of liver dispersion, resulting in stone formation.

Chief manifestations: Distending pain of right hypochondrium, bitter taste of mouth, throat dryness, dysphoria with inclination to anger, epigastric discomfort, nausea, anorexia, with frequent belching. All the symptoms exacerbated with anger. Tongue coat thin and yellow. Pulse taut and fine.

Therapeutic principle: To disperse the liver and regulate the *qi*, to promote biliary excretion and expel the stones.

1. Patent drug: *Shu Gan He Wei Wan* 6g, t.i.d. and oral intake of powder of chicken's gizzard membrane and lysimachia 5g, t.i.d.

2. Decoction recipe: *Chai Hu Shu Gan San* with modifications:

Bupleurum root 12g, Stir-fried immature bitter orange 12g, Curcuma root 15g, Cyperus tuber 10g, White peony root 15g, Lysimachia 30g, Climbing fern spore 30g, Chicken's gizzard membrane 12g, Licorice root 3g, for oral administration after being decocted in water, one dose a day.

Plus-minus: With fever plus honey-suckle flower, forsythia fruit; for constipation plus rhubarb, mirabilite; weak constitution and malaise, add Dangshen, poria, white atractylodes root, licorice root.

3. Acupoints: *Ganshu, Danshu, Taichong, Riyue, Yanglingquan* (all with reducing technique).

4. Ear acupoints: Biliary zone, Sympathetic, Duodenum, Liver.

(II) Damp heat of liver and biliary tract

Key points of pathogenesis: Liver and spleen stasis with inability to resolve water dampness, heat production after prolonged stasis, the cooking and decoction of body fluid finally with stone formation.

Chief manifestations: Chill and fever in alternation, acute pain over right hypochondrium, sclera yellow, bitter taste of mouth, dryness of throat, nausea and anorexia, even profuse sweat, pallor of face, urine dark colored, stool constipated. Tongue coat yellowish slimmy, pulse taut and rapid.

Therapeutic principe: To clear up the heat and remove dampness with diuretics, to expel the stones with dispersion and purgation.

1. Patent drug: *Long Dan Xie Gan Wan* 10g, t.i.d. and *Da Huang Pain* 5 tab. t.i.d.

2. Decoction recipe: *Yin Chen Hao Tang* with modifications:

Bupleurum root 15g, Curcuma root 15g, Lysimachia 30g, Oriental worm wood 30g, Capejasmine fruit 12g, Honeysuckle flower 30g, Talc 15g, Rhubarb 10g, Stir-fried immature bitter orange 12g, Mirabilite 6g, for oral administration after being decocted in water, one dose daily.

Plus-minus: Nausea and vomiting, plus ginger treated pinellia tuber, ginger treated bamboo shavings; high fever add moutan bark, antelope's horn; chronic illness with weak constitution, add Dangshen, poria, white peony root.

3. Acupoints: *Ganshu, Danshu, Zhangmen, Qimen, Zhongwan, Taichong, Yanglingquan* (all with reducing

technique).

4. Ear acupoints: Pancreas, Biliary tract, Liver, Sympathetic, *Shenmen*, Subcortex, Duodenum, Small intestine.

I. Case report

Mr. Li, 38 years old, worker, came to the clinic on May 25, 1981, with chief complaint of acute paroxysmal pain and fullness over right hypochondrium for 8 hours, accompanied with fever, bitter taste in mouth, nausea, vomiting dark urination and stool constipated. Tongue proper red, tongue coat yellow thick and slimmy. Pulse taut and rapid. B type ultrasonic examination revealed stone in the neck of gall bladder, diameter 1.0×0.8 (cm) Blood transpeptidase 88 units.

TCM syndrome differentiation: Accumulate heat in liver and biliary tract, stone obstruction in interior. The therapeutic principle should be to disperse the liver and attain cholecystagogic action, to clear up the heat and expel stones.

Recipe: Bupleurum root 15g, Curcuma root 12g, Capejasmine fruit 12g, Honey suckle flower 30g, Rhubarb 10g, Stir-fried immature bitter orange 12g, Lusimachia 21g, Chicken's gizzard membrance 12g, Ginger treated bamboo shaving 10g, Mirabilite 6g, for oral administration after being decocted in water, one dose daily. The simulataneus use of ear acupuncture: *Dan* (biliary tract), sympathetic, subcortesx, duodenum.

After 10 recipe doses, sudden exacerbation of right

hypochondriac pain, and other symptoms also aggravated. The pain disappeared half a day later, and all symptoms disappeared with expelling of bile stones two pieces as the size of soybean. The above recipe with the removal of rhubarb and mirabilite, add Dangshen and pinellia tuber, continued for 10 doses, all the symptoms disappeared. B type ultrasonic examination again bile stones already expelled out. The blood transpeptidase returned to normal.

Ⅲ. Personal experience

(I) Though the manifestations of cholelithiasis may be classified into two types according to TCM as above, yet they are closely correlated, thus in the treatment may be summarized into six methods which should be used in combination with one another. The first is *Qing*, that is to clear the heat, the commonly used drugs are capejasmine fruit, honey- suckle flower, bupleurum root, forsvthia fruit and others. The second is *Li*, that is to remove dampness, oriental worm wood, lophatherum and talc are usually used. The third is *Rong* that is to dissolve the stones, lysimachia, chicken's gizzard membrane, climbing fern spore, mirabilite, walnut seed and others. The fourth is *You*, that is to induce contraction of biliary duct, such as using cooked pig's foot one or two to induce seizure of attack, in order to induce contraction of bile duct and the expelling of stones. The fifth *Dao* is to disperse the commonly used drugs are bupleurum root, curcuma root, immature bitter orange, cyperus tuber and others; the sixth *Pai* is to expel the stones, the frequently used drugs are rhubarb, mirabilite and magnolia bark and others.

(Ⅰ) Ear acupuncture or medicine press over the ear points: specific effect in treating cholelithiasis, equal portions of bupleurum root, curcuma root, stir-fried immature bitter orange and grass-leaved sweetflag rhizome, all ground into fine powder, flood with water to make pill as the size of vaccaria seed or using the vaccaria seed pressing over the ear points, once daily after meal.

(Ⅱ) In stubborn cases, stones not expelled after repeated treatment, with manifestations of *qi* and blood deficiency, in the recipe, Dangshen, white atractylodes root, walnut seed, astragalus root, white peony root, poria and coix seed may be added.

Nephrolithiasis

Nephrolithiasis is a term for calculus or stone formation in kidney pelvis or calyx. In clinic it may induce renal colic and hematuria, sometimes obstruction in urinary passage and secondary infections, and renal failure in late stage. This disease pertains to the category of 'lumbago','stone stranguria' and others. Nephrolithotony has the defect of recurrences, and at present there remains a problem for radical cure. TCM the syndrome differentiation and treatment of this disease has comparatively better therapeutic effects.

I. TCM syndrome differentiation and treatment

Pathogenesis in brief: The damp heat in the lower burner affects the steaming function of kidney, the sediments of urine on decoction result in formation of calculi which retain in kidney.

(I) Damp heat in the lower burner

Key points of pathogenesis: The stagnation of damp heat, which steam heat the urine, with calculi formation in the kidney.

Chief manifestations: Paroxysmal lumbar pain, awling or twisting in character, associated with frequent micturation, unbearable pain, even chilliness and fever, nausea, vomiting, hematuria, sandy stone passed off with the urine. Tongue proper red, tongue coat yellow, thick and slimmy, pulse taut slippery and rapid.

Therapeutic principle: To clear up heat and remove dampness with diuretics; to treat the stranguria and expel the stones.

1. Patent drug: *Zhi Bai Di Huang Wan* one bolus, t.i.d. Lysimache, plantain seed each 30g, the bolus swallowed with decocted fluid of lysimachia and plantain seed.

2. Decoction fluid: *Ba Zheng San* with modifications:

Common knot grass 15g, Chinese pink herb 15g, Akebia stem 6g, Rehmannia root 18g, Phellodendron bark 12g, Vaccaria seed 12g, Abutilon seed 12g, Talc 30g, Plantain herb 30g, Lysimachia 30g, Cyathula root 12g, Licorice root 3g, for oral administration after being decocted in water, one dose a day.

Plus-minus: Hematuria marked, plus biota top, cogongrass rhizome, small thistle; nausea, vomiting add ginger treated bamboo shaving; chill and fever in alternation, add bupleurm root, scutellaria root.

3. Acupoints: *Zhongji, Yinlingquan, Qihai, Sanyinjiao, Taixi, Pangguangshu* (all with reducing technique).

4. Ear acupoints: Kidney, Sympathetic, Urinary bladder, Liver.

(II) Insufficiency of kidney *yin*

Key points of pathogenesis: The persistent stagnation of damp heat with impairment and exhaustion of *yin* fluid. The obstruction of urinary calculi results in stranguria.

Chief manifestations: Soreness and weakness of loin and knee; vague aching, mild at day time, severe at night. Urination short and dark, even stranguria, mouth and throat dry, dysphoria with hotness over palms, soles and in the chest, insomnia and dreamfulness, stool constipated. Tongue proper red with little coating, pulse taut, fine, rapid. In case *yin* damage extending to *yang* with chilliness and cold limbs, edema of lower limbs, tongue proper light colored, with white moist coating. Pulse deep and slow and others.

Therapeutic principle: To nourish and replenish the

kidney *yin*; to expel the stones with diuretics.

1. Patent drug: *Liu Wei Di Huang Wan* one bolus, t.i.d. swallowed with the water decoction of lysimachia 30g.

2. Decoction recipe: *Yi Shen Pai Shi Tang* with modifications:

> Rehmannia root 30g, Prepared fleece-flower root 20g, Chinese angelica root 12g, Eucommia bark 12g, Mulberry mistletoe 15g, Moutan bark 15g, Alismatis rhizome 30g, Pyrrosia leaf 30g, Talc 30g, Climbing fern spore 20g, Grass leaved sweetflag rhizome 12g, for oral administration after being decocted in water, one dose a day.

Plus-minus: In case constipated plus anemarrhena rhizome, phellodendron bark, cinnamon bark; dysphoria with feverishness over palms, soles and in the chest, add capejasmine fruit, asparagus root; calculi of long standing without being resolved, add lysimachia, chicken's gizzard membrane, walnut kernel; *yin* damage with extension to involve *yang*, add psoralea fruit. Curculigo rhizome, epimedium, walnut kernel.

3. Acupoints: *Shenshu, Taixi, Kunlun, Zhishi* (all with reinforcing technique), *Zusanli, Yinlingquan, Qihai, Zhongji* (all with reducing technique).

4. Ear acupoints: Kidney, Urinary bladder, Subcortex, Sympathetic, *Shenmen*.

II. Case report

Ms. Zhang, 24 years old, worker, came to clinic on Jan. 25, 1981, with chief complaint of lumbar pain, fever, and painful micturation, frequency and urgency for 3 days, aggravated for one day, associated with nausea, vomiting, hematuria, stool constipated, dysphoria, easy to lose temper. Tongue proper red, tongue coat thick, yellow and slimmy, pulse taut, slippery and rapid. T38.5°C, Urine WBC a few, RBC four plus. X-ray plain film revealed calculus 0.2×0.15(cm) size in kidney calyx, 0.15× 0.21(cm) calculus in ureter.

TCM syndrome differentiation: Damp heat in the lower burner, stone retention. The therapeutic principle selected to clear up the damp heat and to expel the stone with diuretics. A diagnosis of nephrolithiasis made.

Recipe: Common knot-grass 15g, Chinese pink herb 21g, Rhemannia root 30g, Akebia stem 6g, Phellodendron bark 10g, Talc 30g, Plantain herb 30g, Vaccaria seed 12g, Lysimachia 30g, Cogongrass rhizome 30g, Honeysuckle flower 20g, Licorice root 3g, for oral administration after being decocted in water, one dose daily.

After 15 doses, symptoms relieved. Tongue proper red, tongue coat thin and yellow, pulse moderate. From the above recipe akebia stem and phellodendron bark removed, walnut kernel 15g and climbing fern spore 12g for another ten doses, then sudden attack of acute intolerable pain of the loin, blood in the urine. One hour later sudden disappearance of pain, a few sandlike stones expelled out, X-ray film revealed the disappearance of stone shadow in kidney and ureter.

II. Personal experience

(1) Exercise and expelling stones: During the course of treatment, encourage patient run and leap, in order to facilitate the expelling of stones, no need to confine to bed.

(2) Pain and expelling stones: During the course of treatment the sudden appearance of acute pain from the loin radiating to the lower abdomen and the external genitalea, on and off, accompanied by hematuria, nausea, vomiting. This is the predromal sign of stone expelling, no need to be frightened badly.

(3) After the expelling of stones, frequent use of kidney bolus of six drugs including rehmannia root, the walnut kernel and others for the purpose of prophylaxis of formation of new stones are beneficial.

Hypertrophy of prostate gland

Hypertrophy of prostate gland is a benign proliferous pathological change, but the micturation may be affected on account of the obstruction at the prostatic urethra, and often complicated with secondary infections and vague dragging pain over the perineum, drippling of urine, white sticky mucoid substance at the end of micturation, and even retention of urine. At present operative surgery is the chief method of choice, but in old aged usually the coexistence of essential hypertension, the cardiac and cerebral vascular disease, or pulmonary dysfunction and others. Such an operation is really a heavy burden to them. This disease pertains to 'stranguria' 'uroschesis' in TCM, and its syndrome differentiation and treatment usually can obtain satisfactory results.

I. TCM syndrome differentiation and treatment

Pathogenesis in brief: Aged, weak constitution, stagnation of damp heat in the lower burner, the deficiency of spleen and kidney, and lingering, obstinate to treatment.

(I) Downward flow of damp heat

Key points of pathogenesis: Senile, weak, easily attacked by exopathogen, heat accumulation in the lower burner, the impaired *qi* function.

Chief manifestations: Dragging and distending pain over the perineum, consciousness of some urine not expelled out, cloudy urine at the end of micturation, some prickling and itching over the urethra, or pain, frequency and urgency of micturation, fever, dryness of mouth, lumbar pain, stool constipated. Tongue proper red, coat thin and yellow. Pulse fine and rapid.

Therapeutic principle: To clear up heat and remove dampness with diuresis.

1. Patent drug: *Long Dan Xie Gan Wan*, 10g t.i.d. after meal.

2. Decoction recipe: *Ba Zheng San* with modifications:

Chinese pink herb 12g, Common knot grass 12g, Phellodendron bark 10g, AKebia stem 10g, Mother wort 30g, Dandelion herb 24g, Honeysuckle flower 24g, Pyrrosia leaf 20g, Plantain herb 24g, Licorice 3g, for oral administration after being decocted in water, one dose a day.

Plus-minus: Acute episode with high fever, plus small thistle, forsythia fruit, gypsum; *yin* damage due to extreme heat, plus rehmannia root, anemarrhena rhizome.

3. Acupoints: *Shenshu, Pangguanshu, Zhongji, Ququan, Yinlingquan, Fuliu* (all with reducing technique).

(II) The combination of stasis and turbid pathogen

Key points of pathogenesis: The accumulation of damp heat and stasis formation, the stagnation of stasis and turbidity results in the impeded water passage.

Chief manifestations: Dragging and distending vague pain of perineum and testicle, the impeded urine passage and drippling of urine, frequent urination and feeling of imcomplete evacuation, turbidity of urine, white mucoid fluid flows out from the urethra during defecation. Tongue proper light red or with ecchymosis, with thin, white coating. Pulse fine, slippery and rapid.

Therapeutic principle: To resolve stagnation and purge the turbidity; to clear up heat and promote diuresis.

1. Patent drug: *Long Dan Xie Gan Wan* 10g, t.i.d. and *Fu Fang Dan Shen Pian* 4 tablets, t.i.d.

2. Decoction recipe: *Kun Cao Fang* with modifications:

Motherwort 30g, Honey suckle flower 30g, Lophatherum 10g, Rhubarb 6g, Phellodendron bark 10g, Peach kernel 12g, Hypoglauca yam 15g, Bugleweed 12g, Pyrosia leaf 21g, Rehmannia root 15g, Plantain herb 21g, Licorice root 6g, for oral administration after being decocted in water, one dose a day.

3. Acupoints: *Shenshu, Pangguangshu, Yanglingquan, Ququan, Sanyinjiao, Xuehai* (all with reducing technique).

(II) Insufficiency of spleen and kidney

Key points of pathogenesis: Stasis and turbidity for long time, with invasion of spleen and kidney, the asthenia of the lower *jiao*, spermatorrhea results.

Chief manifestations: Soreness and weakness of loin and knees, frequency of urination, drippling of urine, white mucus at the end of micturation, spermatorrhea, early ejaculation and impotence, dizziness, insomnia, dreamfulness, general malaise. Tongue coat thin and white, pulse fine weak and rapid.

Therapeutic principle: To replenish spleen and kidney, to resolve turbidity and stagnation.

1. Patent drug:

(1) *Gui Pi Wan* one bolus, t.i.d. and *Du Qi Wan* one

bolus, t.i.d.

(2) *Bu Yi Zi Sheng Wan* one bolus. t.i.d.

2. Recipe decoction: *Si Jun Zi Tang* and *Liu Wei Di Huang Tang* with modifications:

Dangshen 15g, Astragalus root 15g, Stir-fried white atractylodes rhizome 12g, Poria 15g, Prepared rehmannia root 12g, Chinese yam 12g, Dogwood fruit 10g, Moutan bark 12g, Peach kernel 12g, Hypoglauca yam 12g, Bitter cadamon 12g, Mulberry mistletoe 15g, Alismatis rhizome 15g, for oral administration after being decocted in water, one dose a day.

Plus-minus: Damp heat not cleared, add phellodendron bark, motherwort; inclination to *yin* deficiency, add tortoise plastron, rehmannia root, eclipta; inclination to *yang* deficiency, add indian mulberry root, epimedium, antler; with stagnation, add bugleweed, safflower, red peony root, burreed tuber, zedoary.

3. Acupoints: *Shenshu, Pishu, Pangguangshu, Zusanli, Sanyinjiao, Mingmen* (all with reinforcing technique).

Plus-minus: With blood stasis, add *Xuehai, Yinlingquan* (both with reducing technique); inclined to *yang* deficiency add *Qihai, Guanyuan* (both moxibustion).

I. **Case report**

Mr. Cui, 71 years old, Cadre, came to our clinic on May 18, 1971. Patient had history of essential hypertension, coronary artery disease. Recently on account of fatigue, he got dull dragging pain over the perineum and lower abdomen, drippling of urine with gradual development to not a single drop passed, associated with dizziness, chest oppression, paroxysmal episode of chest pain. Tongue proper light red with ecchymosis, tongue coat thin white and slimmy. Pulse fine, rapid and slippery. He was diagnosed hypertrophy of prostate gland in a hospital and catheterization done with a retained catheter left in the bladder. B.P. 190/120mmHg, EKG showed chronic coronary insufficiency, at that time surgical operation not indicated, so came to search for help in traditional medicine.

TCM syndrome differentiation, this pertains to *yin* deficiency of liver and kidney, with stagnation turbidity in the interior, the impeded passage of urine.

Recipe: Rehmannia root 30g, Anemarrhena rhizome 12g, Phellodendron bark 12g, Honeysuckle flower 30g, Motherwort 20g, Peach kernel 12g, Bugleweed 12g, Red sage root 30g, White and red peony root each 12g, Poria 15g, Licorice root 5g, for oral administration after being decocted in water, one dose a day.

Acupuncture: *Shenshu, Pangguangshu, Yanglingquan, Xinshu, Sanyinjiao, Xuehai* (all with reducing technique) once daily.

The second visit on May 22. After three doses of the above prescription, acupuncture for three times, all the symptoms alleviated. The catheter removed after the second dose, he can pass urine, with drippling. The increased frequency of micturation and a sensation still having residual urine not evacuated. Urine turbid and white mucoid fluid flowed out from the urethra during defecation. Tongue proper light red with ecchymosis, tongue coat white. Pulse fine and weak. B.P. 180/110 mmHg.

Recipe: On the above recipe with further addition of eclipta 15g, mulberry mistletoe 20g, eucommia bark 12g.

The third visit on June 10. Another 15 doses taken, the above symptoms basically disappeared, dizziness, suffocating pain in the chest, soreness and weakness of loin and knees. Tongue proper light red, coat thin and white. Pulse deep and weak. B.P. 175/100 mmHg.

He was told to take *Zhi Bai Di Huang Wan* one bolus t.i.d. and *Fu Fang Dan Shen Pian* 4 tablets, t.i.d., to fortify the results.

II. Personal experience

This disease most frequently occurred in senile patient and often coexisting with other gerontal diseases such as essential hypertension, coronary artery disease, cerebral vascular disease and others. During prescription, these conditions should be kept in mind and drugs used dealing with all these diseases.

At onset of the disease, the pathogen of excess to be dealt with mainly, aiming at the damp-heat and turbidity stagnation, the therapeutic principle is to clear heat and remove dampness, to resolve turbidity and remove stagnation, and assisted with drugs of reinforcing spleen and replenishing kidney in order to consolidate the fundamental, and drugs to resolve stagnation, clear heat and promote diuresis as an adjuvant, in order to prevent too much astringincy and enhance the force of pathogen.

Nephrosis syndrome

Nephrosis syndrome is a group of kidney diseases of different etiological factors, being characterized with clinical manifestations of large amount of albuminuria, edema of gradual development, hypoproteinemia and hypercholesterolemia. This syndrome pertains to the catogory of 'edema', 'consumptive disease' and others in TCM.

I. TCM syndrome differentiation and treatment

Pathogenesis in brief: The mechanish of edema, with its fundamental at kidney, its incidental at lungs, and its control at spleen, asthenia of *yang qi*, impaired resolution of water dampness. The stagnation of the triple burner, and the retention of water with edema formation.

(I) Flood of wind and water

Key points of pathogenesis: The invasion of lung with wind pathogen, the impeded function of water regulation of lung. The colition of wind and water with the sudden appearance of edema.

Chief manifestations: Puffiness of eyelids followed by edema of the whole body, the rapid development of the edema, marked over the face. The edema with pitting on pressure, but easy recovery to the original on release of pressure. Skin color bright. usually associated with chilliness and fever, general aching, urination not smooth. Tongue proper normal or with inclination to red color, tongue coat thin and white or yellow, pulse floating tense or rapid.

Therapeutic principle: To disperse the wind and remove edema with diuresis.

1. Patent drug: *Fang Feng Tong sheng Wan* 6g, t.i.d. swallowed with fluid of 30g plantain herb decocted in water.

2. Decoction recipe: *Ma Huang Lian Qiao Chi Xiao Dou Tang* with modifications:

Honey fried ephedra 12g, Forsythia fruit 15g, Red bean 30g, Poria 24g, Alismatis rhizome 24g, White atractylodes rhizome 12g, Tetrandra root 12g, Fresh ginger 6g, Chinese date 3 pieces, for oral administration after being decocted in water, one dose a day.

Plus-minus: Inclination to excess of wind-heat, painful reddish swelling of throat, plus gypsum, honeysuckle flower, reed rhizome, isatis root, platycodon root; inclined to excess of wind cold, severe aversion to cold, pulse floating and tense, add spirodela, perilla leaf, ledebouriella root, cinnamon twig; severe cough, add peucedanum root, bitter apricot kernel.

3. Acupoints: *Lieque, Yinlingquan, Fuliu, Xiaochangshu, Shuigou, Pangguangshu* (all with reducing technique).

(Ⅱ) Soaking of noxious dampness

Key points of pathogenesis: Insufficiency of spleen

yang, uncontrollable water retention due to spleen asthenia. Be swamped with edema.

Chief manifestations: Generalized edema, beginning from the inferior, pitting on press, with slow recovery to original, accompanied by skin wound, chest suffocation and abdominal distension, malaise, urine scanty in amount and turbid. tongue plump with tooth imprint over the margin, tongue coat white thick and slimmy; pulse soft and relaxed.

Therapeutic principle: To replenish spleen *yang*, to resolve dampness with diuresis.

1. Patent drugs: *Yin Chen Wu Ling Wan* 10g, t.i.d.
2. Decoction recipe: *Wei Ling Tang* with modifications:

Cinnamon twig 12g, Poria 20g, Atractylodes rhizome 12g, White atractylodes rhizome 12g, Alismatis rhizome 20g, Plantain seed 20g, Fresh ginger peel, Tangerine peel, Shell of areca nut 15g, Coix seed 30g, Licorice root 3g, for oral administration after being decocted in water, one dose a day.

Plus-minus: The middle *jiao* disturbed with dampness, the appearance of abdominal distension, nausea, vomiting, plus magnolia bark, pinellia tuber, pepper plumule, deficiency of superficial *yang*, aversion to wind and easy to catch cold, add astragalus, ledebouriella root; exuberance of noxious heat with skin infections and dysphoria, add honey-suckle flower, forsythia fruit, flavascent sophora root, dandelion herb; urine deeply colored, stool constipated, add rhubarb, black and white pharbitis seed, Beijing spurge root.

3. Acupoints: *Pishu, Sanyinjiao, Lieque, Yinlingquan, Xiaochangshu, Fuliu, Pangguangshu, Shuigou* (all with reducing technique).

(Ⅱ) *Yang* decline of spleen and kidney

Key points of pathogenesis: Impaired transportation due to spleen deficiency with accumulation of dampness in the interior, *yin* exuberance and *yang* decline, edema of long duration, severe below the loin.

Chief manifestations: Edema of long duration, with repeated recurrences, severe below the loin, pitting on pressiong, suffocation and distension of epigastrium and abdomen. Anorexia and loose stool, soreness and cold pain at the lumbar region, spirit-less, aversion to cold, cold limbs, grey and stagnation of facial appearance. Tongue proper light colored and plump, with white and slimmy coating. Pulse deep slow and weak.

Therapeutic principle: To warm up the kidney and replenish the spleen, to promote *qi* circulation and to eliminate edema with diuresis.

1. Patent drug: *Jin Gui Shen Qi Wan* one bolus, t.i.d. and simultaneous intake of *Ren Shen Jian Pi Wan* one bolus t.i.d.

2. Decoction recipe: *Ji Sheng Shen Qi Wan* and *Zhen Wu Tang* with modifications:

Prepared aconite root 12g, Cinnamon twig 12g,
White atractylodes rhizome 12g, Poria 15g, Alismatis

rhizome 20g, Pepper plumule 10g, Epimedium 12g, Indian mulberry root 12g, Plantain seed 20g, White peony root 12g, for oral administration after being decocted in water, one dose a day.

Plus-minus: *Yin* consumption due to *yang* damage, minus epimedium, plus prepared rehmannia root, dog wood fruit, asparagus root; *qi* deficiency of spleen and kidney, add astragalus root, Dangshen; complicated with blood stasis, skin grey color and with stagnancy, tongue proper purple and dark, add motherwort, bugleweed, red sage root, peach kernel, safflower; in cases water-*qi* invasion of heart and lung, the inspiration impaired due to kidney dysfunction, dyspnea and sweat, rapid administration of ginseng, dogwood fruit,gecko and others in order to prevent from the dyspnea developing into collapse.

3. Acupoints: *Shenshu, Pishu, Zusanli* (all with reinforcing technique), *Qihai, Shuifen* (both moxibustion).

II. **Case report**

Ms. Chi, 23 years old, worker, admitted into the hospital on Jan. 7, 1980, with chief complaint of generalized edema for 50 days, aggravated in 5 days. 50 days ago after fatigue and catching cold, the puffiness of eyelids followed by generalized edema of the whole body, lumbar pain, malaise and anorexia, she was diagnosed acute nephritis and admitted in the local hospital. The treatment consisted of penicillin and streptomycia and Chinese herb medicine for one month, edema subsided, and other symptoms relieved, later on after catching cold, the disease had relapse, then the treatment became less effective. Recently after cold, all the symptoms aggravated, generalized edema of the whole body, with deep pitting on press, it required long time to return to its original condition on release of pressure, the other accompanied symptoms were lumbar soreness and lumbar aching, general malaise, discomfort in the throat, cough with scanty sputum, nausea, anorexia, urination short and scanty. Stool loose. Tongue proper light white, with thin yellowish coating. Pulse deep and fine.

On examination B.P. 130/90mmHg, shifting dullness present in the abdomen, signs of ascites positive, percussion tenderness over the both lumbar regions. Generalized pitting edema, especially over the lower limbs, laboratory examination. Blood routine:hemoglobin 12g, blood potassium 5.3milliequivalent, sodium 130 milliequivalent. Calcium 3.4 milliequavalent, chloride 109 milliequivalent. Creatinine 1.4mg%, creatine 5.9mg%, nonprotein nitrogen 50mg%, CO_2 combining power 14.6milliequivalent, urea nitrogen 20mg%. Urine routine: albumin 4 plus, RBC 0~1, WBC 1~2, granular cast 0~1. Blood lipids: Cholesterol 350mg%, triglyceride 275 mg%, β lipo-protein above 1150mg%. ESR 69mm/h.

TCM syndrome differentiation and treatment: This pertained to flood of wind-and water, noxious pathogen disturbance in the interior. The proper treatment should be directed to the incidental, namely to disperse the lung and eliminate edema with diuresis, to clear up the heat and remove toxic material.

Recipe: Honey-fried ephedra 15g, Tetrandra root 12g, Red bean 30g, Astragalus root 30g, Tetrandra root 12g, Cogongrass rhizome 30g, Motherwort 30g, Plantain seed 15g, Honeysuckle flower 30g, Cicada slough 10g, Lindera root 8g, for oral administration after being decocted in water, one dose daily.

The socond visit on Jan. 13. After six doses, edema gradually diminished, large amount of urine passed, nausea and vomiting, anorexia and malaise, spontaneous sweating pronounced, stool still loose, tongue proper light white, with white slimmy coating. Pulse deep fine and weak. Blood non-protein nitrogen 38mg%, CO_2 combining power 20.8 milli equivalent, urea nitrogen 13mg%, urine routine: albumin two plus, RBC 1~3, WBC 0~1. EKG showed strain of right ventricle, suggesting low blood potassium. The principle of treatment adopted was to treat the fundamental when the condition permitted, namely to reinforce kidney and replenish spleen, to warm up *yang* and eliminate edema with diuresis.

Recipe: Prepared aconite root 21g, Chinese yam 21g, Respberry fruit 30g, Prepared rehmannia root 18g, Dogwood fruit 12g, Poria 15g, Schisandra fruit 10g, Wolfberry fruit 12g, Plantain seed 12g, Dodder seed 15g, Alismatis rhizome 12g, Pharbitis seed 12g, Motherwort 21g,

White peony root 12g, Tangerine peel 6g, for oral administration after being decocted in water, one dose daily.

After 22 recipe doses, all the symptoms gradually disappeared, no albumin in the urine, blood lipids, EKG all returned to normal, other laboratory examinations all normal. Tongue proper light red, tongue coat thin and white. Pulse moderate, she was told to continue oral intake of *Jin Gui Shen Qi Wan* and *Ren Shen Jian Pi Wan* one bolus each, twice a day, consecutively for two months to strengthen the therapeutic effects.

Follow-up one year later she enjoyed healthy life.

II. Personal experience

The main symptoms of nephrosis syndrome are edema, albuminuria. Its TCM syndrome differentiation and treatment usually is in accordance with 'edema'. From the above mentioned three types are given, yet clinically there may be simultaneous presenting of two types or more than two types, such as flooding of wind and water for long duration with involvement of spleen damage or stagnation of the triple burner; the impairment of spleen *yang* for long time the kidney *yang* may be also involved with the formation *yang* deficiency of both spleen and kidney. In clinical application, the transmission or transfer from one type to another, the associated or complicated types should be taken into consideration and the corresponding treatment adopted.

After the disappearance of edema, it is not unusual

to find out the depletion of *yin* after the damage of *yang*, and the deficiency of both *yin* and *yang* as mentioned in the case report. At that time the treatment of the fundamental should be punctuate in time, the adoption of tonifying lung, replenishing spleen and reinforcing kidney and astringency of the essence and others may be selected. In cases generalized edema, not eliminated after diuresis, or with repeated remissions, the total plasma protein, especially the albumin low, mutton 200g, Chinese angelica root 12g, astragalus root 30g, donkey's hide glue 10g (melted and added to the decocted fluid), fresh ginger peel 9g, for oral administration after being decocted in water with removal of residue, one recipe dose for two days.

As to the treatment of edema, if ineffective with ordinary methods, one way is that drugs with dispersion of lungs such as ephedra, platycodon root, bitter apricot kernel and others may be added, this method is symbolized 'to lift the cover of a pot'. The second is addition of drugs to activate the blood and remove stasis, such as motherwort, bugleweed, peach kernel, safflower, sweetgum fruit and others in case with symptoms of blood stasis. The third is using aromatic drugs to promote the circulation of *qi* such as aucklandia root, areca, magnolia bark, shell of areca nut, eagle wood and others.

Primary thrombocytopenic purpura

Primary thrombocytopenic purpura is a common hemorrhagic disease with clinical manifestations of petechiae and ecchymosis in the skin, bleeding of mucosa and internal organs. The occurrence of the disease may be related to immune defect but up to now the mechanism of immunology to the disease has not been completely clarified. In TCM the disease is categoried as 'blood troubles','*yin* macules' and others.

I. TCM syndrome differentiation and treatment

Pathogenesis in brief: Deficiency of both *qi* and *yin* responsible for blood-dryness, impairment of blood collateral; deficiency of *qi* concerned with dysfunction of transportation, disability to keep the blood flowing within the blood vessels, thus give rise to the bleeding from ruptured collaterals.

(I) Blood-heat due to deficiency of *yin*

Key points of pathogenesis: Insufficiency of *yin* blood, dryness of the blood producing heat which induces damage of the blood collateral, causing external hemorrhages.

Chief manifestations: Frequent presence of purple red

ecchymosis on the skin. Bruise readily after trauma, accompanied by bleeding from the gum, nose, dizziness and blurred vision, hot sensations in chest, palms and soles, tidal fever, night sweat, flushed cheeks, dry mouth, dark urine, constipation, massive menstruation purple in colour, red tongue proper with little coating, fine and rapid pulse.

Therapeutic principle: To nourish *yin* and replenish blood, to cool blood and stop bleeding.

1. Patent drug:
    (1) *Liu Wei Di Huang Wan* 1 bolus, t.i.d.
    (2) *Da Bu Yin Wan* 1 bolus, t.i.d.
2. Decoction recipe: *Zuo Gui Wan* and *Er Zhi Wan* with modifications:

Dried rehmannia root 30g, Dogwood fruit 12g, Tortoise-plastron glue 12g, Eclipta 15g, Glossy privet fruit 15g, Capejasmine fruit 10g, Scrophularia root 15g, Red sage root 12g, Donkey-hide gelatin 12g (melted and mixed into decoction), for oral administration after being decocted in water, one dose a day.

Plus-minus: In case with heat of deficient type stirring up blood flow and causing continuous bleeding, the recipe should include arnebia or lithosperm root, carbonized madder root, node of lotus, ophiopogon root and powder of notoginseng; in case with tidal fever and night sweat, fresh-water turtle shell, sweet wormwood, wolfberry bark, and honey-fried loquat leaf included.

3. Acupoints: *Shenshu, Pishu, Houxi, Sanyinjiao* (all

with reinforcing technique), *Xuehai*, *Dadun* (both with reducing technique).

(II) *Qi* being insufficient to keep the blood circulation within the vessels

Key points of pathogenesis: *Qi* is the 'commander' of blood, while blood is the 'mother' of *qi*. Deficiency of *qi* is insufficient to keep the blood flow within the vessels and causes massive loss of blood.

Chief manifestations: Frequent presence of blue yellowish purpura on the skin with dim colour, or in the shape of spider's web, purpura in patches after bruise, accompanied by bleeding from the nose and gum, dizziness, mental fatigue, palpitation, shortness of breath, pallor of complexion, poor appetite, pale tongue proper, with thin whitish coating, fine feeble pulse.

Therapeutic principle: To replenish *qi* and invigorate the spleen, to enrich blood and keep blood circulating in the vessels.

1. Patent drug:

(1) *Ren Shen Jian Pi Wan* 1 bolus, t.i.d.

(2) *Bu Zhong Yi Qi Wan* 1 bolus, t.i.d. along with the intake of notoginseng powder 2g, t.i.d.

2. Decoction recipe: *Bao Yuan Tang* and *Gui Pi Tang* with modifications:

Ginseng 10g, Astragalus root 20g, white atractylodes rhizome 12g, Chinese angelica root 12g, Prepared rehmannia root 12g, Tangerine peel 6g, Honey-fried licorice root 3g, Chinese date 5 ones (split), Notoginseng powder 3g (swallow with boiled water or decocted solution), Hairy vein agrimony 24g, Honey-fried loquat leaf 10g, Cinnamon bark 3g, for oral administration after being decocted in water, one dose a day.

Plus-minus: Supplementary ingredients such as antler and powder of placenta are for cases with *yang* deficiency of the spleen and kidney manifested by soreness of loins, aversion to cold, pale complexion; stir-baked carbonized-ginger, carbonized eucommia bark, hyacinth bletilla and Yunnan white drug for cases with extravasation of blood and massive hemorrhage.

3. Acupoints: *Pishu, Shenshu, Qihai, Guanyuan, Sanyinjiao, Xuehai* (all with reinforcing technique). Additional acupoints *Mingmen, Baihui* (both with moxibustion) for cases with deficient cold of the spleen and kidney.

Ⅱ. **Case report**

Miss Li, 22 years old, came to seek medical advice on Nov.5, 1968.

The patient complained of grey purple ecchymosis for half a year, and was diagnosed in our hospital as primary thrombcytopenic purpura, medication with prednisone and others for more than one month but without effect. The presenting symptoms and signs: Bluish purple eccymosis in the skin, more concentrated on the extremities, dark colour, some as big as a coin, some as small as spider's webs, menstruation lasting half a month and continued dripping, dizziness, blurred vision, mental fatigue, palpitation, tongue plump, tongue proper pale with teeth prints at its borders, tongue coating white, pulse fine and feeble. Blood platelet count done with the average value of 67000.

According to TCM syndrome differentiation and treatment, the disease is ascribable to the deficiency and weakness of the spleen-*qi* leading to the failure of the spleen to regulate the blood. The treatment should be directed at keeping blood flow in the vessels and stopping bleeding by strengthening the spleen.

Recipe: Ginseng 10g, Astragalus root 30g, Prepared rehmannia root 15g, Siberian solomonseal rhizome 15g, Chinese angelica root 12g, Donkey-hide gelatin 12g, White atractylodes rhizome 12g, Poria 12g, Notoginseng powder 2g (swallowed with boiled water or decocted fluid), Chinese dates 5 ones (split), Hairy vein agrimony 15g, Madder root 12g, Amomum fruit 6g, Honey-fried licorice root 3g, for oral administration after being decocted in water, one dose a day.

Acupoints: *Pishu, Yinbai, Zusanli, Qihai, Sanyinjiao* (all with reinforcing technique), once a day.

The second visit on Dec, 6. After ten times of acupuncture and 30 doses of decoction recipe many symptoms were relieved, only abdominal distension and fullness were more obvious than before. Her tongue proper pink with its coating thin, whitish and greasy, pulse fine and soft. Recipe: Continuous prescription above recipe with ginseng, and prepared rehmannia root with-drawn, at the same time with addition of 15g Dangshen and hawthorn fruit. For oral administration after being decocted in water, one dose a day.

The third visit on Feb. 10, 1969. After another 51 doses of medication, all the symptoms subsided. The menstruation of that month lasted 3 days with its colour and amount moderate. Her tongue and pulse normal. Platelets increased to 130 thousand.

Follow-up three years later, she was found in good condition, giving birth to a boy baby.

II. Personal experience

As observed clinically, every case, that has recurrence following recovery or not at all response to treatment with adrenocortical hormones, is listed among those knotty ones. Thus, it's better not to treat this disease with hormones therapy. If the case is severe, it is preferable to deal with by administration of traditional Chinese drugs and simultaneously giving fresh blood transfusion or infusion of suspension of concentrated platelets. In this way, not only the severity can be relieved, but therapeutic course can be shortened as well.

While bleeding occurs, blood stasis causing obstruction in the interior often coexists. Therefore, notoginseng, which possesses double actions of both arresting blood and resolving stasis, plays an important role in the treatment of the disease, no matter which syndrome it pertains.

Leukopenia of unknown origin

Leukopenia exists whenever the number of the white blood cells in the peripheral blood is continuously lower than 4000 cells per cu mm. The treatment of leucopenia of unknown origin is to be dealt with in this passage. This disease is comparatively common and chiefly manifested as lassitute, weakness, soreness of loins and knees, insomnia, dizziness, low-grade fever, night sweat and others. It pertains to the category of 'consumptive disease' in TCM.

I. TCM syndrome differentiation and treatment

Pathogenesis in brief: Asthenia and deficiency of the spleen and kidney, insufficiency of *qi* and blood, weakness of *wei* (the defensive function), to protect the integument and musculature leads to the weak resistance to the exopathogen.

(I) Weakness of *qi* and blood

Key points of pathogenesis: Failure of transportation arising from deficiency of the spleen, responsible for the insufficiency of source of nutrients resulting in failure to produce vital essence and deficiency of both *qi* and blood.

Chief manifestations: Lassitute and weakness, palpitation, shortness of breath, dizziness, insomnia, dim complexion, low fever, restlessness, pale colour of tongue proper with teeth prints on its border, fine and feeble pulse.

Therapeutic principle: To invigorate the spleen and stomach, to replenish *qi* and blood.

1. Patent drug:

(1) *Ren Shen Jian Pi Wan*, 1 bolus t.i.d.

(2) *Gui Pi Wan*, 1 bolus t.i.d.

(3) *Shi Quan Da Bu Wan* 1 bolus, t.i.d.

2. Decoction recipe: *Ba Zhen Tang* with modifications:

Dangshen 15g, Astragalus root 15g, White atractylodes rhizome 12g, Siberian solomonseal rhizome 12g, Prepared rehmannia root 12g, Wolfberry fruit 15g, Chinese angelica root 12g, Amomum fruit 6g, Spatholobus stem 21g, Honey-fried licorice root 3g, for oral administration after being decocted in water, one dose a day.

Plus-minus: In case with insomnia, arborvitae seed and honey-fried lily bulb are included in the recipe; in case with low fever and restlessness, ophiopogon root and Chinese mahonia leaf included.

3. Acupoints: *Pishu, Zusanli, Neiguan, Shenmen* (all with reinforcing technique).

(Ⅱ) Deficiency of both spleen and kidney

Key points of pathogenesis: Deficiency of the spleen

and kidney, insufficiency of essence and blood, malnourishment of mind, mal-replenishment of the bone.

Chief manifestations: Listlessness, soreness of loins and weakness of the legs, dizziness, blurred vision, dificiency of *qi*, disinclination to talk, tinnitus, impairment of memory, anorexia, plump fresh tongue proper with thin whitish coating, deep and fine pulse.

Therapeutic principle: To nourish the kidney and invigorate the spleen.

1. Patentdrugs: *Liu Wei Di Huang Wan* and *Ren Shen Jian Pi Wan*, 1 bolus of each, t.i.d.

2. Decoction recipe: *You Gui Wan* and *Si Jun Zi Tang* with modifications:

Prepared rehmannia root 15g, Chinese yam 15g, Psoralea fruit 12g, Antler 12g, Powder of human placenta 10g (swallow with boiled water or decocted fluid), Ginseng 6g, White atractylodes rhizome 12g, Tangerine peel 10g, Chinese ange-lica root 12g, Licorice root 3g, Germinated barley 30g, for oral administration after being decocted in water, one dose a day.

Plus-minus: Prepared fleece-flower root and tortoise plastron are employed provided the case exhibits more signs of *yin* deficiency complicated with low-grade fever and night sweat; epimedium and cinnamon bark supplemented provided the case exhibites more signs of *yang* deficiency complicated with aversion to cold and cold limbs.

3. Acupoints: *Shenshu, Pishu, Zusanli, Sanyinjiao, Houxi, Neiguan, Mingmen* (all with reinforcing technique).

I. **Case report**

Mr. Li, 36 years old, cadre, first consultation on May 4, 1974.

The patient complained of general debility for three months, accompanied by dizziness, palpitation, shortness of breath, anorexia, insomnia, disturbed sleep by dreams, pale tongue proper with teeth prints on its borders, thin and whitish coating, deep, fine and feeble pulse. He had no other disease in his history. Chest X-ray fluoroscopy, liver function, composite examination of cardiac function, stool test, urine test and others are all normal Blood routine: WBC 1900 per cu mm, neutrophil: 38%, lymphocyte 62%, myelogram: chronic granulocytopenia. He often took much medicines as vitamins, batyl alcohol, *Shi Quan Da Bu Wan*, *Gui Pi Wan* and others but the curative effect was not marked.

TCM syndrome differentiation and treatment: This disease is attributable to the weakness of the spleen and stomach, giving rise to debility of transportation, insufficiency of the source of nutrients for growth and development. The treatment should be aimed at invigorating the spleen and regulating the stomach, enriching the source of nutrients.

Recipe: Dangshen 24g, Astragalus root 18g, White atractylodes rhizome 12g, Poria 12g, Chinese angelica root 12g, Siberian solomonseal rhizome 15g, Wolfberry fruit 15g, Aucklandia root 6g, Amomum fruit 6g,

Honeyfried licorice root 3g, for oral administration after being decocted in water, one dose daily.

Therapeutic effect: After administration of 104 doses, various symptoms disappeared, tongue proper and pulse become normal. Blood count WBC: 4800 per cu mm, neutrophil 68%, lymphocyte 32%. The patient was advised to keep taking *Ren Shen Jian Pi Wan*, 1 bolus, t.i.d. for 2 months in succession for the sake of strengthening the curative effect.

Follow-up two years later found that the patient was healthy.

III. Personal experience

Leukopenia of unknown origin is a common chronic desease. It is ascribed to deficiency and is easily be affected by external pathogen. If such affection occurs, it is strictly prohibited to abuse antibiotics, especially antipyretic and analgesic agents. Most of these drugs possess side effects to white blood cells. In case noxious heat is overabundant, it is preferable to prescribe traditional Chinese drugs with heat clearing and detoxicating actions. In case with impairment of body fluid caused by excess of heat, heat clearing and yin nourishing drugs should be used together.

At ordinary time, frequent administration of powder of placenta is encouraged, 10g, t.i.d. Or it is recommended to take boiled bone morrow of ox mixed with stir-fried flour of wheat, 30g, each time, b.i.d., to be taken after being mixed with boiling water. Keeping doing so is certainly beneficial to complete cure of the disease.

Aplastic anemia

Aplastic anemia is a clinical syndrome of hemopoietic system marked by distinct decrease of red bone marrow and gradual declination of blood-manufacturing function. It is clinically characterized by panhematopenia. In view of its unknown origin, the curative effect is poor. In western medicine, the disease has once been called 'knotty anemia'. In TCM the disease pertains to the category of 'consamptive disease', 'blood troubles' and others. Only can syndromes be properly differentiated and treated, will the ideal therapeutic effect be yielded.

I. TCM syndrome differentiation and treatment

Pathogenesis in brief: Accumulation of noxious pathogen in the interior, exhausting qi and impairing the blood, deficiency of qi resulting in its disability to take the guiding rule of blood, deficiency of blood resulting in its disability to carry qi, debility and decline of the spleen and kidney, exhaustion of blood source, consequently breaking out of various symptoms.

(I) Acute comsumption due to blood-heat

Key points of pathogenesis: Prolonged accumulation of noxious pathogen in the interior producing heat, overabundance of noxious heat leading to bleeding.

Chief manifestations: Palpitation, shortness of breath, vertigo, fatigue, epistaxis, hemoptysis, hematemesis, bleeding from rectum, hematuria, high fever, restlessness, dark urine, constipation, red tongue proper with ecchymosis or hemorrhagic blister, dry and yellowish tongue coating with scanty saliva, rapid, deficient and large pulse.

Therapeutic principle: To clear away heat and toxic material; to remove heat from blood and arrest bleeding.

1. Patent drugs:

(1) *Zi Xue San* 3g (to be taken priorly), *Yun Nan Bai Yao* 2g, q.d. or b.i.d. for the sake of relieving high fever.

(2) *Shi Hui San*, 10g each time, t.i.d.

2. Decoction recipe: *Qing Wen Bai Du Yin* with modifications:

Dried rehmannia root 30g, Coptis root 15g, Gypsum 45g, Capejasmine fruit 12g, Honey suckle flower 30g, Forsythia fruit 15g, Scrophularia root 30g, Scutellaria root 15g, Anemarrhena rhizome 15g, Red sage root 12g, Red peony root 12g, Cogongrass rhizome 30g, Rhinoceros horn 12g (or buffalo horn 30g instead), Rhubarb 12g, for oral administration after being decocted in water, one dose a day.

Plus-minus: In case high fever severe at night, gypsum and scutellaria root are with-drawn, while wolfberry bark, and phellodendron bark supplemented. In case with massive epistaxis, madder root and hairy vein agrimony employed, for cases with *yin* deficiency of the kidney, eclipta and glossy privet fruit included.

3. Acupoints: *Xinshu, Ganshu, Quze, Weizhong, Hegu, Xuehai, Dadun* (all with reducing technique), *Yongquan* (with reinforcing technique).

(Ⅱ) *Yin* deficiency syndrome of the heart and kidney

Key points of pathogenesis: *Yin* deficiency of the heart and kidney, fire of deficient type produced in the interior, giving rise to damage of blood collateral, blood stasis obstruction in the interior.

Chief manifestations: Soreness and weakness of loins and knees, vertigo, tinnitus, hot sensation on palms and soles, low-grade fever in the afternoon, dry mouth and throat, bleeding from the nose gums and skin, palpitation, restlessness, irritability, insomnia, dark urine, constipation, red tongue proper sometimes with ecchymosis, fine, rapid and feeble pulse.

Therapeutic principle: To nourish the kidney and remove heat, to tonify the heart and tranquilize the mind.

1. Patent drugs:

(1) *Zhi Bai Di Huang Wan*, 1 bolus, t.i.d.

(2) *Er Zhi Wan*, 10g, b.i.d.

2. Decoction recipe: *Zhi Bai Di Huang Tang* with modifications:

Anemarrhena rhizome 12g. Phellodendron bark 10g, Dried rehmannia root 30g, Dogwood fruit 6g, Chinese yam 15g, Red sage root 12g, Poria 12g, Chinese angelica root 12g, Notoginseng powder 3g (swallow with boiled water or decoction fluid), Capejasmine fruit 10g, for oral administration after being decocted in water, one dose a day.

Plus-minus: Tortoise plastron and prepared fleece-flower root are supplemented for cases with marked vertigo and tinnitus; sweet wormwood, wolfberry bark and fresh-water turtle shell supplemented for those with tidal fever and night sweat; coptis root and stir-fried wild jujuba seed for distinct insomnia; rhubarb 12g (decocted later) for prominent constipation; amomum fruit and rice sprout for anorexia.

3. Acupoints: *Shenshu, Xinshu, Taixi, Sanyinjiao* (all with reinforcing technique) *Xingjian, Taichong Yinlingquan* (all with reducing technique).

(Ⅱ) *Yang* deficiency of the spleen and kidney

Key points of pathogenesis: *Yang* deficiency of the spleen and kidney, insufficiency of the source of nutrients for growth and development, deficiency and want of *qi* and blood, accumulation of excessive fluid.

Chief manifestations: Abdominal distension, anorexia, bloody stool, cold and pain of loins and knees, chill and cold limbs impotence, spermatorrhea, shortness of breath, fatigue, listlessness, pallor and puffiness of the face, pale tongue proper with teeth prints on its borders, whitish and slippery coating of the tongue, deep, slow and feeble pulse.

Therapeutic principle: To warm the kidney and invigorate the spleen, to replenish *qi* and resolve fluid retention.

1. Patent drugs: *Jin Gui Shen Qi Wan* 1 bolus each time, t.i.d.

2. Decoction recipe: *Zhen Wu Tang* and *Ling Gui Zhu Gan Tang* with modifications:

Prepared aconite root 6g, Morinda root 10g, Stir-fried white peony root 12g, Poria 15g, Stir-fried white atractylodes rhizome 12g, Ginseng 6g, Cinnamon twig 6g, Licorice root 3g, for oral administration after being decocted in water, one dose a day.

Plus-minus: Stir-fried immature bitter orange 10g and stir-fried rice sprout 30g are added for cases with prominent abdominal distension and anorexia; donkey-hide gelatin 10g, notoginseng powder 3g and rhubarb 10g for those having bloody stool; epimedium 10g for those having chills and cold limbs.

3. Acupoints: *Mingmen, Shenshu, Guanyuan, Qihai, Pishu, Sanyinjiao* (all with moxibustion), *Yinlingquan, Yongquan, Ganshu* (all with reducing technique).

II. Case report

Ms. Chang, 56 years old, because of bloody stool for 20 days, was diagnosed as aplastic anemia (chronic), and then transfered to our hospital. Examination revealed: Extremely anemic appearance and complexion, heart rate regular, 96 times per minute, systolic murmur of the third grade could be heard from the region of cardia capex. Lung:

negative, abdomen soft without distinct tenderness or rebound tenderness. Laboratory examination found Hb 3.5g (10.5g before bleeding), WBC 2800, platelet number: 35 thousand. Since bleeding per rectum, 3300ml of blood transfusion had been given and styptic medicines such as dicynone, PAMBA (p-aminomethy-benzoic acid) had been administered for two days but without effect. The patient was still haunted with fatigue, palpitation, dizziness, bleeding per rectum with its colour dark and amount massive (every time 1500~2000ml), pink tongue proper and fine weak pulse. All the above were differentiated as: *qi*-deficiency of the spleen and kidney resulting in disability to keep blood flow in the vessels. The treatment should be directed at reinforcing *qi* to keep blood circulation in the vessels, and warming *yang* to resolve stagnancy. The preferalbe drugs: Dangshen, white atractylodes rhizome, astragalus root, Chinese angelica root, donkey-hide gelatin, amomum fruit, red peony root, white peony root, sanguisorba root, poria, licorice root, large dosage of rhubarb powder 15~30g per day(for oral administration in 2~3 portions, one portion each time). The administration of drugs was coordinated by blood transfusion (twice, the total amount 600ml). Three days later, bleeding was arrested. Rhubarb was withdrawn. Over half month, bloody stool did not occur. Going on with administration of the above recipe with addition of prepared rehmannia root and morinda root, the patient's symptoms were relieved and then dischanged from hospital with Hb 11g, WBC

4000, platelet count 100000.

II. Personal experience

(I) In TCM, acute aplastic anemia is differentiated as 'acute comsumption due to blood heat', while chronic aplastic anemia is differentiated as '*yin*-deficiency of the liver and kidney' and '*yang*-deficiency of the spleen and kideny'. Although there is a difference between the acute and the chronic, a difference between deficiency and excess, they can be mutually transformed from one another, associated and complicated. Accordingly, attention should be paid when the principle is acertained and the prescriptions given.

(II) Acute consumption due to blood heat is chiefly manifested as sudden onset, severe condition and rapid progress of the disease. Therefore, careful observation, precise and punctuate prescriptions are required. In case bleeding is acute and massive, blood transfusion is necessary.

(III) The syndromes of aplastic anemia are complex and changeable, but the deficiency of both spleen and kideny covers the whole course of the disease. Since the spleen is the source of nutrients for growth and development of *qi* and blood, the kideny dominates the bone, supplies bone with marrow and stores the essence of life, and vital essence and blood can be transformed mutually, nourishing the kidney and invigorating the spleen is the fundamental principle and the major link to be grasped firmly, so doing, ideal therapeutic effect can be expected.

Epidemic hemorrhagic fever

Epidemic hemorrhagic fever is an acute infections disease, its pathogenic organism is not confirmed yet, probably virus in origin. High fever, hypotension, hemorrhage, kidney damage and electrolytes disturbances are the chief characteristics of the disease. In typical course, there are 5 stages, the fever, hypotension, oligouria, polyuria and convalescence stage. This disease pertains to the category of 'epidemic febrile disease', 'grape pestilance', 'epidemic rash' and others in TCM.

I. TCM syndrome differentiation and treatment

Pathogenesis in brief: Invasion of noxious heat widespread involving the three burners, lungs, heart, liver and kidney, resulting in exhaustion of *yin* fluid and damage of *yang qi*.

(I) Exuberance of noxious heat (fever stage)

Key points of pathogenesis: The invasion of epidemic noxious heat, spread all over the three burners, during the attack of *qi* and *ying* system.

Chief manifestations: High fever, thirsty, profuse sweating, headache, lumbar pain, face reddened as if drunken, congested eyes, blurred vision, skin rash, epistaxis, spitting blood. In the early stage, there may be chill, general aching and others belonging to superficial syndrome, urine deep colored, stool constipated, impaired consciousness and delirium, convulsions, opisthotonus. Tongue proper deep red, tongue coat yellowish and dry, even with prickles. Pulse slippery and rapid.

Therapeutic principle: To clear up *qi* and cool the *yin*: to resolve stasis and remove toxic material.

1. Patent drug:
(1) *Xi Ling Jie Du Pian*, 12 tab. t.i.d.
(2) *Yin Qiao Jie Du Pian*, 12 tab. t.i.d.
(3) *Da Qing Ye He Ji*, three tubes oral take, each time, t.i.d.

2. Decoction recipe: *Qing Wen Bai Du Yin* with modifications:

Gypsum 45g, Anemarrhena rhizome 15g, Honeysuckle flower 30g, Forsythia fruit 15g, Scutellaria root 15g, Coptis root 12g, Moutan bark 12g, Red peony root 12g, Paris rhizome 15g, Fresh reed rhizome 45g, for oral administration after being decocted in water, one dose a day.

Plus-minus: With manifestations of superficial syndrome plus schizonepeta, peppermint; with severe noxious heat add buffalo's horn, isatis leaf, arnebia root; high fever, coma, further addition of *An Gong Niu Huang Wan*; extreme heat with wind production, the appearance of convulsions, add antelope horn powder, uncaria stem with hooks, earthworm; for constipation, rhubarb and mirabilite added.

3. Acupoints: *Shixuan, Waiguan, Hegu, Ganshu, Xinshu* (all with reducing technique). High fever, coma, add *Shierjing* (puncture to bleed), *Laogong, Yanglingquan* (both with reducing technique), *Yongquan* (with reinforcing technique).

(II) Exuberance of the pathogenic evil, and the weakness of the vital energy (hypotension shock stage)

Key points of pathogenesis: The exuberance of pathogenic evil in the interior, exhaustion of *qi* and *yin*, the vital energy can not conquer the pathogenic evil, the appearance of cold limbs and collapse.

Chief manifestations: Still feverish or the sudden drop of high fever, dysphoria, profuse sweat, thirsty, spiritless, malaise. Skin cruptions vaguely seen. In severe condition, coma and delirium, coldness of four limbs, drop of blood pressure. Tongue proper deep red, pulse fine, rapid and without force.

Therapeutic principle: To clear up the heat and cool the blood, to support the vital energy to eliminate the pathogenic evils.

1. Patent drug: *Niu Huang Qin Xin Wan* one bolus, t.i.d., and *Mai Wei Di Huang Wan* one bolus, t.i.d.

2. Decoction recipe: *Qing Gong Tang* and *Shen Mai San* with modifications:

American ginseng 12g, Gypsum 30g, Anemarrhena rhizome 12g, Coptis root 10g, Honey-suckle flower 30g, Forsythia fruit 15g, Scrofularia root 20g, Ophiopogon root 30g, Fresh rehmmania root 30g, Bamboo leaflet 12g, Licorice root 3g, Schisandra fruit 10g, for oral administration after being decocted in water, one dose a day.

Plus-minus: Noxious heat blockage of the interior, add Zi Xue Dan; with cold limbs and collapse, emergency use of prepared aconite root, ginseng, Dogwood fruit, ophiopogon root, schisandra fruit, Dragon's bone, oyster shell to rescue the *yang* from collapse, to supplement the *qi* and promote the production of body fluid.

3. Acupoints: *Shenshu, Ganshu, Xinshu, Yongquan* (all with reinforcing technique), *Hegu, Waiguan, Xingjian* (all with reducing technique), with the appearance of cold limbs and collapse, *Qihai, Guanyuan, Baihui, Zusanli, Shenshu.* (all moxibustion).

(Ⅲ) Heat accumulation and *yin* deficiency (oligouria stage)

Key points of pathogenesis: Long standing fever, with exhaustion of *yin* fluid, heat accumulation in the lower burner, the disturbance in *qi* transformation.

Chief manifestations: Urine scanty, deep colored, and unsmooth passage, dysuria, even anuria. Or with hematuria, distending pain in the lower abdomen, thirsty and dysphoria, soreness and aching over the loin and back, listless, stool constipated. Tongue proper deep red, tongue coat yellow. Pulse fine and rapid.

Therapeutic principle: To nourish the kidney and clear away the heat; to promote the production of body fluid and urination.

1. Patent drug: *Zhi Bai Di Huang Wan* each time one bolus, three or four times a day.

2. Decoction recipe: *Ba Zheng San* and *Zeng Ye Tang* with modifications:

Rehmannia root 30g, Scrofularia root 24g, Ophiopogon root 24g, Anemarrhena rhizome 12g, Common knotgrass 10g, Chinese pink herb 10g, Plantain seed 20g, Moutan bark 12g, Cogongrass rhizome 30g, Licorice root 3g, for oral administration after being decocted in water, one dose a day.

Plus-minus: Cough, dyspnea, constipated, plus lepidium seed, rhubarb, glehnia; for hematuria, add capejasmine fruit, small thistle, Japanese thistle.

3. Acupoints: *Shenshu, Pangguangshu, Yinlingquan, Zhongji* (all with reducing technique), *Sanyinjiao, Houxi* (both with reinforcing technique).

(Ⅳ) Unconsolidation of the kidney-*qi* (polyuria stage)

Key points of pathogenesis: Struggle of vital energy and pathogenic evil, successful removal of pathogenic evil and the decline of vital energy, the unconsolidation of kidney *qi* and the loss of control of urinary bladder.

Chief manifestations: Frequent micturation, urine large amount and clear, even in-continence of urine, dizziness and spiritlessness, lumbar soreness, malaise, mouth dryness, thirsty. tongue proper light colored, with thin, white coating. Pulse fine and weak.

Therapeutic principle: To reinforce the kidney to

consolidate and astringe the *qi*, to nourish *yin* and promote the formation of body fluid.

1. Patent drug: *Du Qi Wan* one bolus, t.i.d.

2. Decoction recipe: *Liu Wei Di Huang Tang* with modifications:

Prepared rehmannia root 18g, Chinese yam 15g, Dogwood fruit 12g, Danshen 15g, Respberry fruit 12g, Mantis egg case 15g, Poria 12g, Chinese date 3 pieces, for oral administration after being decocted in water, one dose a day.

Plus-minus: Inclined to kidney *yang* deficiency, plus psorales fruit, galangal fruit, minus cinnamon bark, lindera root; inclined to kidney *yin* deficiency, add siberian solomonseal rhizome, schisandra fruit, eclipta.

3. Acupoints: *Guanyuan, Shenshu, Qihai, Baihui* (all with reinforcing technique).

(V) Evil pathogens removed, weakness of vital energy left (convalescent stage)

Key points of pathogenesis: During convalescence, depletion of both *yin* and *yang*, weakness of viscera organs, insufficiency of *qi* and blood.

Chief manifestations: Low grade fever not cleared yet, spontaneous sweating, dryness of mouth and throat, Dizziness and lumbar aching, malaise, anorexia, loose stool. Tongue proper light, tongue coat thin and white. Pulse fine and weak.

Therapeutic principle: To support the vital energy and consolidate the fundamental, to replenish the spleen and open the source of generation and transmission.

1. Patent drugs:

(1) *Ren Shen Jian Pi Wan* one bolus t.i.d.

(2) *Shen Ling Bai Zhu San* 10g, t.i.d.

2. Decoction recipe: *Yi Wei Tang* with modifications:

Pseudostellaria root 24g, Glehnia root 20g, Ophiopogon root 12g, Chinese yam 12g, Stir fried white atractylodes rhizome 12g, Poria 12g, Barley sprout 30g, Licorice root 3g, for oral administration after being decocted in water, one dose a day.

Plus-minus: Asthenia of *wei qi*, spontaneous sweating, plus astragalus root, cinnamon twig, white peony root; *yin* deficiency with dryness of mouth and throat, add rehmannia root, wolfberry fruit; low grade fever add swallwort root, turtle shell.

3. Acupoints: *Pishu, Shenshu, Zusanli, Qihai, Guanyuan* (all with reinforcing technique).

I. **Case report**

Mr. Qin, 19 years old, peasant, had his first visit on Jan. 5, 1988, with the chief complaint of fever for 4 days. 4 days ago after exposure to cold, he had headache, fever, slight aversion to wind and cold, general aching, no sweat, dysphoria, nausea, vomiting. He was treated with penicillin, stretomycin, hydrocortisone in a hospital at his home town without effect. Body temperature around 40°C. The symptoms at our clinic consisted of fever, headache, facial flush, dysphoria, thirsty but no desire to drink, no sweat, nausea, vomiting, impaired appetite, urine deep colored, stool loose, tongue proper deep red with yellow thick coating. Pulse fine and rapid. B.P. 100/80mmHg. Laboratory examination: Urine routine albumin two plus. Blood routine: Hgb 11g, WBC 11000 neutrophil 80%, lymphocyte 20%, platelet count 100 thousands, urea nitrogen 26.6mg%, immune-fluorescence test, enzyme linked-SPA test, antibody titre were correspondingly 1:20, 1:80, and 1:320. IgG + + +, + +, and +. Diagnosis of western medicine: Epidemic hemorrhagic fever.

TCM syndrome differentiation and treatment: Noxious heat invasion of the interior, spreading all over the three burners, exhaustion of body fluids, disturbance of stomach and intestine. The therapeutic principle adopted was to clear up heat and toxic material. *Qin Wen Bai Du Yin* with modifications:

Recipe: Honeysuckle flower 30g, Forsythia fruit 15g, Gypsum 30g, Anemarrhena rhizome 12g, Rehmannia root 15g, Scrofularia root 30g, Ophiopogon root 15g, Moutan bark 12g, Capejasmine fruit 10g, Pueraria root 30g, Bupleurum root 15g, Licorice root 8g, for oral administration after being decocted in water, one dose daily, to be associated with infusion therapy and others in western medicine.

After 12 recipe doses, all the symptoms disappeared, diet and drink, urination and defecation all normal. Body temperature normal. Blood and urine routine all normal.

II. Personal experience

Epidemic hemorrhagic fever usually gives an acute onset, severe symptoms, rapid transmissions, the involvement of many viscera, in TCM so called the dissemination all over the three burners. During the course of the illness, the appearance of bleeding, shock, renal failure, heart failure, pulmonary edema are critical signs and the combination of western and TCM therapy is necessary for emergent disposal.

The typical course consists of 5 stages as described, and the TCM syndrome differentiation and treatment selected accordingly. As the difference of constitution of patients and the severity of infection vary, the manifestations of the disease also vary. In severe patients the anterior three stages may follow rapidly one after another and may coalesce into one. In mild cases also not all the five stages presenting. In some cases after suitable treatment the disease may be interrupted and aborted at the fever stage. The above case is an example.

During the stage of exuberance of noxious heat, the punctuate diagnosis and treatment with big dosage of drugs of clearing away heat and toxic material is the clue of the matter. In case to grasp this hinge in hand, the course of the disease can be greatly shortened, the visceral damage lessened, and the rate of cure elevated.

In accordance with the clinical observation, *Qing Kai Ling* injection 20ml added to 10% glucose water 500ml intravenuous drip, once daily, consecutive use for 5～7 days, and in association with TCM syndrome differentiation and treatment will give comparatively good therapeutic effects.

Cervical spondylopathy

Cervical spondylopathy occurs often after middle age, especially frequent in those persons constantly bending over one's desk reading or working. Over 90% the lesion occurs between the 5th and 6th, or between the 6th and 7th cervical vertebrae. On account of the protrusion of inter-vertebral fibrous ring or narrowing of intervertebral foramen and spur formation, with compression of the spinal nerve root or the vertebral artery causing blood insufficiency of basilar artery. The main clinical manifestations are pain or numbness of neck and shoulder, and over the distributed area of affected nerve root, and dizziness due to vertebral-basilar arterial insufficiency. This pertains to the category of 'dizziness', 'stiffness of neck', 'shoulder pain', 'arm pain' and others in TCM.

I. TCM syndrome differentiation and treatment

Pathogenesis in brief: *Yin* deficiency of liver and kidney, the insufficiency of brain, the collateral obstruction with phlegm-stagnation, the stasis of *qi* and blood.

(I) *Yin* deficiency of liver and kidney

Key points of pathogenesis: Brain insufficiency due to insufficiency of liver and kidney, and upward perversion of phlegm and fluid, with stagnation of collaterals.

Chief manifestations: Stiffness and pain of the neck, dizziness, blurred vision, nausea, vomiting, soreness or numbness of shoulder and arm, associated with lassitude in loin and knees, dysphoria and feverishness over palms, soles and in the chest, insomnia and forgetfulness. Tongue proper red with little coating, pulse taut and fine.

Therapeutic principle: To nourish the kidney and fill in the marrow, to resolve phlegm and activate the collaterals.

1. Patent drug: *Liu Wei Di Huang Wan* one bolus, t.i.d., swallowed with the water decoction fluid of ginger treated pinellia tuber 12g, fresh ginger 10g.

2. Decoction recipe: *He Shou Wu Wan* and *Er Chen Tang* with modifications:

Prepared fleece flower root 30g, Cibot rhizome 15g, Achyranthes root 12g, Ginger treated pinellia tuber 12g, Tangerine peel 10g, Alismatis rhizome 30g, Poria 24g, Pueraria root 24g, Siegesbeckia herb 20g, for oral administration after being decocted in water, one dose a day.

Plus-minus: For prominent dizziness, vomiting, plus fresh ginger, white atractylodes root, drink frequently; with severe shoulder and arm pain, plus notopterygium root, gentian root, clematis root.

3. Acupoints: *Shenshu* (reinforcing technique), *Zhongwan, Zusanli, Neiguan, Shanzhong, Fenglong* (all with reducing technique). For shoulder and arm pain add *Dazhui, Jianyu, Quchi, Shousanli* (all with reducing technique).

(II) Phlegm stagnation obstruction of collaterals

Key points of pathogenesis: Collateral obstruction with phlegm stagnation, stasis and stagnation of *qi* and blood. Stiffness of neck, arm pain, severe on motion.

Chief manifestations: Stiffness and pain of posterior collum, spread to back, pain or numbness of shoulder and arm, even referred to finger. Paroxysmal dizziness, even syncope may occur. Tongue proper red, or with ecchymosis, pulse taut.

Therapeutic principle: To activate blood and remove stagnation, to resolve phlegm and activate the collaterals.

1. Patent drug:

(1) *Qu Zeng Sheng Pian* 5 tablets, t.i.d.

(2) *Gu Ci Wan* one bolus, t.i.d.

2. Decoction recipe: *Tao Hong Si Wu Tang* and *Ge Gen Tang* with modifications:

Peach kernel 10g, Safflower 10g, Chinese angelica root tail 12g, Chuanxiong rhizome 12g, White peony root 10g, Red peony root 10g, Bile-treated arisaema tuber 10g, White mustard seed 10g, Pueraria root 24g, Honey-fried ephedra 10g, Siegesbeckia herb 15g, Licorice root 3g, for oral administration after being decocted in water, one dose a day.

Plus-minus: shoulder and arm pain severe, plus turmeria, batryticated silkworm, whole scorpion; the hind neck soreness, add cibot rhizome, notopterygium root, numbness or pain of fingers, add earthworm, stir-fried mulberry twig, finger citron.

3. Acupoints: *Dazhui, Jianyu, Tianzong, Jianliao, Binao, Quchi, Waiguan, Lieque, Hegu* (all with reinforcing technique).

I. Case report

Mr. Qiu, 50 years old, cadre, came to clinic on June 21, 1987, with a history of soreness of neck and pain of right arm for 3 months, X-ray film revealed hypertrophic changes of the 6th and 7th cervical vertebrae, narrowed intervertebral foramen, and a diagnosis of cervical spondylopathy made. Through traction, vitamin B_1, B_{12} acupoint injection and other treatment no much effect. The complaint at that time consisted of numbness and pain, over shoulder, arm and referred to thumb and index fingers' Stiffness and pain of neck, soreness and heaviness of both shoulders, aggravated with turning of head, after exposur to cold. Tongue proper light colored, with thin, white wet coating. Pulse taut. This was considered due to collateral obstruction with wind-phlegm, cold condensation and blood stasis. The therapeutic principle was to warm up the channel and resolve phlegm, to activate blood and collaterals.

Recipe: Honey-fried ephedra 12g, Cinnamon twig 10g,

Puerarum root 24g, Notopterygium root 10g, White mustard seed 12g, Typhonium tuber 10g, Gastrodia tuber 10g, Chinese angelica root tail 12g, Chuanxiong rhizome 12g, Peach kernel 10g, Safflower 10g, Finger citron 12g, Licorice root 3g, for oral administration after being decocted in water, one dose a day.

In the same time acupuncture *Dazhui*, *Jianyu*, *Tianzong*, *Binao*, *Quchi*, *Lieque*, *Hegu* (all with reducing technique). After acupuncture topical application of *She Xiang Hu Gu Gao* on *Dazhui*, *Jianjing*, *Jianyu*.

The second visit on July 10. After 15 doses, acupuncture 10 times, all the symptoms basically disappeared except soreness and discomfort of neck, slight weakness of right arm. Tongue proper light red, with thin and white coating. Pulse fine.

Recipe: Prepared fleece-flower root 24g, Cibot rhizome 20g, Astragalus root 24g, Chinese angelica root 12g, Chuanxiong rhizome 12g, Siegesbeckia herb 24g, Gastrodia tuber 12g, Stir-fried mulberry twig 24g, Honey treated licorice root 3g, for oral administration after being decocted in water, one dose every other day, consecutively for 15 doses, to strengthen the therapeutic effects. Half year later follow up, no discomfort over the neck.

Ⅲ. Personal experience

This is a disease of deficiency in fundamental and excess of incidental. The upward perversion of phlegm-fluid, the collateral obstruction due to phlegm and stagnation, the stasis of *qi* and blood contribute to the symptoms of excess. The *yin* deficiency of liver and kidney with insufficiency of brain (considered as sea of marrow) constitute the insufficiency of fundamental. In acute state, to treat the incidental first, when the acute state is over, shift to treat the fundamental should be the principle of choice.

This is a stubborn disease, the combination of internal medication, acupuncture and external use of plaster is necessary, especially the external application of plaster to the acupoints after acupuncture usually give satisfactory results. The recipe of plaster given below is commonly used: Drynaria rhizome 30g, Speranskia 45g, Dahurian angelica root 15g, Chinese angelica root tail 30g, Chuanxiong 60g, Ground beetle 30g, Pangolin scales 30g, Honey fried ephedra 15g, Musk 0.5g (put in after other drugs).

All ground into coarse powder, decoct with small fire for one hour with water and vinegar each 1500ml added. After removal of the residue, the decocted fluid concentrated to make a drug paste, prior to the removal of paste from pot add musk in, and preserved in porcelain container ready for use. Each time 10g paste spread upon the gauze, apply to *Dazhui* point (after acupuncture or moxibustion), change once in two days.

Neck training is also important. Bending anteriorly and posteriorly, with head up or low, head turn or deviate to left or right. The velocity, frequency and time of exercise should be increased in order gradually from slow to rapid, time from short to long.

Brachial plexus neuritis

Brachial plexus neuritis is commonly met in adults. It frequently occurs in the convalescent stage of a number of infectious diseases and in serum disease. In another portion of patients its etiology remains obscure. With an acute onset, the disease begins from the shoulder pain of one side or both sides, and spreads to the neck and upper extremity. Abduction or anterior extension of the upper arm aggravate the pain. It pertains to the catetory of 'shoulder pain', 'limited shoulder motion', and others in TCM.

I. TCM syndrome differentiation and treatment

Pathogenesis in brief: Shoulder pain of wind, cold dampness and heat. The stasis of qi and blood, inability to raise the arm.

(I) Wind-cold stagnation

Key points of pathogenesis: Wind, cold and dampness are the causes to induce shoulder pain, inability to raise the arm due to qi stagnation and blood stasis.

Chief manifestations: Pain of shoulder and arm, some difficulty in elevation of shoulder, pain may be referred to back or to arm, accompanied by weakness of the affected limb, swelling of fingers, chillness and cold limbs, or alternate attacks of chill and fever. Tongue proper light red, with thin and white coating, pulse taut and tense.

Therapeutic principle: To promote blood circulation and remove obstruction in the collaterals; to warm up the channels and disperse the cold.

1. Patent drug:

(1) *Xiao Huo Luo Dan* one bolus, t.i.d. and *Yuan Hu Zhi Tong Pian* 4 tab. t.i.d.

(2) *Yi Li Zhi Tong Dan* each time 3~5 pills, once daily.

2. Decoction recipe: *Wu Tou Tang* with modifications:

Prepared sichuan aconite root 10g, Astragalus root 20g, Chinese angelica root, Chuanxiong rhizome 12g, Honey-fried ephedra 12g, White peony root 10g, Red peony root 10g, Siegesbeckia herb 15g, Notopterygium root 10g, Erythrina bark 12g, Turmeria 12g, Honey fried licorice root 3g, for oral administration after being decocted in water, one dose a day.

Plus-minus: Pain in connection with back, add puerarum root, cibot rhizome, antler glue; pain referred to arm and fingers, add spatholobus stem; obstruction of channels and collaterals with damp phlegm and occult blood, add cinnamon bark, bile treated arisaema tuber, earthworm, safflower, peach kernel, batry-ticated silkworm, scorpion, black tail snake and others.

3. Acupoints : *Jianyu, Jianliao, Jianzhen* (all with

reinforcing technique or moxibustion). Shoulder and back pain, add *Dazhui, Tianzong*; shoulder pain and referred to arm add *Binao, Quchi, Waiguan, Lieque*.

(II) Collateral obstruction with wind-heat

Key points of pathogenesis: Heat stagnation in channels and collaterals, stasis of *qi* and blood, accumulated in the shoulder and inability to lift the arm.

Chief manifestations: Shoulder pain, burning hot, redness, swelling, alleviated after exposure to cold, afraid to be touched, pain linked to back or arm and hand, accompanied by fever, aversion to wind, dysphoria. Tongue proper red, coat yellow and slimmy. Pulse slippery rapid.

Therapeutic principle: To clear away heat and activate the collaterals, to expel the wind and dampness.

1. Patent drug: *She Xiang Hu Gu Gao* external application.

2. Decoction recipe: *Bai Hu Jia Gui Zhi Tang* with modifications:

Gypsum 30g, Anemarrhena rhizome 12g, Cinnamon twig 10g, Honey suckle stem 30g, Erythrina bark 12g, Clematis root 12g, Moutan bark 12g, Red peony root 12g, Trilobus root 10g, Licorice root 3g, for oral administration after being decocted in water, one dose a day.

Plus-minus: Shoulder pain involving back, plus puerarum root, notopterygium root, cibot rhizome; arm pain too, add turmeria, mulberry twig; complicated with dampness add silkworm excrement, red bean, coix seed;

exuberance of heat with *yin* exhaustion, add rehmannia root, ophiopogon root.

3. Acupoints: *Jianyu, Jianliao, Jianzhen, Dazhui, Tianzong, Quchi, Lieque* (all with reducing technique).

I. Case report

Mr. Suo, 48 years old, cadre, came to attend clinic on Oct. 25, 1978. Five days ago after catching cold, he had a sudden attack of shoulder and arm pain, with limitations in motion such as lifting. The pain not relieved with prednisone and analgesic tablets. Also associated with aversion to cold and inclination to warm, the pain exacerbated with exposure to cold, general aching. Tongue proper light red, with thin, white moist coating. Pulse floating and tense. This indicated the obstruction of collaterals with wind-cold, the stagnation of *qi* and blood in shoulder. The principle of treatment was to warm up the channels and expel the cold, to activate the blood circulation and remove obstructions in the collaterals.

Recipe: Honey fried ephedra 10g, Asarum herb 3g, Prepared sichuan aconite root 10g, Chuanxiong rhizome 12g, Chinese angelica root 12g, Puerarum root 15g, Notopterygium root 10g, Turmeria 12g, Clematis root 10g, Honey-fried licorice root 6g, for oral administration after being decocted in water.

In the same time apply moxibustion to *Jianyu, Jianliao, Jianzhen,* acupuncture *Dazhui, Quchi, Lieque* using reinforcing technique at first, and reducing technique later,

After 15 doses of the above decoction and acupuncture 14 times, the shoulder pain disappeared, and the shoulder movement returned to normal.

II. Personal experience

At onset the punctuate proper treatment is very important, in case not on time or treatment improper, the disease become procrastinate and not healed, the impaired vital energy and the pathogenic evils still prevailing. The stagnancy and phlegm obstruction of collateral, with shoulder pain mild at a certain times, and severe at another, shoulder movement impeded. Tongue proper purple, pulse thin and unsmooth. The the rapeutic principle of resolving phlegm and removing stagnation, expelling wind and activating the collateral circulation, selected for gradual recovery with no hurry. The commonly adopted recipe is the following: Chinese angelica root tail 12g, Chuanxiong rhizome 12g, Peach kernel 10g, Safflower 10g, Clematis root 10g, Pangolian scale 10g, White mustard seed 10g, Scorpion 10g, Honeyfried ephedra 6g, Honey fried licorice root 3g, for oral administration after being decocted in water, one dose a day.

Besides the internal medication, acupuncture and moxibustion, massage therapy may be also adopted. Digital acupoint pressure method, with thumb, index finger and middle fingers press on *Jianyu*, *Jianchen*, *Jianliao* seperately. The manipulation technique of pointing, pinching, massaging, and pressing from heavy pressure first, then change to light pressure, each time 5~10 minutes, satisfactory effect usually obtained.

Chronic recurrent urticaria

Urticaria, also called wheal, is characterized with fresh red or white colored wheal, of various size, rapidly erupted and rapidly fading, usually with itching or burning sensation, in some cases there may be fever, vomiting, abdominal pain and others. This pertains to *pei lei* (swelling on the skin), 'wind eruption', 'chronic recurrent eruption' and others in TCM. In some chronic cases, the recurrent epizode and lingering course are very annoying.

I. **TCM syndrome differentiation and treatment**

Pathogenesis in brief: With damp heat retention in the interior, the exopathogen as an inducing factor. Blood deficiency in prolonged illness, and there by the production of wind which stays and accumulates in the skin and muscle bringing about the repeated recurrence of the disease.

(I) Retention of damp heat in the interior

Key points of pathogenesis: The retention of damp heat in the interior, and stir-up with wind as an inducing factor. The pathogens accumulated in the skin and muscle with the formation of skin eruption or pimple.

Chief manifestations: The eruption red in color and elevated, itching, accompanied by epigastric oppression, anorexia, belching of foul breathing, regurgitation of acids, abdominal pain and constipation, urination short, urine dark colored. Tongue proper red, tongue coat yellow and slimmy, pulse deep and unsmooth.

Therapeutic principle: To relieve exterior with diaphoresis; to clear the interior. To activate the blood circulation and expel the wind.

1. Patent drug:

(1) *Fang Feng Tong Sheng Wan* 10g t.i.d.

(2) *Qiang Li Yin Qiao Pian* and *Da Huang Pian* each 6 tablets, t.i.d.

2. Decoction recipe: *Fang Feng Tong Sheng Wan* with modifications:

Ledebouriella 10g, Schizonepeta 10g, Honeysuckle flower 30g, Forsythia fruit 15g, Honey fried ephedra 10g, Scutellaria root 12g, Red peony root 12g, Moutan bark 10g, Wine treated rhubarb 10g, Mirabilite 8g, Licorice root 3g, Broom cypress fruit 12g, for oral administration after being decocted in water, one dose a day.

Plus-minus: Exuberance of dampness in middle burner, epigastric oppression and anorexia add atractylodes rhizome, poria, magnolia bark; food stagnancy and abdominal pain add hawthorn fruit, fermented leaven, barley sprout; with helminthiasis add quisqualis fruit, black plurn, chinaberry bark, pepper.

3. Acupoints: *Fengchi, Hegu, Quchi, Yanglingquan, Sanyinjiao, Xuehai* (all with reducing technique), edema of larynx, further add *Shanzhong, Shaoshang*.

(Ⅱ) Wind production due to blood deficiency

Key points of pathogenesis: Urticaria for long time, deficiency of *qi* and blood, wind production and stagnation in skin and muscle.

Chief manifestations: Eruption color light red, itch severe at night, frequent recurrence, accompanied by no brilliance, dry skin, malaise, dysphoria, insomnia, dizziness, lumbar aching, easy recurrence during mens. Tongue proper light red, exfoliation. Pulse fine and weak.

Therapeutic principle: Reinforce *qi* and nourish the blood to expel the wind and quench the wind.

1. Patent drug: *Gui Pi Wan* one bolus, t.i.d. and *Yu Ping Feng San* 6g, t.i.d.

2. Decoction recipe: *Dang Gui Yin Zi* with modifications:

Chinese angelica root 12g, Astragalus root 30g, Prepared fleece flower root 30g, Chuanxiong rhizome 12g, White peony root 10g, Red peony root 10g, Rehmannia root 15g, Cicada slough 10g, Schizonepeta 12g, Ledebouriella 10g, Licorice root 6g, for oral administration after being decocted in water, one dose a day.

Plus-minus: With prominent blood-heat, plus moutan bark, scrofularia root, cimicifuga rhizome, peppermint; *qi* deficiency evident, add white atractylodes root, Chinese date; persistent case without healing, add batryticated silkworm, earthworm, epimedium.

3. Acupoints: *Fengchi, Quchi, Hegu, Yanglingquan* (all with reducing technique), *Xuehai, Sanyinjiao, Zusanli* (all with reinforcing technique).

II. Case report

Ms. Wang, 23 years old, peasant, had her first visit to our hospital on Dec. 5, 1978. Complained of wheal for 3 years, with repeated recurrences, the recurrence at a definite time, quite certain after menstrual period, had been treated with western and chinese herbal medicine without effect, The wheal all over the body, light red in color, coalesced into patches, very itching, especially at night, skin dry, no facial brilliance, soreness and weakness of loin and legs. Spiritless and malaise, insomnia and plenty dreams, dysphoria. Tongue proper light red with scanty coating. Pulse fine and weak.

TCM syndrome differentiation: This pertained to both deficiency of *qi* and blood wind production due to blood asthenia *qi* asthenia and weak resistence of *wei* with wind stagnation in skin and muscles, the therapeutic principle adopted was to replenish blood and reinforce *qi*, to strengthen *wei* and expel or eliminate the wind.

Recipe: Astragalus root 45g, Atractylodes rhizome 12g, White atractylodes rhizome 12g, Ledebouriella 10g, Schizonepeta 10g, Chinese angelica root 15g, Chuanxiong rhizome 12g, Red peony root 12g, White peony root 12g, Prepared fleece flower root 30g, Batryticated silkworm 15g,

Tribulus fruit 12g, Cicada slough 10g, Licorice root 6g, Arborvitae seed 15g, for oral administration after being decocted in water, one recipe dose daily.

After 15 doses, no recurrence after the subsidence of the eruption. She was told to continue the oral intake of *Bu Zhong Yi Qi Wan*, one bolus, t.i.d., continued for one month to strengthen the therapeutic effect.

2 years later, a follow-up study revealed no recurrence from then.

II. Personal experience

At the time of initial episode of wheals, it is easy to arrest the condition, but in longstanding, chronic cases with repeated recurrences which caused the *qi* and blood deficiency, then it is a knotty problem to deal with. Clinically the use of astragalus root, prepared fleece flower rhizome, and batryticated silkworm with big dosage should be emphasized. On this basis, with further addition of other drugs usually satisfactory results can be obtained.

Besides, be cautious in the observation of inducing factors, such as weather, pollen, lacquer, sea foodstuff of fishes, lobsters and mutton preparations, helminthesis in the body. In the light of this, to perform prophylactic measure and give treatment for radical cure is a good scheme.

Functional metrorrhagia

Functional metrorrhagia is a kind of uterine bleeding without inflammation, tumor, pathologic pregnancy or other abnormal findings on detailed physical and gynecological examinations. It pertains to the category of 'beng lou' (metrorrhagia and metrostaxis) in TCM.

I. TCM syndrome differentiation and treatment

Pathogenesis in brief: Qi stagnation and blood stasis, damp-heat, blood heat, asthenia of spleen and kidney are all causes to induce impairment of *chong* and *ren* channels, unable to consolidate the channels to arrest bleeding.

(I) Qi stagnation and blood stasis

Key points of pathogenesis: Stagnation of the liver *qi* and impeded *qi* function with blood stais, as a result, damage of *chong* and *ren* channels.

Chief manifestations: Sudden uterine bleeding, large amount, purple dark in color and with clots, lower abdomen distending pain, resistent to palpation, relieved after the expel of the clots. Distension and fullness of the chest and hypochondria, swelling and pain of breasts, dysphoria and ready loss of temper. Tongue proper dark red, tongue coat thin and white. Pulse deep and unsmooth.

Therapeutic principle: To regulate the *qi* and arrest pain; to activate blood and remove stasis.

1. Patent drug:

(1) *Bao Kun Dan*, 6 g, t.i.d.

(2) *Jian Xue Ning*, 4 tablets t.i.d.

2. Decoction recipe: *Shi Xiao San* and *Tao Hong Si Wu Tang* with modifications:

Stir-fried cat-tail pollen 12 g, Trogopterus dung 10g, Peach kernel 10 g, Safflower 10 g, Red peony root 10 g, White peony root 10 g, Chinese angelica root 12 g, Rehmannia root 15 g, Prepared cyperus tuber 12 g, Notoginseng powder 3 g (swallowed with boiled water or decocted fluid), for oral administration after being decocted in water, one dose a day.

Plus-minus: For severe bleeding, plus madder root, small thistle (both carbonized); for *qi* stagnancy, add bupleurum root.

3. Acupoints: *Guanyuan, Sanyinjiao, Yinbai, Baihui* (all moxibustion), *Taichong, Xuehai, Qichong* (all with reducing technique).

(II) Metrorrhagia due to blood heat

Key points of pathogenesis: Accumulated heat in blood, perversion of blood flow due to blood heat, debility of *chong* and *ren* channels, metrorrhagia results.

Chief manifestations: Profuse menstrual flow like landslide, the mens blood deep red in color, with purple black clots, associated with facial flush, dryness of mouth, thirst, inclined to cold drink, tongue proper red, tongue coat yellow, pulse full and rapid.

Therapeutic principle: To clear heat and nourish *yin*; to cool the blood and arrest bleeding.

1. Patent drug:

(1) *Long Dun Xie Gan Wan*, 6 g t.i.d. and *Yun Nan Bai Yao*, 2 g t.i.d.

(2) *Zhi Zi Yan Qin Gao Pian*, 3 tab. t.i.d.

2. Decoction recipe: *Qing Re Gu Jing Tang* with modifications:

Rehmannia root 30 g, Wolfberry bark 12 g, Scutellaria root 10 g, Stir-fried black capejasmine fruit 10 g, Prepared tortoise plastron 20 g, Sanguisorba root 12 g, Lotus node 30 g, Carbonized palmae bark 10 g, Donkey hide glue 10 g (add to the decoction after melting), Ophiopogon root 20 g, Licorice root 3 g, for oral administration after being decocted in water, one dose a day.

Plus-minus: Incessant bleeding add carbonized small thistle, carbonized eucommia bark, notoginseng powder, complicated with dampness, in ordinary time leucorrhea, puffiness of face, epigastric oppression, anorexia, remove tortoise plastron, rehmannia, add atractylodes tuber, phellodendron bark, coix seed, poria, calcined oyster shell.

3. Acupoints: *Guanyuan, Sanyinjiao, Baihui, Shenshu* (all with reinforcing technique), *Xuehai, Dadun* (both with reducing technique).

(Ⅲ) Asthenia of spleen and kidney

Key points of pathogenesis: Insufficiency of both spleen and kidney, debility of *chong* and *ren* channels, depletion of *qi* and *yin*, incessant flow of mens.

Chief manifestations: Incessant dripping of menstrual flow, blood light red in color, dilute and thin in consistency, accompanied by soreness and weakness of loin and knees, malaise, cold sensation and pain of lower abdomen, aversion to cold, cold limbs, abdominal distension and anorexia, urine clear and stool loose, tongue plump with teeth imprints over the margins. Tongue proper light, tongue coat thin and white, pulse deep fine and weak.

Therapeutic principle: To tonify kidney and reinforce spleen, to regulate menstruation and arrest bleeding.

1. Patent drugs: *You Gui Wan* and *Ren Shen Jian Pi Wan* each one bolus, t.i.d.

2. Decoction recipe: *Gu Ben Zhi Beng Tang* with modifications:

Prepared rehmannia root 15 g, Dogwood fruit 12 g, Prepared fleece flower root 15 g, Dangshen 20 g, Astragalus root 20 g, Carbonized madder root 12 g, Carbonized palmae bark 12 g, Calcined dragon's bone 24 g, Vinegar-fried tortoise plastron 20 g, Calcined oyster shell 24 g, Baked black ginger 10 g, Amomum fruit 6 g, Honey-fried licorice root 6 g, Cimicifuga rhizome 6 g, for oral administration after being decocted in water, one dose a day.

Plus-minus: For abdominal distension and loose stool with predominance of spleen asthenia, plus white atractylodes rhizome, poria, bupleurum, tangerine peel; with predominance of asthenia of kidney *yang*, plus prepared aconite root, carbonized argyi leaf; with predominant kidney *yin* deficiency, the expelled blood bright red, dizziness and tinnitus, minus prepared rehmannia root, plus rehmannia root, eclipta. Sudden incessant bleeding with syncope, weak respirations, pulse feeble with impending stoppage, promptly giving red ginseng 30 g decocted in water, with this decocted fluid swallow *Yun Nan Bai Yao* 3 g and the red pill enclosed inside the white drug bottle.

3. Acupoints: *Shenshu, Pishu, Zusanli, Sanyinjiao, Yinbai, Baihui* (all moxibustion). With *yang* insufficiency predominant, add moxibustion of *Mingmen* and *Zhongji*; with inclination to *yin* deficiency, add *Houxi, Ganshu* (both with reinforcing technique).

I. Case report

Ms. Ni, 44 years old, cadre, came to clinic for the first time on Nov. 25, 1977. In the last three months she had menstruation twice in a month, each lasting 10 days, large amount and light in color, exacerbated after motion, accompanied by palpitation, shortness of breath, malaise, impaired appetite, stool dry. Tongue plump with teeth imprint over the margin. Tongue coat thin and white, pulse fine relaxed and weak. Blood routine Hgb 7 g, RBC 2750 thousands, WBC 5000.

TCM syndrome differentiation and treatment: Overstrain and over-fatigue with impairment of spleen *qi*, inability to govern the blood, the debility of *chong* and *ren* channels. The therapeutic principle adopted was to reinforce spleen and stop bleeding.

Recipe: Honey fried astragalus root 18 g, Dangshen 15 g, White atractylodes rhizome 12 g, Poria 10 g, Earth fried Chinese angelica root 10 g, Longan aril 10 g, Donkey's hide glue beads 10 g, Calcined magnetite 12 g, Arborvitae seed 12 g, Amomum fruit 6 g, Aucklandia root 6 g, Barley sprout 15 g, Fresh ginger 2 slices, Chinese date 3 ones (split), for oral administration after being decocted in water, one recipe dose daily.

The second visit on Dec. 15, 19 doses taken, all the symptoms disappeared, no menstruation for more than 20 days. The diet, urine and stool, sleep all returned to normal. Tongue proper light red, tongue coat thin and white, pulse moderate. Blood routine: Hgb 13g. She was advised to continue the intake of *Gui Pi Wan* one bolus, t.i.d. for one month to strengthen the therapeutic effect.

Follow-up 6 months later, menstruation was normal since then.

III. Personal experience

Since 'beng lou' (metrorrhagia and metrostaxis) has many etiologic factors, but the main one is the debility of *chong* and *ren* channels, inability to keep the blood inside the vessels, liver unable to store the blood, spleen unable to hold the blood within. The principle of treatment is to manage to reinforce spleen, to regulate liver and consolidate the *chong* and *ren* channels. It's important to pay attention to the use of carbonized drugs, such as eucommia, rehmannia, palmae bark, sangui sorba root, madder root in accordance with the clinical alternations of symptoms, and good therapeutic effects usually obtained.

Metrorrhagia incessant and patient in critical condition on the verge of death, at one hand the immediate oral intake of *Du Shen Tang* (Decoction of ginseng alone) and simultaneous dripping per rectum of 200~300 ml placental blood of healthy woman. With this measure, good hemostatic effect usually obtained in most cases.

Habitual abortion

Habitual abortion denotes premature delivery of fetus not reaching full term without apparent inducing factors for at least two times. It belongs to the category of '*hua tai*' (abortion), '*tai lou*' (vaginal bleeding during pregnancy) and others in TCM.

I. TCM syndrome differentiation and treatment

Pathogenesis in brief: The deficiency of spleen and kidney, the debility of *chong* and *ren* channels, the insufficiency of *qi* and blood leading to malnourishment of fetus.

(I) The asthenia of kidney *qi*

Key points of pathogenesis: The asthenia of kidney *qi*, the debility of *chong* and *ren* channels, loss of restraint of *dai* channel, loss of protection of fetus.

Chief manifestations: Consecutive habitual abortion, soreness and weakness of loin and legs, spiritless and malaise, leucorrhea, decreased sexual desire, dizziness and blurred vision, aggravated after fatigue. Tongue proper light in color, tongue coat white and moist, pulse deep and weak.

Therapeutic principle: To reinforce kidney and consolidate the fundamental; to tonify *qi* and prevent abortion.

1. Patent drug: *Tai Chan Jin Dan* 2 boli, two or three times a day.

2. Decoction recipe: *You Gui Yin* with modifications:

Prepared rehmannia root 15 g, Stir-fried Chinese yam 12 g, Wolfberry fruit 12 g, Dogwood fruit 12 g, Eucommia bark 12 g, Astragalus root 15 g, Mulberry mistletoe 12 g, Psoralea fruit 10 g, Stir fried white atractylodes rhizome 12 g, Honey-fried licorice root 3 g, for oral administration after being decocted in water, one dose a day.

Plus-minus: Threatened abortion, plus Chinese angelica root, perilla stem; much leucorrhea, add poria, calcined dragon's bone, calcined oyster shell; for anorexia, add amomum fruit, fermented leaven, tangerine peel. In cases with dysphoria, insomnia, minus astragalus root, licorice root, plus scutellaria root, phellodendron bark, stir fried wild jujuba seed.

3. Acupoints: *Shenshu, Pishu, Guanyuan, Qihai, Mingmen, Zusanli, Sanyinjiao, Baihui* (all with reinforcing acupuncture or moxibustion).

(II) Deficiency of spleen and kidney

Key points of pathogenesis: Deficiency of spleen and kidney, insufficiency of *qi* and blood, malnourishment of fetus, debility of *chong* and *ren* channels.

Chief manifestations: Continuous abortion, malaise, anorexia, loose or liquid stool, soreness and weakness of loin and knees, pallor of face, spiritlessness, aversion to cold, leucorrhea profuse, clear and dilute. Tongue plump with teeth imprint over margins, tongue proper light, with white smooth coating. Tongue coat deep fine and weak.

Therapeutic principle: To replenish kidney and reinforce spleen.

1. Patent drug:

(1) *Bao Tai Wan*, one bolus t.i.d.

(2) *Nü Jin Dan*, one bolus b.i.d.

2. Decoction recipe: *You Gui Wan* and *Gui Pi Wan* with modifications:

Prepared rehmannia root 12 g, Stir-fried Chinese yam 15 g, Wolfberry fruit 12 g, Antler glue (stir-fried into beads) 12 g, Cinnamon bark 6 g, Honey-fried astragalus root 12 g, Ginseng 10 g, Stir-fried white atractylodes rhizome 12 g, Earth-fried Chinese angelica root 12 g, Poria 12 g, Perilla stem 10 g, Tangerine peel 12 g, Honey-fried licorice root 3 g, for oral administration after being decocted in water, one dose a day.

Plus-minus: With predominance of water flood due to *yang* deficiency, the presence of much leucorrhea, add epimedium, prepared aconite root, plantain seed; with predominance of *yin* deficiency and the manifestation of internal heat, ginseng and astragalus root to be withdrawn, and tortoise plastron, turtle shell, sweet wormwood, swallowwort root, scutellaria root added; with *qi* stagnancy ginseng to be withdrawn, and bupleurum root, curcuma root, cyperus tuber; complicated with blood stasis, antler glue removed, red sage root, peach kernel, safflower, motherwort to be added; for anorexia the addition of amomum fruit and medicated leaven.

3. Acupoints: *Shenshu, Pishu, Guanyuan, Qihai, Zusanli, Sanyinjiao, Mingmen, Xuehai* (all moxibustion or acupuncture with reinforcing technique). Internal heat with *yin* deficiency, add *Taixi* (reinforcing), *Rangu, Xinjian* (both reducing); *yang* deficiency with cold

manifestation, add *Zhongji* (moxibustion), complicated with stagnation, the addition of *Taichong, Qichong* (both reducing).

II. Case report

Ms. Guo, 31 years old, cadre, came to the clinic on Dec. 15, 1977, with history of abortion for 3 times, mostly at the time of 1~3 month pregnancy without evident inducing factors. This time already pregnant for 40 days, much leucorrhea, loose or liquid stool, Tongue proper light white. Pulse deep, fine and weak. This pertained to deficiency of spleen and kidney, malnourishment of fetus, depletion of *chong* and *ren* channels. The therapeutic principle adopted was to replenish the kidney amd reinforce the spleen, to nourish the blood and prevent abortion.

Recipe: Prepared rehmannia root 12 g, Dogwood fruit 10 g, Stir-fried Chinese yam 15 g, Wolfberry fruit 12 g, Ginseng 10 g, Astragalus root 15 g, White atractylodes rhizome 15 g, Poria 15 g, Chinese angelica root 12 g, Longan aril 12 g, Donkey hide glue 10 g (stir-fried into beads), Amom fruit 6 g, Perilla stem 10 g, Tangerine peel 10 g, Licorice root 3 g, for oral administration after being decocted in water, one recipe dose daily, and simultaneous moxibustion of *Zusanli, Sanyinjiao, Guanyuan,* once daily.

The second visit on Dec. 26, after nine doses, all symptoms alleviated, no leucorrhea, appetite increased, tongue proper light red, with thin, white coating. Pulse deep and fine.

Recipe: 5 times the dosage of the above recipe, ground into fine powder, thoroughly mixed with heated honey to make pill, each bolus weighed 10 g, one bolus, t.i.d. to fortify the therapeutic effect.

On Sept. 1988, she delivered a female baby at full term, the mother and the daughter both healthy and the good news reported.

II. Personal experience

This condition is due to deficiency of spleen and kidney, the insufficiency of qi and blood. As ren channel is chiefly responsible for uterine pregnancy, uterus linked to kidney. Deficiency of kidney induces depletion of chong and ren channels. Blood feeds the fetus, qi consolidated the fetus, spleen is the source of production and transformation of qi and blood, insufficiency of spleen leads to insufficiency of qi and blood, and thus depletion of nutrition and consolidation of fetus. The therapeutic principle of tonifying the kidney and reinforcing the spleen assisted by soothing the liver and regulating qi, by activating the blood and removing stasis, resolving dampness and arresting leucorrhea, clearing heat and preventing miscarriage.

Beside the delighted spirit and proper ratio of work and rest, the increase of nutrition, sexual intercourse should be strictly forbidden.

Myoma of uterus

Uterine myoma is a comparative common benign tumour of female genital organs. The tumors growing out from the uterine muscular fibre are usually multiple and of various size, most frequently found in middle aged women over 30 years of age. Its etiology is not well known at present. The chief clinical manifestations are metrorrhagia, leucorrhea, abdominal pain, dysmenorrhea and others. It belongs to the category of *'zheng jia'* (mass in the abdomen), *'beng lou'* (metrorrhagia and metrostaxis), 'leucorrhea', 'sterility' and others in TCM.

I. TCM syndrome differentiation and treatment

Pathogenesis in brief: Emotional upset, *qi* stagnation and blood stasis, asthenia and decline of internal organs, debility of *chong* and *ren* channels.

(I) Deficiency of spleen and kidney

Key points of pathogenesis: Deficiency of spleen and kidney, debility of *chong* and *ren* channels, blood not along the usual pathway, stagnation with abdominal tumor mass formation.

Chief manifestations: Abdominal pain during menstruation, menstrual blood large in amount, light colored, incessant drippling of mens blood, mass in lower abdomen, spiritless, malaise, impaired appetite, soreness of loin, weakness of legs, leucorrhea white colored, large in amount. Tongue proper ight colored, with thin and white coat. Pulse deep fine and weak.

Therapeutic principle: To reinforce spleen and replenish kidney; to resolve stagnation and arrest uterine bleeding.

1. Patent drug: *Jian Nao Bu Shen Wan*, one bolus t.i.d. and notoginseng powder 3g, t.i.d.

2. Decoction recipe: *Ba Zhen Tang* with modifications:

Prepared rehmannia root 15g, Chinese angelica root 12g, Oyster shell 30g, Astragalus root 20g, Dangshen 15g, Motherwort 20g, Stir-fried peach kernel 12g, Biota tops 12g, Notoginseng 3g (swallow with boiled water or decocted fluid of the above drugs), for oral administration after being decocted in water, one dose a day.

Plus-minus: With prominent anorexia, plus amomum fruit, white atractylodes rhizome, chicken's gizzard membrane; loin soreness and leg weakness, plus eucommia bark, achyranthes root; mass in lower abdomen, add zedoary, burreed tuber; profuse leucorrhea add Chinese yam, poria, cuttle bone; leucorrhea yellowish fishy stinky, minus prepared rehmannia root, plus honey suckle flower, dandelion herb, plantain herb, alismatis rhizome and others.

3. Acupoints: *Pishu, Shenshu, Guanyuan, Diji* (all moxibustion), *Xuehai Taichong, Qichong* (all with reducing technique).

(Ⅱ) Stagnation of the liver *qi*

Key points of pathogenesis: Emotional depression or melancholia, *qi* stagnation and blood coagulation, stagnation in the uterus, blood not along the normal pathway.

Chief manifestations: To regulate *qi* and activate the blood; to soften the hardness and eliminate the stagnation.

1. Patent drug: *Qi Zhi Xiang Fu Wan*, 6g t.i.d.

2. Decoction recipe: *Da Qi Qi Tang* with modifications:

Green tangerine orange peel 10g, Tangerine peel 10g, Bupleurum root 12g, Burreed tuber 10g, Zedoary 10g, Peach kernel 12g, Stir-fried corydalis tuber 10g, Licorice root 3g, Sichuan chinaberry 10g, Cyperus tuber 12g, for oral administration after being decocted in water, one dose a day.

Plus-minus: Large mass in abdomen, plus red peony root, chuanxiong rhizome, moutan bark; anorexia severe, add *Xiang Sha Liu Jun Zi Wan*; profuse leukorrhea, add atractylodes rhizome, cuttle bone; yellow fishy stinky leucorrhea, add phellodendron bark, red poria, honey-suckle flower, dandelion herb, plantain herb.

3. Acupoints: *Taichong, Qichong, Zhongji* (shallow puncture), *Diji, Xuehai* (all with reducing technique).

Ⅱ. Case report

Ms. Zhao, 49 years old, cadre, came to the clinic on March 12, 1974, with a history of menostaxis with incessant drippling for 8 years. Menstrual cycle 20~23 days, mentrual period 8 days, menstrual blood light purple, with large amount and blood clots, associated with loin pain, dragging pain of lower abdomen, abdomen mass, profuse leucorrhea, spiritless, malaise. Tongue proper light, thin and white coat. Pulse deep fine and unsmooth. She had parturation of five fetus, artificial abortion 4 times. Since June 1973, she was examined in many hospitals; all agreed that her uterus enlarged as the size of 50 days pregnancy, nodular feeling, with eminence at the anterior, a diagnosis of uterine myoma made. Methyltestosteron, propyl testosteron, durabolin used without much effect. As the patient refused to be operated so came for TCM treatment.

TCM syndrome differentiation and treatment: History of many pregnancies, over fatigue, with the damage of spleen and kidney, *qi* losing the power being a guide and control the blood, debility of the *chong* and *ren* channel, the blood unable to circulate in its ordinary way, the stagnanted blood accumulated in the interior, metrorrhagia and metrastaxis result. The principle of treatment adopted was to replenish spleen and reinfore kidney, to resolve stagnation and arrest blooding.

Recipe: Astragalus root 24g, Dangshen 12g, stir-fried gordon euryale seed 30g, Poria 12g, White atractylodes rhizome 18g, Cuttle bone 15g, Chinese angelica root 10g, Rehmannia root 20g, Lotus leaf 30g, Biota top 3g, Argyl leaf 2g, Auricular fungus 3g, Notoginseng 3g (to be swallowed with boiled water or decocted fluid), for oral administration after being decocted in water.

The second visit on April 24, 28 doses of the above recipe taken. After 5 recipe doses, the bleeding stopped, and other symptoms alleviated. The next mens came more than 40 days later, and the blood not much, no other discomfort. Tongue proper light in color, with thin and white coating, pulse deep and fine.

From the above recipe dangshen altered to 24g, continued for another dose.

The third visit on May 5, slight pain of the lower abdomen. On gynecological examination done in the provincial hospital (one of the three hospitals confirmed the diagnosis before) revealed no tumour found, the tongue and pulse findings as before. The above recipe with black auricular fungus added to 6g for oral administration after being decocted in water, one recipe daily for another 6 days.

The fourth visit on May 16, after medication, the lower abdominal pain arrested, no much leucorrhea, with slight rigidity of loin and legs. Tongue proper light with thin white coating, pulse deep fine. The above recipe with further addition of deglued antler powder 10g for three doses to strengthen the therapeutic effect.

Ⅱ. Personal experience

For the treatment of uterine myoma, hysterectomy is the main treatment in western medicine, but this kind of treatment is difficult to be accepted by young patient, according to TCM syndrome differentiation and treatment, not a few patient acquired satisfactory therapeutic results. During therapy, it is important to notice the relationship between 'bu' (reinforcing) and 'hua' (resolving), 'hua' (resolving) and 'zhi' (arresting). Reinforcing is to reinforce spleen and kidney; resolving is to resolve stagnation and activate the blood, arresting is to arrest bleeding. As menorrhagia is a common symptom of uterine myoma, and is due to stagnation. To resolve stagnation will arrest bleeding. Therefore be not afraid to use drugs to soften the hardness, to activate the blood and resolve stagnation, such as zedoary, burreed tuber, peach kernel and cat-tail pollen, assisted with some hemostatic drugs. Notoginseng is very precious because of its effect, combining activating blood, resolving stagnation and hemostasis. In chronic cases with deficiency of spleen and kidney, *qi* unable to control blood flow, be brave to use reinforcing in those cases, that is to restore the vital energy and the capacity to resolve stagnation thereby. TCM syndrome differentiation and treatment is the central core of TCM, especially in dealing with difficult knotty diseases.

Dysmenorrhea

Dysmenorrhea is one of the common gynecological

disease, characterized with lower abdominal pain before or during menstruation, or both before and during menstruation ensues. It pertains to the categories of *'tong jing'* (painful menstruation) and *'xing jing fu tong'* (abdominal pain during mens) in TCM.

I. TCM syndrome differentiation and treatment

Pathogenesis in brief: Condensation of cold dampness, *qi* stagnation and blood stasis, asthenia of *qi* and blood, depletion of liver and kidney.

(1) Cold condensation and blood stasis

Key points of pathogenesis: Invasion of cold pathogen, *qi* stagnation and blood stasis, abdominal pain during menstruation, aggravated after exposure to cold.

Chief manifestations: Cold pain in the lower abdomen before and during mens, thermophile and aversion to cold, tenderness on palpation, mens blood dark red, scanty in amount with clots, associated with chilliness, loose stool, limbs not warm, tongue proper bluish purple, tongue coat white and moist. Pulse deep and tense.

Therapeutic principle: To warm the channel and promote the flow of mens blood.

1. Patent drug:

(1) *Ai Fu Nuan Gong Wan* 10g, t.i.d.

(2) *Fu Zi Li Zhong Wan* one bolus, t.i.d.

2. Decoction recipe: *Dang Gui Si Ni Tang* with modifications:

Chinese angelica root 12g, White peony root 12g, Asarum herb 3g, Cinnamon twig 10g, Honey-fried licorice root 6g, Lindera root 10g, Chinese date 3 pieces, for oral administration after being decocted in water, taken 10 days prior to the coming menstruation, one recipe dose daily.

Plus-minus: Heavy infection with cold pathogen, plus evodia fruit, common fennel fruit, fresh ginger; cold limbs add prepared aconite root, cinnamon bark; abdominal pain and tenderness with blood clots add cat-tail pollen, trogopterus dung; fatigue and malaise, anorexia and loose stool, add Dangshen, white atractylodes rhizome, amomum fruit.

3. Acupoints: *Guanyuan* (moxibustion), *Pishu*, *Shenshu*, *Sanyinjiao* (all with reinforcing technique).

(II) *Qi* stagnation and blood stasis

Key points of pathogenesis: Stagnation of the liver *qi*, inability to guide the blood which accumulated in the uterus, distending pain during menstruation.

Chief manifestations: Distending pain over the lower abdomen, before or during mens, with tenderness on palpation, mens blood scanty in amount, dark in color with blood clots, associated with distending pain of breast, referred to both hypochondria. Tongue proper dark purple with petechie at the margin, pulse deep and taut.

Therapeutic principle: To activate *qi* and resolve stagnation, to activate the blood flow and arrest pain.

1. Patent drug: *Qi Zhi Xiang Fu Wan* 10g, t.i.d. or q.i.d.

2. Decoction recipe: *Xue Fu Zhu Yu Tang* with modifications:

Chinese angelica root tail 12g, Red peony root 10g, Peach kernel 10g, Safflower 10g, Cyathula root 15g, Prepared cyperus tuber 12g, Motherwort 15g, Chuanxiong 6g, Bupleurum root 6g, Stir fried bitter orange 6g, Licorice root 3g, for oral administration after being decocted in water.

3. Acupoints: *Hegu* (reinforcing), *Xingjian*, *Qihc, Xuehai, Sanyinjiao, Guilai* (all reducing).

(III) Yin deficiency of liver and kidney

Key points of pathogenesis: Asthenia of *yin* and blood, improper filling of the uterus, devoid of source of the menstrual blood, incessant dull pain.

Chief manifestations: Mens blood scanty in amount, light colored, dull pain in the lower abdomen, accompanied by soreness and weakness of loin and legs. Dizziness and tinnitus, dysphoria and feverishness over the palms, soles and in the chest. Tongue proper light colored, with thin and white coating, pulse deep and fine

Therapeutic principle: To nourish and tonify the liver and kidney.

1. Patent drug: *Bai Feng Wan* one bolus, t.i.d.

2. Decoction recipe: *Tiao Gan Tang* with modifications:

Prepared rehmannia root 18g, Stir fried Chinese yam 18g, Chinese angelica root 12g, white peony root 12g, Dogwood fruit 10g, Cyperus tuber 10g, Donkey hide glue 10g (melted and added to the decocted fluid), Licorice root 3g, for oral administration after being decocted in water, one dose a day.

Plus-minus: Prominent lumbar pain, plus eucommia bark, dipsacus root; hypochondriac pain, add curcuma tuber, sichuan chinaberry fruit; lower abdominal pain, add common fennel fruit, complicated with qi deficiency, general malaise, anorexia, Dangshen, astragalus root, white atractylodes rhizome, amomum fruit.

3. Acupoints: *Shenshu, Ganshu, Zusanli, Qihai, Xuehai, Guilai, Sanyinjiao* (all with reinforcing technique).

II. Case report

Ms. Zhang, 25 years old, peasant, came first to the clinic on May 25, 1968, with a history of dysmenorrhea for 4 years, aggravated for half an year. One day before mens she began to have lower abdominal pain, increase in severity during menstruation, restlessness unable to sit down or sleep at ease, perturbed, tenderness over the lower abdomen, mens blood scanty and black, with blood clots. After the expelling of the clots the pain became less severe, distention of both breasts. All the above aggravated after anger. Tongue proper purple and dark, pulse deep and taut. She was married 3 years ago, she had no pregnacy since then. TCM syndrome differentiation and treatment: This was a case of *qi* stagnation and blood stasis. The suitable principle of treatment should be to activate the flow of *qi* and blood, and remove stagnation.

Recipe: Bupleurum root 12g, Cyperus tuber 10g,

Curcuma root 10g, Peach kernel 10g, Safflower 10g, Chinese angelica root tail 12g, Chuanxiong rhizome 10g, Red peony root 10g, White peony root 10g, Asarum herb 3g, Licorice root 3g, Cyathula root 12g, for oral administration after being decocted in water, to begin the intake 10 days before the mens, continued to the initiation of mens, continue the medication for three months.

One month after medication pain alleviated, the second month pain greatly reduced. The third month no pain. The fourth month she became pregnant.

Ⅲ. Personal experience

For the treatment of dysmenorrhea, in (Ⅰ) (Ⅱ) these two types the medicine should be given 10 days before mens, and continue the intake for 10 doses, continue this schema for 2~3 months. In type (Ⅲ) the time to recieve treatment should be given after menstruation is over, one recipe dose daily continuously for 1~2 month, this may be related to this saying, purge excess should be given befor mens, in deficiency the reinforcing drugs should be given following the mens.

Impotence

Impotence is mostly due to sexual neuroasthenia, with clinical manifestations of no or poor erection of penis and interference of normal sexual life.

I. TCM syndrome differentiation and treatment

Pathogenesis in brief: Decline of the fire of vital gate, consumption of essence and *qi*; down-ward flow of the damp heat, softness and relaxation of penis, the deficiency at the anterior, the excess at the posterior.

(I) Decline of the fire of vital gate

Key points of pathogenesis: Fire decline of the vital gate, consumption of essence and *qi*, decline of the kidney *yang*, impotence as the result.

Chief manifestations : Debility of penis erection, semen thin, dilute and cold, pallor of face, dizziness and tinnitus, soreness and weakness of loin and knees. Aversion to cold and cold limbs, spiritless, malaise, forgetfulness or poor memory, dreamfulness. Tongue proper light white. Pulse deep fine and weak.

Therapeutic principle: To reinforce the vital gate using drugs with warm or hot property; to replenish the semen and promote erection.

1. Patent drug:

(1) *Jin Gui Shen Qi Wan* one bolus, t.i.d.

(2) *Chu Feng Jing* 5~10g each time, two or three times a day.

2. Decoction recipe: *Huan Shao Wan* with modifications:

Prepared rehmannia root 12g, Prepared fleece-flower root 15g, Dogwood fruit 12g, Chinese yam 12g, Indian mulberry root 12g, Epimedium 12g, Wolfberry fruit 15g, Pilose antler slice 10g, Honey fried ephedra 8g, Prepared polygala root 10g, Grass-leaved sweetflag rhizome 6g, for oral administration after being decocted in water, one dose a day.

Plus-minus: Prominent *qi* deficiency, plus ginseng, astragalus root; deficiency of heart *qi* forgetfulness, and dreamfulness, add American ginseng, schisandra fruit, arborvitae seed.

3. Acupoints: *Shenshu, Mingmen, Guanyuan, Shangliao, Ciliao* (all moxibustion).

4. Ear acupuncture: Kidney, *Mingmen*, Endocrine, Sympathetic.

(Ⅱ) Downward flow of damp heat

Key points of pathogenesis: Damp heat in the lower burner, where *yang qi* can't reach, penis flabby and soft.

Chief manifestations: penis soft and flabby, sorotum wet and foul, heaviness of body, especially the lower limbs, urine short and deep colored. Mouth sticky and foul. Tongue coat yellow slimmy, pulse without strength and rapid.

Therapeutic principle: To clear the heat and remove dampness with diuresis, to strengthen *yang* and treat impotence.

1. Patent drug: *Zhi Bai Di Huang Wan* one bolus, t.i.d. and *Long Dan Xie Gan Wan* 10g, t.i.d.

2. Decoction recipe: *San Miao San* with additional ingredients:

Phellodendron bark 10g, Atractylodes rhizome 12g, Gentian root 12g, Hypoglauca yam 12g, Capejasmine fruit 10g, Alismatis rhizome 21g, Achyranthes root 12g, Plantain seed 15g, Chinese angelica root 12g, Rehmannia root 15g, Honey-fried ephedra 6g, for oral administration after being decocted in water, one dose a day.

Plus-minus: *Yin* damage by damp heat, thirsty with preference to drinks, add dendrobium, Chinese yam; exuberance of heat evil, minus ephedra, plus gypsum, scutellaria root.

3. Acupoints: *Zhongji*, *Yinlingquan*, *Qihai*, *Sanyinjiao*, *Taixi* (all with reducing technique).

I. Case report

Mr. Hu, 34 years old, cadre, came to attain the clinic on May 15, 1978, with history of impotence for 8 years. The patient had the bad habit of masturbation since he was a youngster. He married at 24 years old. After marriage he suffered from early ejaculation during coupling. Two years later, he became impotent, associated with dizziness and tinnitus, loin soreness, legs weakness, no spirit, poor memory, liquid stool, urine clear, amount not scanty, tongue proper slight white, pulse deep, fine and weak. He received various treatment without much effect. This was considered to belong to the type of declination of fire of vital gate, depletion of kidney *yang*. To warm and tonify the vital gate, to enhance its fire and strengthen the *yang*.

Recipe: Prepared rehmannia root 120g, Chinese yam 150g, Prepared fleece flower root 100g, Dogwood fruit 60g, Wolfberry fruit 120g, Morinda root 90g, Epimedium 90g, Pilose antler 30g, American ginseng 30g, Honey-fried ephedra 30g, Amomum fruit 30g, Chives seed 60g, Honey fried licorice root 30g, Safflower 15g, Chinese angelica root 60g. The above ground into fine powder, flood with water and made into pill the size of parasol, each time 10g, t.i.d. and simultaneous application of ear acupuncture of *mingmen*, kidney, endocrine, sympathetic, masturbation should be strictly forbidden.

After taking the above pill recipe for three recipe doses, the impotence cured, yet early ejaculation (5~10 min) still existed. Another dose of the pill recipe given to strengthen the therapeutic effects.

Ⅲ. Personal experience

Majority of impotence pertains to asthenia, few of excess, the therapy should use warm tonic, on the basis of replenishing essence and nourishing *yin* drugs for strengthening kidney *yang* should be added, such as epimedium, chives seed, morinda root, wolfberry fruit and others, pilose antler, testicle of fur seal, penis of deer and other animal preparations are of special importance. Though the pill preparation has gradual effect and yet it is the preparation of choice (the case of damp heat should receive different disposal), as large doses of drugs to stimulate erection may have rapid effect, but afterwards the impotence will become more severe than before and form a knotty problem resist to further treatment. In the mean while masturbation should be strictly forbidden, and the sexual life should be restricted. The husband and wife should cooperate to accomplish this aim, to insist on comparatively long term treatment. Besides, proper physical training, breathing exercise, acupuncture and moxibustion may also be helpful and may be coordinated into the entire scheme of treatment.

Climacteric syndrome

Climacteric syndrome is a kind of involutionary psychosis with its first occurrence at the climacterium namely the transition period from the middle age to the old age, corresponding in women the period around menopause, so also called menopausal syndrome. But the term of climacteric syndrome is better, because it occurs also in men as well, and it relates to endocrine and metabolic disorder. The symptoms consist of anxiety, melancholy, insomnia, being nervous, suspicious and other emotional disorders. It pertains to the category of 'zang zao' (hysteria),'insomnia', 'melancholia' and others in TCM.

1. **TCM syndrome differentiation and treatment**

Pathogenesis in brief: At or coming to the old age

kidney debility, disharmoney of *yin* and *yang*, disorder of *chong* and *ren* channels.

Chief manifestations: Abrupt alternation of chilliness and feverishness, malar flush, paroxysmal feverishness and sweating, dizziness and tinnitus, dysphoria and feverishness over the palms, soles and in the chest. Palpitation and insomnia or sorness and weakness of loin and knees, aversion to cold, and cold limbs, puffiness of face, edema of limbs. Melancholia, irritability, extreme dysphoria. Tongue proper red with teeth imprints over the margin. Pulse taut and fine.

Therapeutic principle: To nourish the kidney and regulate the liver *qi*, keep the balance of *yin* and *yang*.

1. Patent drug:

(1) *Liu Wei Di Huang Wang* one bolus, t.i.d. and *Xiao Yao Wan* 6g, t.i.d. (used for predominance of *yin* deficiency.

(2) *Jin Gui Shen Qi Wan* one bolus, t.i.d. and *Ren Shen Jian Pi Wan* one bolus, t.i.d. used for predominance of *yang* deficiency.

2. Decoction recipe: *Zi Shui Qing Gan Yin* with modifications:

Rehmannia root 10g, Prepared rehmannia root 10g, Chinese yam 12g, Dogwood fruit 10g, Moutan bark 10g, Alismatis rhizome 12g, Poria 15g, Bupleurum root 12g, Stir-fried wild jujuba seed 30g, Epimedium 12g, Honey-fried lily bulb 21g, for oral administration after being decocted in water, one dose a day.

Plus-minus: with preponderance of *yin* deficiency of liver and kidney, plus anemarrhena rhizome, scrofularia root, dragon's teeth, magnetite, tortoise plastron; with predominence of *yang* deficiency of spleen and kidney, plus Indian mulberry fruit, Dangshen, amomum fruit and others. Fire exuberance due to *yin* deficiency with irritability, unsteadiness of mind, add phello-dendron bark, ophiopogon root, polygala root, cinnamon bark; profuse sweating, add calcined dragon's bone, calcined oyster shell and floating barley.

3. Acupoints; *Shenshu, Ganshu, Xinshu, Taixi* (all reinforcing), *Xingjian, Taichong, Daling* (all reducing). With predominence of *yang* deficiency, add *Guanyuan* (moxibustion), *Zusanli, Pishu, Shenmen* (all reinforcing), *Xingjian, Taichong, Daling* to be removed.

II. Case report

Ms. Cui, 51 years old, peasant, came to the clinic the first time on March 6, 1988. In recent two months, due to emotional upset she had distending sensation of the whole body, sudden feverishness at a time, chilliness-at another, palpitation, full of suspicion, irritability and vexation, oppression in chest and shortness of breath, dizziness and insomnia, soreness of loin, softness of legs, much leucorrhea, with paroxysmal exaggeration, three to five times a day. Tongue proper light red, with tooth imprint over the margin. Tongue coat white and slimmy. Pulse taut rapid and without strength. Laboratory examinations of blood. Urine and stool no abnormal finding, EKG examination, fluoroscopy of chest nothing abnormal, a diagnosis of climacteric syndrome made in western medicine, and on TCMa diagnosis of deficiency of kidney essence, disharmony of *yin* and *yang* made, and the therapeutic principle to reinforce the kidney and strengthen the will, to harmonize *yin* and *yang*.

Recipe: Rehmannia root 10g, Prepared rehmannia root 10g, Dogwood fruit 10g, Chinese yam 15g, Moutan bark 12g, Poria 12g, Alismatis rhizome 12g, Bupleurum root 10g, Stirfried wild jujuba seed 30g, Capejasmine fruit 6g, Honey fried lily bulb 24g, White peony root 10g, Epimedium 12g, for oral administration after being decocted in water, one recipe dose daily.

In the meanwhile, acupuncture *Shenshu, Xinshu, Taixi* using reinforcing technique, *Taichong, Daling* with reducing technique.

After 10 recipe doses, and acupuncture seven times, all the symptoms mainly eliminated, she was told to take *Liu Wei Di Huang Wan* one bolus, t.i.d. and *Xiao Yao Wan* 6g, t.i.d. continuous intake for half month to strengthen the therapeutic effect.

III. Personal experience

This disease should not be treated with medicine only, psychic treatment is also quite important, advise patient to establish correct attitude to the symptoms, and related psychic elements, to get rid of bad psychic stimuli.

Besides, it is found that high valence negative ion generator is beneficial to patient, each time inspiration 50 minutes, twice a day. There was such a case of female patient with dysphoria, insomnia, general vague discomfort, with western and herb medicine given the therapeutic effect not evident, she received negative ion treatment for 10 days with pretty good effects.

Senile hyperthyroidism

The clinical characteristics of senile hyperthyroidism may be grouped into two kinds: one kind is concerning with typical manifestations such as over excitement, restlessness, aversion to heat, profuse sweat, polyphagia, loss of weight, palpitation, exophthalmos, thyroid enlargement and others that are related to increased excitability and metabolism; the other kind concerned with non-typical manifestations and signs as the patient with hyperthyroidism would produce, and frequently marked by prominent symptoms of one particular system, especially cardiovascular system such as congestive heart-failure, paraxysma arrhythmia, loss of weight with unknown origin, chronic diarrhea, and long-standing low-grade fever. Some other patients, produced no nervous excitement, but conversely, presented nervous depression that is called apathetic hyperthyroidism with following clinical features: 1. neuropsychic state: apathy, depression, slowness to reaction and lethargy. 2. wan and sallow complexion, dry and cold skin with corrugation. 3. absence of exophthalmos, but presence of dull look in the eyes. 4. slight thyroid enlargement often with node. 5. thinned muscles. 6. slight or moderate speed up of pulse, frequently accompanied with heart failure and auricular fibrillation. 7. indistinct but definite abnormal change of thyroid function. In short, in comparison with other common hyperthyroidism, senile one involves more cases with atypical features, and its pathogenesis still not well known, recently, it is considered to be related to the lack of magnesium. In TCM the disease pertains to the category of 'consumptive disease', 'palpitation', 'spontaneous sweat', and others.

I. TCM syndrome differentiation and treatment

Pathogenesis in brief: *Yin*-deficiency of the liver and kidney, flaming upward of deficient fire, impairment of *yang* affecting *yin*, deficiency of both *yin* and *yang*.

Chief manifestations: Restlessness, irritability, hectic fever, spontaneous sweat, polyphagia with tendency to hunger, progressive emaciation, exophthalmos, swollen and enlarged laryngeal protuberance, severe palpitation, insomnia, sleep disturbed by dreams, pantalgia aggravated during night, thinned tongue, deep red colour of tongue proper with scanty coating. In chronic cases, the impairment of *yin* affects *yang* with symptoms such as set face expression, lassitude, somnolence, wan and sallow complexion, dry and squamous skin, loose stool, deep red colour of tongue proper with little coating, fine and weak pulse.

Therapeutic principle: To nourish the kidney and liver, and to purge pathogenic fire and tranquilize the mind.

1. Patent drug: *Liu Wei Di Huang Wan* 1 bolus,t.i.d. together with *Long Dan Xie Gan Wan* 3g, t.i.d.

2. Decoction recipe: *Zi Shui Qing Gan Yin* with modifications:

Dried rehmannia root 30g, Dendrobium 20g, Glehnia root 20g, Dogwood fruit 10g, Poria 12g, Moutan bark 12g, White peony root 15g, Bupleurum root 6g, Capejasmine fruit 10g, Burreed tuber 6g, Stir-fried wild jujuba seed 20g, Zedoary 6g, Japanese sea tangle 15g, Coptis root 6g, Pueraria root 15g, for oral administration after being decocted in water, one dose a day.

Plus-minus: The above recipe should include dragon's teeth and sepium periploca bark in case with comparatively more severe palpitation and edema; black plum in case with marked diarrhea; red sage root, spatholobus stem and tetrandra root in case with distinct pantalgia. Provided night sweat and hectic fever are prominant, pueraria root and bupleurum root are to be excluded while stellaria root and tortoise plastron included.

In case the impairment of *yin* affects *yang*, exhibiting deficiency of both *yin* and *yang*, the treatment should be directed at supplementing *qi* and restoring *yang*, nourishing *yin* and removing obstructions from collateral. It is preferable to prescribe modified *Shen Fu Tang* and *Sheng*

Mai San, with following ingredients: American ginseng 10g, Cinnamon twig 10g, Honey-fried licorice root 6g, Ophiopogon root 18g, Red peony root 12g, White peony root 12g, Moutan bark 12g, Poria 12g, Bupleurum root 6g, White atractylodes rhizome 12g. All the drugs are for oral administration after being decocted in water. Furthermore, if the case marked by cold sweat, American gingseng and bupleurum root are to be with-drawn while amomum fruit, black plum and hawthorn fruit added.

3. Acupoints: *Guanyuan, Shenshu, Mingmen* (all with reinforcing technique), *Yongquan, Shuidao, Feishu, Chize, Xingjian* (all with reducing technique). In case with impairment of *yin* affecting *yang*, to select acupoints: *Guanyuan, Qihai, Mingmen, Shenshu* (all with moxibustion), *Zusanli, Zhongwan, Taixi, Xuehai, Xinshu* (alll with reinforcing technique), *Shuidao, Xingjian, Yongquan* (all with morderate reinforcing reducing technique).

II. Case report

Ms. Wang, 65 years old, retired worker, first consultation on May 20, 1988.

Her chief complaints: Palpitation, fatigue and progressive emaciation for a year or more, aggravation of the symptoms three month.

Six months before, all the symptoms were aggravated in relation to tiredness and anger. The patient went to a hospital for medical advice and there her disease was identified as hyperthyroidism. Carbimazolum was administered for treatment. Consequently, all the symptoms were aggravated rather than relieved. The present symptoms: pallor and sallow complexion, emaciation, deficiency of *qi*, fatique, restlessness, insomnia, severe palpitation, low-grade fever in the afternoon, dry skin with profuse sweat, thirst, polydipsia, loose stool, anorexia with tendency to hunger, red tongue proper with little coating, fine, rapid and weak pulse.

Physical examinations: T 37.2°C, P 88 beats per minute, R 22 beats per minute, B.P. 120/70 mmHg.

Senile female, mentally clear, listlessness, wan and sallow complexion, emaciation, dry and cold skin with corrugation, pigmentation, slight exophthalmos, a little bit large and hard thyroid but without node, soft abdomen with a bit of tenderness, liver and spleen not palpable, regular heart rate, 88 beats per minute, no murmur, lung no positive finding, muscular atrophy of the extremities. Laboratory test: serum T_3 309 ng%, serum T_4 4.4 ug% thyroid ^{131}I uptake higher than normal value.

Diagnosis: palpitation, consumptive disease in TCM, senile hyperthyroidism in western medicine.

Therapeutic principle: To nourish the kidney and heart, to invigorate the spleen and arrest diarrhea.

Recipe: *Zi Shui Qing Gan Yin* with modifications: Dried rehmannia root 20g, Dendrobium 20g, Glehnia root 15g, Poria 15g, White peony root 12g, Coptis root 6g, Amomum fruit 6g, Dangshen 12g, White atractylodes rhizome 12g, Burreed tuber 6g, Zedoary 6g, Pueraria root 20g, Hawthorn fruit 15g, for oral administration after being decocted in water, one dose a day.

Therapeutic effect: After 28 doses of the above recipe with a bit of modifications, almost all the symptoms disappeared, with tongue proper pink, tongue coat thin and white, and pulse moderate. Serum T_3, serum T_4 were within normal range, thyroid ^{131}I uptake normal.

III. Personal experience

(I) Throughout the course, the pathogenesis of the disease is the *yin*-deficiency of the liver and kidney, but sometimes manifests itself as *yin*-deficiency of the heart and kidney, and sometimes as deficiency of both *qi* and *yin*. Attention should be paid specially to the stage at which the impairment of *yin* affects *yang*. On the basis of deficiency of kidney-*yin* some cases exhibit *yang*-deficiency of the heart and kidney, others exhibit *yang*-deficiency of the spleen and kidney, and still others exhibit *yang*-deficiency of the heart, spleen and kidney. All these should be noticed specially when a prescription is to be composed.

(II) As for the treatment, it is recommended to administer decoction for nourishing the kidney and removing heat from the liver combined with drugs for softening masses and resolving stasis such as laminaria or ecklonia, sargassum, oyster shell, burreed tuber and zedoary. In addition if the case is complicated with *qi* deficiency, drugs for invigorating *qi* should be added, if complicated with *yang*-deficiency, drugs for warming *yang* added. However, no matter what drugs are used, be sure to avoid drugs of over-greasy and over dry property and to avoid too large dosage. Administration in small portions at frequent intervals should be suggested.

(III) Take care to have good rest, being patient in doing things, give up smoking and avoid peppery and stimulating foodstuffs.

Postconcussional syndrome of the brain

Postconcussional syndrome of the brain is concerned, with a syndrome after concussion of the brain including disturbance in memory, somnolence, bradycardia, headache, perspiration and others which do not disappear within a short time after concussion, and influence normal life and work. In TCM, the syndrome pertains to 'impairment of memory', 'headache', 'palpitation' and others.

I. TCM syndrome differentiation and treatment

Pathogenesis in brief: Injury of the brain, concussion of the brain, primordial *qi* and mental activities out of control, disturbance of blood circulation, damage of brain, blood stasis in the brain.

(I) Blood stasis in the brain

Key points of pathogenesis: Injury of the brain concussion of the sea of marrow, stagnancy of blood stasis, primordial *qi* and mental activities out of control.

Chief manifestations: Brain trauma in previous week, responsible for present symptoms such as headache, somnolence, amnesia, palpitation, spontaneous perspiration, being easily scared, red tongue proper with ecchymosis and whitish greasy coat, fine and hesitant pulse.

Therapeutic principle: To promote blood circulation and remove blood stasis; to arouse mind and induce resuscitation.

1. Patent drug:

(1) *Fu Fang Dan Shen Pian* 4 tablets, t.i.d.

(2) *Die Da Wan* 1 bolus, t.i.d.

2. Decoction recipe: *Tong Qiao Huo Xue Tang* with modifications:

Bupleurum root 12g, Chuanxiong rhizome 15g, Peach kernel 12g, Safflower 10g, Red peony root 12g, Prepared polygala root 10g, Pueraria root 18g, Stir-fried bitter orange 6g, Musk 0.5g (wrapped in cloth and decocted later), for oral administration after being decocted in water, one dose a day.

Plus-minus: The above recipe should include capejasmine fruit for cases with restlessness; grassleaved sweetflag rhizome and curcuma root for those with obvious somnolence; dragon's bone and oyster shell for those having spontaneous sweat and being easily scared.

3. Acupoints: *Ganshu, Xinshu* (with moderate reinforcing-reducing technique), *Xuehai, Xingjian, Laogong* (all with reducing technique).

(II) Consumption of the sea of marrow

Key points of pathogenesis: Concussion of the sea of marrow, insufficiency of primordial *qi*, prolonged consumption causing the loss of determination for primordial *qi* and mental activities.

Chief manifestations: Listlessness, forgetfulness, aphasia, dreamfulness, easily scared, or accompanied by headache, palpitation, restlessness, pink tongue proper, sometimes with ecchymosis, thin, whitish and greasy coat on the tongue, fine and weak pulse.

Therapeutic principle: To tonify the marrow of the brain, to remove blood stasis and arouse mind.

1. Patent drug: *Qi Ju Di Huang Wan* 1 bolus, t.i.d. along with *Fu Fang Dan Shen Pian* 3 tablets, t.i.d.

2. Decoction recipe: *Zuo Gui Yin* with modifications: Prepared rehmannia root 15g, Antler glue 12g, Prepared fleece-flower root 20g, Dogwood fruit 12g, Chinese yam 12g, Chuanxiong rhizome 15g, Stir-fried wild jujuba seed 24g, Pueraria root 15g, Prepared polygala root 10g, Amomum fruit 6g, Poria with hostwood 12g, for oral administration after being decocted in water, one dose a day.

Plus-minus: In case with obvious headache, plus eclipta, glossy privet fruit and moutan bark; with aphasia, plus grassleaved sweetflag rhizome, bile treated arisaema tuber and amber powder.

3. Acupoints: *Shenshu, Xinshu, Mingmen, Zusanli* (all with reinforcing technique), *Dazhui, Baihui, Laogong, Shenmen*(all with moderate reinforcing-reducing technique). For the case with headache, add acupoint *Ashi* (with reducing technique).

II. Case report

Mr. Yan, 34 years old, worker, came to seek medical advice on March 5, 1978.

The patient had his head injuried in a traffic accident ten days before. At that moment, he lost consciousness and, after regaining consciousness, he had somnolence, headache, forgetfulness of past things. Through treatment, the wound healed but he was still haunted with headache, forgetfulness, insomnia, irritability, palpitation, restlessness, poor appetite, constipation, pink tongue proper with ecchymosis, yellowish and thick coat on the tongue, taut and rapid pulse.

Syndrome differentiation and treatment: Injury of the brain, concussion of the sea of marrow resulted in the obstruction of blood stasis in the interior. Fright brought on the disturbance of the vital energy flow and the dysfunction of conduction. It is fit to direct the treatment at relieving spasm, removing blood stasis, invigorating functions of bowels and regulating the flow of vital energy.

Recipe: Bupleurum root 12g, Peach kernel 15g, Chuangxiong rhizome 15g, Rhubarb 10g, Amber powder 2g (swallowed with boiled water), Pangolin scales 10g, Cinnabar powder 1g (swallowed with boiled water or decocted fluid), Stir-fried bitter orange 10g, Cyperus tuber 10g, Prepared polygala root 10g, for oral administration after being decocted in water. One dose a day. Moreover, intake of *Si Chong Wan* 3g, t.i.d.

The second visit on March 15, after medication, various symptoms took a turn for the better. At the beginning of administration, stool became loose, bowels moved three times a day accompanied with a slight pain in the abdomen. Now, stool became less loose with bowels moved two times a day, and disappearance of abdominal pain. Appetite was improved, headache vanished and sleep sound, but amnesia was persistant. Tongue proper pink with thin and white coat, pulse fine and feeble.

Recipe: *Qi Ju Di Huang Wan* 1 bolus, t.i.d. *Xiao Yao Wan* 6g, t.i.d. two weeks in succession for strengthening the curative effect.

Follow-up half a year later revealed a good recovery.

III. Personal experience

As concerns the pathogenesis of postconcussional syndrome, generally, blood stasis stagnated in the interior is dominant within three months; damage and consumption of the marrow dominant after three months. Hence, it is advisable to focus the treatment at promoting blood circulation and removing blood stasis at the onset of the disease; if the disease is prolonged, to tonify the marrow of the brain should dominates the treatment. However, the two principles can not be seperated from each other completely. Particularly, while the drugs prescribed mean to tonify the marrow of the brain, such ingredients as are used for eliminating stasis, dispelling phlegm and removing obstruction from collaterals should also be listed in the recipe to serve as adjuvant and conductant drugs. Provided the disease becomes chronic and resistant to the treatment, which suggests that the illness invades collateral, the additional administration of drugs for plundering the collateral should be given emphatically, such as *Da Huang Zhe Chong Wan* (rhubarb and ground beetle pill), pangolin, scorpion, earthworm, ground beetle, leech, gadfly, etc.

Index of Prescriptions

Ai Fu Nuan Gong Wan, Argyi-cyperus pill for warming the uterus (《Yang's collections of formularies》): Argyi leaf, cuperus tuber, Chinese angelica root, astragalus root, evodia fruit, chuanxiong rhizome, white peony root, rehmannia root, cinnamon bark, dipsacus root.

An Gong Niu Huang Wan, Bezoar bolus for resurrection (《Treatise on differentiation and treatment of epidemic febrile diseases》): Bezoar, curcuma root, rhinoceros horn, scutellaria root, coptis root, capejasmine fruit, realgar, cinnabar, borneol, pearl, musk.

Ba Li Ma injection, Chinese azalea fruit injection fluid (《Chinese pharmacopia》1977 edition): each ml contains andromedotoxin 1mg.

Ba Zhen Tang, Eight precious ingredients decoction (《Zheng Ti Lei Yao》): Ginseng, poria, white atractylodes rhizome, licorice root, Chinese angelica root, chuanxiong rhizome, white peony root, prepared rhemannia root, fresh ginger, Chinese date.

Ba Zheng San, Eight health restoring powder(《Formularies of peaceful benevolent dispensary》): Akebia stem, Chinese pink herb, plantain seed, common knot grass, talc, rhubarb, capejasmine fruit, licorice root.

Bai Feng Wan, White feathered chicken pill («A dictionary of Chinese medicine»): White feathered cock (with black bone), cyperus tuber, rehmannia root, prepared rehmannia root, Chinese angelica root, white peony root, astragalus root, achyranthus root, bupleurum root, Sichuan fritillary tuber, moutan bark, anemarrhena rhizome, coptis tuber, dried ginger, wolfberry bark, corydalis tuber, poria, large leaf gentian root, carbonized argyi leaf, sweet worm wood.

Bai Hu Jia Gui Zhi Tang, White tiger decoction with addition of cinnamon twig («Synopsis of prescriptions of the golden chamber»): Gypsum, anemarrhena rhizome, good rice, licorice root, cinnamon twig.

Bai Hu Tang, White tiger decoction(«Treatise on febrile diseases»): anemarrhena rhizome, gypsum, good rice, licorice root.

Bai Zi Yang Xin Wan, Mindeasing tonic pill with arborvitae seed (proved recipe): Arborvitae seed, dangshen, astragalus root, chuanxiong rhizome, Chinese angelica root, poria, polygala root, wildjujuba seed, cinnamon bark, schisandra fruit, pinellia leaven, cinnabar, licorice root.

Ban Liu Wan, Pill of pinellia and sulfur («Formularies of peaceful benevolent dispensary»): pinellia tuber, sulfur, fresh ginger juice.

Ban Xia Bai Zhu Tian Ma Tang, Decoction of pinellia, white atractylodes and gastrodia («Medicine comprehened»): Pinellia tuber, gastrodia tuber, poria, white atractylodes rhizome, red tangerine peel, licorice root.

Ban Xia Xie Xin Tang, Pinellia decoction for purging stomach fire (《Treatise on febrile diseases》): Pinellia tuber, scutellaria root, dried ginger, ginseng, coptis root, licorice root, Chinese date.

Bao Kun Dan, Powder for the health of woman (proved recipe): Chinese angelica root, chuanxiong, prepared rehmannia root, red peony root, peach kernel, safflower, cyperus tuber, corydalis tuber, moutan bark, poria, evodia fruit, tangerine peel, licorice root, scutellaria root, motherwort, deglued antler powder.

Bao Tai Wan, Bolus for preventing abortion (《Prescriptions worth a thousand gold for emergencies》): Poria, prepared rehmannia root, carbonized argyi leaf, astragalus root, white atractylodes rhizome, white peony root, Chinese angelica root, dodder seed, mulberry mistletoe, chuanxiong rhizome, bitter orange, Sichuan fritilliary bulb, schizonepeta spike, dangshen, Notopterygium root, licorice root.

Bao Yuan Tang, Decoction for reinforcing the primordial *qi* (《The benevolent hearty book》): Astragalus root, ginseng, cinnamon bark, licorice root, fresh ginger.

Bie Jia Jian Wan, Decocted turtle shell pill (《Synopsis of prescriptions of the golden chamber》): Prepared turtle shell, belamcanda rhizome, scutellaria root, pillb driedug, cinnamon twig, dried ginger, rhubarb, pyrrosia leaf, magnolia bark, donkey hide glue, bupleurum root, peony root, moutan bark, lepidium seed, pinellia tuber, ginseng, peach kernel, Chinese pink herb, ground beetle, wasp's nest, dung beetle and others.

Bu Sui Jian Nao Tang, Decoction to replenish the marrow and reinforce the brain (proved recipe): Prepared fleece flower root, siberian solomonseal rhizome, ginseng, antler glue, alismatis rhizome, pueraria root, lotus plumule cinnamon bark.

Bu Xin Dan, Heart reinforcing powder (《*Chi Shui Xuan Zhu*》 a mysterious pearl of medicine): Ophiopogon root, polygala root, grass-leaved sweetflag rhizome, cyperus tuber, asparagus root, trichosanthes root, white atractylodes rhizome, fritillary bulb, prepared rhemannia root, poria with host stem, wolfberry bark, ginseng, Chinese angelica root, achyranthes root, astragalus root, sichuan clematis stem, Chinese date, licorice root.

Bu Yang Huan Wu Tang, Decoction invigorating *yang* for recuperation (《Corrections on the errors of medical works》): Astragalus root, Chinese angelica root tail, red peony root, earthworm, chuanxiong rhizome, peach kernel, safflower.

Bu Yi Zi Sheng Wan, Tonifying and healthy maintaining pill (《Gong's prescription》): Dangshen, white atractylodes rhizome, coix seed, tangerine peel, hawthorn fruit, fermented leaven, poria, licorice root, Chinese yam, euryale seed, barley sprout, hyacinth bean, lotus seed, platycodon root, agastache, coptis root, round cardamon seed, alismatis rhizome.

Bu Zhong Yi Qi Tang (Wan), Decoction (bolus) for reinforcing middle-*jiao* and replenishing *qi* (《Treatise on the spleen and stomach》): Ginseng, astragalus root, Chinese angelica root, tangerine peel, bupleurum root, cimicifuga rhizome, white atractylodes rhizome, licorice root.

Chai Hu Shu Gan San, Bupleurum powder for relieving liver-*qi* (《Jing Yue's complete works》): Bupleurum root, bitter orange, red peony root, cyperus tuber, chuanxiong rhizome, licorice.

Chang Pu Yu Jin injection, Injection fluid of grass-leaved sweetflag and curcuma (proved recipe) 1ml contains grass-leaved sweetflag rhizome 2g and curcuma root 2g.

Chang Pu Yu Jin Tang, Decoction of grass leaved sweetflag and curcuma (《A complete book of epidemic febrile diseases》): Grass leaved sweetflag rhizome, curcuma root, pinellia tuber, bamboo juice, stirfried-capejasmine fruit, forsythia fruit, chrysanthemum flower, lophtharum, talc, arctium fruit, ginger juice, Yu Shu Dan.

Chen Xiang Hua Zi Wan, Pill of eagle wood to resolve stagnation (proved recipe): Eagle wood, pharbitis seed, hawthorn fruit, bitter orange, tangerine peel, cyperus tuber, magnolia bark, zedoary, amomum fruit, burreed tuber, rhubarb and others.

Chu Feng Jing, Chicken's embryo tonic (proved recipe):

Ginseng, chicken's embryo, goat penis, amomum fruit, astragalus root, wolfberry fruit, epimedium, moutan bark, white peony root, Chinese angelica root, desert-living cistanche, eagle wood, pilose antler, prepared rehmannia root, grass leaved sweetflag rhizome.

Chuan Dan injection, Chuanxiong and red sage root injection (proved recipe): 1 ml equavalent to red sage root 0.5g and chuangxiong 0.5g.

Da Bu Yin Wan, Bolus with great *yin* tonifying action (《Medical cases by master *Danxi*》): Anemarrhena rhizome, phellodendron bark, prepared rehmannia root, tortoise plastron, pig's spinal column.

Da Cheng Qi Tang, Major decoction for purging down the stomach *qi* (《Treatise on febrile disease》): Rhubarb, magnolia bark, stir-fried bitter orange, mirabilite.

Da Huang injection, Rhubarb injection fluid (proved recipe): Wine treated rhubarb, licorice root, 1ml. contains wine treated rhubarb 0.1g.

Da Huang Pian, Tablet of rhubarb (proved recipe): rhubarb.

Da Huang Zho Chong Wan, Rhubarb and ground beetle bolus(《Synopsis of prescriptions of the golden chamber》): Rhubarb, rehmannia root, peach kernel, peony root, bitter apricot seed, licorice root, scutellaria root, leech, horsefly, grub, ground beetle, lacquer.

Da Qi Qi Tang, Decoction to treat stagnation (《Elementary medicine》): Green tangerine peel, tangerine peel, platycodon root, agastache, cinnamon bark, licorice root, zedoary, burreed tuber, cyperus tuber, bitter cardamon, fresh ginger, Chinese date.

Da Qing Ye He Ji, Mixture of isatis leaf (proved recipe): Isatis leaf, honeysuckle flower, notopterygium root, polyganum rhizome, rhubarb.

Dan Shen Yin, The drink including red sage (《The golden mirror of medicine》): Red sage root, sandal wood, amomum fruit.

Dang Gui Si Ni Tang, Chinese angelica decoction for restoring *yang* (《Treatise on febrile diseases》): Chinese angelica root, cinnamon twig, peony root, asarum herb, licorice root, rice paper pith, Chinese date.

Dang Gui Yin Zi, Drink of Chinese angelica (《Standards of diagnosis and treatment of six branches of medicine》): Chinese angelica root, white peony root, chuanxiong rhizome, rehmannia root, ledebouriella, schizonepeta, tribulus fruit, fleece-flower root, astragalus root, licorice root.

Dao Chi San, Powder for treating dark urine (《Key to therapeutics of children's diseases》): Rehmannia root, licorice root, lophtharum, akebia stem.

Dao Tan Tang, Decoction for expelling phlegm (《Life preserving prescriptions》): Arisaema tuber, immature bitter orange, pinellia tuber, red tangerine peel, poria, licorice root, fresh ginger.

Di Huang Yin Zi, Rehmannia drink (《Six books of medicine》): Rehmannia root, indian mulberry root, dogwood fruit, dendrobium, desert living cistanche, aconite root, schisandra fruit, cinnamon bark, poria, ophiopogon root, grassleaved-sweetflag rhizome, polygala root.

Di Tan Tang, Phlegm removing decoction («Excellent recipe with marvellous effect»): Pinellia tuber, bile treated arisaema tuber, red tangerine peel, immature bitter orange, poria, ginseng, grass leaved sweetflag rhizome, bamboo shaving, licorice root, fresh ginger.

Die Da Wan, Pill for trauma (proved recipe): Wine treated rhubarb, wine treated curcuma root, notoginseng, safflower, wine treated rhubarb, red peony root, rehmannia root, ground beetle, sappan wood.

Ding Xian Wan, Pill for epilepsy («Medicine comprehended»): Gastrodia tuber, sichuan fritilliary bulb, bile treated arisaema tuber, ginger treated pinellia tuber, tangerine peel, amber, bamboo juice, licorice root, red sage root, ophiopogon root, grass-leaved sweetflag rhizome, scorpion, batryticated silkworm.

Du Qi Wan, All converging bolus («Self duty in medicine»): Rehmannia root, dogwood fruit, Chinese yam, moutan bark, poria, alismatis rhizome, schisandra fruit.

Du Shen Tang, Decoction of ginseng only («A complete book of febrile diseases»): Ginseng.

Er Chen Tang, Decoction including two old drugs («Formularies of peaceful benevolent dispensary»): Pinellia tuber, tangerine peel, poria, licorice.

Er Long Zuo Ci Wan, Deafness curing pill (《Key to therapeutics of children's diseases》): Prepared rehmannia root, dogwood fruit, Chinese yam, moutan bark, poria, alismatis rhizome, schisandra fruit, magnetite.

Er Miao San, Powder of two wonderful drugs (《A medical book by master *Danxi*》): Anemarrhena rhizome, phellodendron bark.

Er Xian Tang, Decoction of curculigo, epimedium and others (proved recipe): Curculigo rhizome, epimedium, Indian mulberry root, phellodendron bark, anemarrhena rhizome, Chinese angelica root.

Er Yin Jian, Shao yin nourishing decoction (《*Jing Yue*'s complete works》): Rehmannia root, ophiopogon root, wild jujuba seed, licorice root, scrofularia root, poria, coptis root, clematis stem, rush pith, lophatherum.

Er Zhi Wan, Bolus of two drugs (《Standards of diagnosis and treatment of six branches of medicine》): Eclipta, glossy privet fruit.

Fang Feng Tong Sheng Wan, Miraculous pill of ledebouriella (proved recipe): Ledebouriella root, ephedra, gypsum, white atractylodes rhizome, chuanxiong rhizome, rhubarb, forsythia fruit, capejasmine fruit, platycodon root and others.

Fu Fang Dan Shen injection, Composite of red sage root injection (proved recipe): 1ml contains red sage root 2g and dalbergia wood 2g.

Fu Fang Dan Shen Pian, Tablet of composite red sage root (proved recipe): Red sage root, notoginseng, borneol.

Fu Fang Dang Gui injection, Injection of composite Chinese angelica root: Chinese angelica root, chuanxiong rhizome, safflower.

Fu Shou Cao Zong Dai, The total alkaloids of adonis injection fluid (proved recipe): each 2ml contains 0.5g total alkaloids.

Fu Zi Li Zhong Tang (Wan), Decoction or bolus of *Li Zhong Tang (Wan)* with addition of aconite root (《Formularies of peaceful benevolent dispensary》): Ginseng, dried ginger, aconite root, licorice root, white atractylodes root.

Fu Zi Li Zhong Wan, Bolus to regulate the middle-burner with addition of aconite (《Formularies of peaceful benevolent dispensary》): Prepared aconite root, ginseng, dried ginger, white atractylodes rhizome, licorice root.

Fu Zi No.1 injection, Higemamine injection (proved recipe): Dl-Demethyl-Coelaurne or higenamine.

Ge Gen Tang, Pueraria root decoction (《Treatise on febrile diseases》): Pueraria root, ephedra, cinnamon twig, peony root, licorice root, fresh ginger, Chinese date.

Gu Ben Zhi Beng Tang, Decoction for arresting uterine bleeding with drugs to consolidate the fundaments (proved recipe): Prepared rehmannia root, prepared fleece-flower root, dogwood fruit, Dangshen, carbonized madder root, carbonized palmae bark, vinegar fried tortoise plastron, calcined dragon's bone, calcined oyster shell, baked black ginger, amomum fruit, cimicifuga rhizome.

Gu Ci Wan, Spur pill (proved recipe): Siberian solomonseal rhizome, pubescent angelica root, clematis root, spatholobus stem, drynaria rhizome, prepared rehmannia root, shiny pricklyash, prepared Sichuan aconite root, cynomorium, cibot rhizome, wolfberry fruit, radish seed.

Gua Lou Xie Bai Ban Xia Tang, Decoction of trichosanthes, pinellia, macrostem onion («Synopsis of prescriptions of the golden chamber»): Trichosanthes fruit, macrostem onion, pinellia tuber, white wine.

Guan Xin Su He Wan, Coronary heart pill including storax (proved recipe): Storax oil, sandal wood, cinnabar, borneol, frankincense, dutchmanspipe root.

Gui Pi Wan (Tang), Bolus (decoction) for invigorating the spleen and nourishing the heart(«Life preserving prescriptions»): Ginseng, honey fried astragalus root, stirfried white atractylodes root, poria, Chinese angelica root, stir-fried wild jujuba seed, longan aril, honeyfried licorice root, fresh ginger, Chinese date, polygala root, aucklandia root.

Hao Qin Qing Dan Tang, Sweet wormwood scutellaria decoction for clearing damp heat from gall bladder («Revised popular explanation of treatise on febrile diseases»): Sweet worm-wood, scutellaria root, bitter orange, prepared pinellia tuber, tangerine peel, red poria, bamboo shaving, *Bi Yu San* (natural indigo, talc, licorice root, enveloped with cloth or silk and decocted).

He Shou Wu Wan, Pill of fleece flower root (proved recipe): Fleece flower root, cibot rhizome, pueraria root, siegesbeckia herb, myrrh.

Hei Xi Dan, Black tin pill (《Formularies of peaceful benevolent dispensary》): Lead, sulphur, Sichuan chinaberry, fenugreek seed, aucklandia root, prepared aconite root, nutmeg, actinolite, eagle wood, fennel fruit, cinnamon bark, psoralea fruit.

Hong Hua injection, Safflower injection fluid (proved recipe): 1ml contains safflower crude drug 1g.

Hou Zao San, Monkey bezoar powder (proved recipe): Monkey bezoar, musk, eagle wood, Sichuan fritillary bulb, chlorite-schist, antelope horn, crystallized juice from waspbite wound of bamboo node, borax.

Hu Qian Wan, Yang subdueing pill including tiger bone (《A medical book by master *Danxi*》): Phellodendron bark, tortoise plastron, anemarrhena rhizome, prepared rehmannia root, tangerine peel, white peony root, tiger bone, cynomorium, dried ginger.

Huan Shao Wan, Pill for restoring youth (《Yang's family preserved formulary》): Chinese yam, achyranthes root, poria, dogwood fruit, paper mulberry fruit, carbonized eucommia bark, schisandra fruit, Indian mulberry root, desertliving cistanche, polygala root, common fennel fruit, grass leaved sweetflag rhizome, prepared rehmannia root, wolfberry fruit.

Huo Xin Dan, Heart stimulating pill (proved recipe):

Ginseng, lucid ganoderma, musk, bezoar, bear gall, safflower.

Ji Chuan Jian, Decoction to increase water in river («*Jing Yue's* complete works»): Chinese angelica root, achyranthes root, desertliving cistanche, alismatis rhizome, cimicifuga rhizome, bitter orange.

Ji Sheng Shen Qi Wan, Life preserving pill for replenishing the kidney *qi* («Life preserving prescriptions»): prepared rehmannia root, poria, dogwood fruit, Chinese yam, moutan bark, alismatis rhizome, achyranthes root, plantain seed, aconite root, cinnamon bark.

Ji Xue Teng Pian, Spatholobus tablet (proved recipe): Spatholobus stem.

Jian Nao Bu Shen Wan, Bolus to reinforce the kidney and replenish the brain (proved recipe): Ginseng, pilose antler, amomum fruit, round cardamon seed, dog's testicle, eucommia bark, honeysuckle flower, wild jujuba seed, white atractylodes rhizome, cyathula root, cinnamon bark, Chinese angelica root, cinnabar, *Jin Niu Cao* (polygala) and others.

Jian Xue Ning, Hemostatic tablet (proved recipe): Japanese thistle root, hyacinth bletilla, loropetal leaf.

Jiang Zhi Tong Mai Yin, Drink for lowering blood lipids and promoting blood circulation (proved recipe): Bupleurum root, curcuma root, oriental worm wood, cassia seed, rhubarb, alismatis rhizome.

Jiao Mu Gua Lou Tang, Decoction of pepper seed and trichosanthes seed («Complement to the refined conception of medicine》): Pepper seed, trichosanthes seed, lepidium seed, mulberry bark, perilla fruit, pinellia tuber, poria, red tangerine peel, tribulus fruit, fresh ginger.

Jin Gui Shen Qi Wan, Bolus for restoring the kidney qi (《Synopsis of prescriptions of the golden chamber》): Rehmannia root, dogwood fruit, Chinese yam, poria, moutan bark, cinnamon twig, prepared aconite root.

Jin Lian Hua injection, Chines globe flower injection fluid (proved recipe): Fluid extract of Chinese globe flower, procaine hydrochloride.

Jin Suo Gu Jing Wan, Golden lock pill for keeping the kidney essence (《Collection of prescriptions with exposition》): Flat stem milk-vetch seed, euryale seed, lotus stamen, dragon's bone, oyster shell.

Jing Fang Bai Du San, Detoxication powder of schizonepeta and ledebouriella (《Theory and case reports on external diseases》): Schizonepeta, ledebouriella root, notopterygium root, pubescent angelica root, bupleurum root, peucedanum root, chuanxiong rhizome, bitter orange.

Jing Fang Jie Du Tang, Antiphlogistic decoction of schizonepeta and ledebouriella root (proved recipe): Schizonepeta, ledebouriella root, bupleurum root, pueraria root, cicada slough, bitter apricot seed, aster root, peucedanum root, platycodon root, licorice root.

Kang Yan injection, Antiphlogistic injection fluid

(proved recipe): Pig bile.

Kong Xian Dan, Controlling phlegm-fluid pill (《A treatise on the three categories of pathogenic factors of disease》): Kansui root, knoxia root, white mustard seed.

Kuan Xiong Wan, Bolus to relieve chest stuffiness (proved recipe): Long pepper, galangal rhizome, sandal wood, borneol, asarum herb, corydalis tuber.

Kun Cao Fang, Recipe of motherwort (proved recipe): Motherwort, honeysuckle flower, lophatherum, licorice root.

Lian Li Tang, Decoction to regulate the middle burner with addition of coptis (《Symptom, etiology, pulse and therapy》): Coptis root, ginseng, white atractylodes root, dried ginger, honeyfried licorice root.

Ling Gui Zhu Gan Tang, Decoction of poria, bighead atratylodes, cinnamom and licorice (《Synopsis of prescriptions of the golden chamber》): Poria, bighead atractylodes rhizome, cinnamon twig, licorice root.

Ling Jiao Gou Tong Tang, Decoction of antelope's horn and uncaria stem (《*Tong Su Shang Han Lun*》): Antelope's horn, mulberry leaf, Sichuan fritillary bulb, rehmannia root, uncaria stem with hooks, chrysanthemum flower, white peony root, bamboo shaving, poria with host stem, licorice root.

Ling Yang Jiao Tang, Antelope's horn decoction (《The remnant meaning of medical refines》): Antelope's horn, tortoise plastron, rehmannia root, moutan bark, bupleurum root, peppermint, chrysanthemum flower, cicada slough, sea-ear shell, white peony root, prunella spike.

Liu Shen Wan, Pill of six drugs with magic effects (proved recipe): Musk, bezoar, pearl, borneol, toad venom, realgar.

Liu Wei Di Huang Tang(Wan), Kidney bolus of six drugs including rehmannia (《Key to therapeutics of children's diseases》): Rehmannia root, dogwood fruit, Chinese yam, moutan bark, poria, alismatis rhizome.

Liu Yi San, Six to one powder (《The incidental and fundamental of febrile diseases》): Talc$_6$, licorice root$_1$.

Long Dan Xie Gan Tang (Wan), Decoction or pill of gentiana for purging the liver fire (《A secret book of the orchids chamber》): Gentian root, capejasmine fruit, scutellaria root, bupleurum root, Chinese angelica root, rehmannia root, clematis stem, plantain seed, alismatis rhizome, licorice root.

Long Hu Wan, Dragon-tiger pill (proved recipe): Cow's bezoar, croton seed frost (removal of oil), arsenic trioxide, cinnabar.

Long Ma Zi Lai Dan, Earthworm and strychnos powder (《Corrections on the errors of Medical works》): Earthworm, prepared strychnos powder.

Ma Huang Fu Zi Xi Xin Tang, Decoction of ephedra, aconite and asarum (《Treatise on febrile diseases》): Ephedra, aconite root, asarum herb.

Ma Huang Lian Qiao Chi Xiao Dou Tang, Decoction of ephedra, forsythia and red bean (《Treatise on febrile diseases》): Ephedra, forsythia fruit, red bean, bitter apricot kernel, Chinese date, fresh ginger, mulberry bark, licorice root.

Mai An Chong Ji, Particle or powdered medicine easily dissolved in boiling water for lowering blood lipids (proved recipe): hawthorn fruit, germinated barley.

Mai Wei Di Huang Wan, Kidney bolus of six drugs including rehmannia with addition of ophiopogon and schisandra (《Stairs to medicine》): Prepared rehmannia, dogwood fruit, Chinese yam, moutan bark, poria, alismatis rhizome, ophiopogon root, schisandra fruit.

Meng Shi Gun Tan Wan, Pill of chlorite-schist for expelling phlegm (《Yang Sheng Zhu Lun》, ethics of hygiene): Chlorite schist, eagle wood, rhubarb, scutellaria root, mirabilite.

Mu Xiang Shun Qi Wan, Aucklandia carminative pills (proved recipe): Aucklandia root, cyperus tuber, bitter orange, radish seed, barley sprout, lindera root, fermented leaven, poria, tangerine peel.

Niu Huang Jie Du Pian, Bezoar antiphlogistic tablet (proved recipe): Cow's bezoare, rhubarb, scutellaria root, platycodon root and others.

Niu Huang Qing Xin Wan, Bezoar sedative bolus (《Formularies of peaceful benevolent dispensary》): Bezoar, cinnabar, coptis root, scutellaria root, capejasmine fruit, curcuma root.

Niu Huang Shang Qing Wan, Bezoar bolus for clearing the heat of upper burner (proved recipe): Cow bezoar, coptis root, scutellaria root, phellodendron bark, chrysanthemum flower, platycodon root, dahurian angelica root, inula flower, peppermint, licorice root, chuanxiong rhizome, rhubarb, frosythia fruit, schizonepeta spike, ledebouriella root, gypsum, chastetree fruit.

Nü Jin Dan, Precious bolus for woman (《*Han*'s general medicine》): Ginseng, white atractylodes rhizome, poria, chuanxiong rhizome, Chinese angelica root, moutan bark, ligusticum root, cinnamon bark, corydalis tuber, myrrh, red halloysite, cyperus tuber, swallowwort root, dahurian angelica root, white peony root.

Qi Ge San, Decoction for treating dysphagia (《Medicine comprehended》): Glehnia root, red sage root, poria, Sichuan fritillary bulb, curcuma root, amomum fruit, lotus leaf stalk, hoe bran.

Qi Ju Di Huang Wan, Kidney bolus of six drugs including rehmannia with addition of wolfberry and chrysanthemum (《*Yi Ji*》 stairs to medicine): Wolfberry fruit, chrysanthemum flower, prepared rehmannia root, dogwood fruit, Chinese yam, moutan bark, alismatis rhizome, poris.

Qi Zhi Xiang Fu Wan, Pill of prepared cyperus (《Elementary medicine》): Prepared cyperus tuber, Chinese angelica root, zedoary, moutan bark, argyi leaf, chuanxiong rhizome, corydalis tuber, burreed tuber, bupleurum root, safflower, black plum, lindera root.

Qian Jin San, Precious Powder (《To keep *yuan qi* and long life for generations》): Scorpion, batryticated silkworm, bezoar, cinnabar, borneol, coptis root, bile treated arisaema tuber, gastrodia tuber, licorice root.

Qian Jin Wei Jing Tang, Reed stem decoction (《Essential prescriptions worth a thousand gold》): Reed stem, coix seed, waxgourd seed, peach kernel.

Qian Zheng San, Powder for treating wry mouth (《Yang's family preserved formularies》): Giant typhonium tuber, batryticated silk worm, scorpion.

Qiang Li Yin Qiao Pian, Strengthened tablet of lonicera and forsythia fruit (proved recipe): Honeysuckle flower, forsythia fruit, reed root, licorice root, platycoden root, schizonepeta, vitamin C, chlorpheniramine maleate, paracetamol.

Qin Jiu Bie Jia San, Large leaf gentian and turtle shell powder (《Precious mirror on hygiene》): Large leaf gentian root, turtle shell, wolfberry bark, bupleurum root, sweet worm wood, Chinese angelica root, anemarrhena rhizome, black plum.

Qing Gong Tang, Decoction to clear away the heart-fire (《Treatise on differentiation and treatment of epidemic febrile diseases》): Scrofularia root (central portion), lotus plumule, bamboo leaflet, ophiopogon root (without removal of the center), forsythia fruit (without removal of the seed), rhinoceros horn tip.

Qing Gu San, Decoction for clearing hectic fever (《Standards of diagnosis and treatment of six branches of medicins》): Stellaria root, picrorhiza rhizome, large leaf gentian root, turtle shell, wolfberry bark, sweet wormwood, anemarrhena rhizome, licorice root.

Qing Kai Ling injection, Bezoar injection for rusurrection (proved recipe): bezoar, buffalo horn, scutellaria root, honeysuckle flower, capejasmine fruit and others.

Qing Re Gu Jing Tang, Decoction to alleviate metrorrhagia with heat clearing drug (proved recipe): Rehmannia root, wolfberry bark, scutellaria root, stir-fried black capejasmine fruit, lotus node, sanguisorba root, carbonized palmae bark.

Qing Wen Bai Du San (Yin), Antipyretic and antitoxic powder (decoction) (《A view of epidemic febrile diseases with rashes》): Gypsum, rehmannia root, rhinoceros horn, coptis root, capejasmine fruit, platycodon root, scutellaria root, anemarrhena rhizome, red peony root, forsythia fruit, scrofularia root, moutan bark, licorice root, lophatherum.

Qing Xin Tang, Decoction for clearing the heart (proved recipe): Rehmannia root, ophiopogon root, coptis root, lotus plumule, red sage root, licorice root.

Qing Ying Tang, Decoction of clearing ying heat (《Treatise on differentiation and treatment of epidemic febrile diseases》): Rhinoceros horn, rehmannia root, scrofularia root, ophiopogon root, red sage root, coptis root, honey-suckle flower, forsythia fruit, bamboo plumule.

Qing Zao Jiu Fei Tang, Decoction for relieving dryness of the lung (《Principle and prohibition for medical prefession》): Mulberry leaf, gypsum, licorice root, ginseng, hemp seed, donkey hide glue, ophiopogon root, bitter apricot seed, loquat leaf.

Qu Zeng Sheng Pian, Tablet to remove hypertrophic degeneration (proved recipe): Prepared rehmannia root, desert living cistanche, epimedium, drynaria rhizome, pyrola, spatholobus stem, radish seed, scorpion, centipede.

Ren Shen Ge Jie San, Powder of ginseng and gecko (《Precious book of eastern medicine》): Ginseng, gecko.

Ren Shen Jian Pi Wan, Bolus for reinforcing the spleen including ginseng (proved recipe): Ginseng, hawthorn fruit, germinated barley, medicated leaven, tangerine peel, white atractylodes rhizome, immature bitter orange.

San Hua Tang, Decoction of three resolving drugs (《Su Wen Bing Ji Qi Yi Bao Ming Ji》): Magnolia bark, rhubarb, immature bitter orange, notopterygium root.

San Miao San, Powder of three wonderful drugs (《Orthodox medical problems》): Atractylodes rhizome, phellodendron bark, achyranthes root.

Sang Xing Tang, Decoction of mulberry leaf, almond seed and others (《Treatise on differentiation and treatment of epidemic febrile diseases》): Mulberry leaf, bitter apricot kernel, capejasmine fruit, fritillary bulb, adenophora root, fermented soya bean, pear pericarpium.

Sha Shen Mai Dong Tang, Decoction of glehnia and ophiopogon (《Treatise on differentiation and treatment of epidemic febrile disease》): Glehnia root, ophiopogon root, fragrant solomon-seal rhizome, mulberry leaf (over winter), trichosanthes root, hyacinth bean, licorice root.

Shao Yao Tang, Decoction of white peony root (《Collection

for life saving》): White peony root, Chinese angelica root, scutellaria root, coptis root, rhubarb, areca seed, aucklandia root, cinnamon bark, licorice root.

She Dan Chuan Bei Me, The powder of snake bile and fritillary bulb (proved recipe): Snake bile, sichuan fritillary bulb.

She Dan Chuan Bei Ye, The fluid of snake bile and fritil lary bulb (proved recipe): Snake bile, Sichuan fritillary bulb, apricot seed fluid, honey, peppermint oil, sucrose.

She Xiang Bao Xin Dan, Musk heart activating powder (proved recipe): Musk, bezoar, berneol.

She Xiang Hu Gu Gao, Musk and tiger tibia bone plaster (proved recipe): Musk, tiger tibia bone, dahurian angelica root, chuanxiong rhizome and others.

Shen Fu injection, The injection fluid of ginseng, aconite and others (proved recipe): Ginseng, aconite root, red sage root.

Shen Fu Tang, The decoctions of ginseng and aconite (《The revisions and expositions of effective prescriptions for diseases of women》): Ginseng, aconite root.

Shen Ling Bai Zhu San, Powder of ginseng, poria and white atractylodes and others (《Formularies of the bureau of pharmacy》): Lotus seed, coix seed, amomum fruit, platycodon root, white hyaciath bean, poria, ginseng, licorice root, white atractylodes rhizome, Chinese yam, Chinese date.

Shen Mai Zhen, Ginseng-ophiopogon injection fluid

(proved recipe): Ginseng, ophiopogon root.

Shen Xi Dan, Marvelous rhinoceros powder (《Compendium on epidemic febrile diseases》): Rhinoceros horn, grass-leaved sweetflag rhizome, scutellaria root, rehmannia root, honeysuckle flower, forsythia fruit, isatis root, prepared soybean, scrofularia root, trichosanthes root, arnebia root.

Shen Ying Yang Zhen Dan, Precious powder to nourish the primordial *qi* (《A complete book on surgery》): Chinese angelica root, chuanxiong rhizome, white peony root, prepared rehmannia root, gastrodia tuber, notopterygium root, chaenomeles fruit, dodder seed, honey.

Sheng Mai San (Zhen), Pulse activating powder or injection fluid (《Discussion of guestionable problems in internal and external injuries》): Ginseng, ophiopogon root, schisandra fruit.

Sheng Tie Luo Yin, Pig iron cinder drink (《Medicine comprehended》): Asparagus root, ophiopogon root, fritillary bulb, bile treated arisaema tuber, red tangerine peel, polygala root, grass leaved sweetflag rhizome, forsythia fruit, poria, poria with host-wood, scrofularia root, uncaria stem with hooks, red sage root, cinnabar, pig iron cinder.

Shi Hui San, Hemostatic powder of ten carbonized drugs (《A miraculous book of ten prescriptions》): Small thistle, Japanese thistle, moutan bark, rhubarb, cogongrass rhizome, lotus leaf, madder root, capejasmine fruit, palmae bark, biota tops, the above ten drugs are all carbonized with preserved property.

Shi Quan Da Bu Wan, Bolus of ten powerful tonics (《Discovery advance in medicine》): Ginseng, poria, white atractylodes rhizome, licorice root, Chinese angelica root, chuanxiong rhizome, white peony root, prepared rehmannia root, astragalus root, cinnamon bark.

Shi Xiao San, Pain relief powder (《Formularies of peaceful benevolent dispensary》): Cat-tail pollen, trogopterus dung.

Shu Gan He Wei Wan, Pill to disperse the liver and regulate the stomach (proved recipe): Ginger-treated pinellia tuber, licorice, tangerine peel, white peony root, lindera root, curcuma root, green tangerine orange peel, magnolia bark, katsumadai seed, medicated leaven, immature bitter orange fruit, Chinese angelica root, areca seed, amomum fruit, bupleurum root, hawthorn fruit, senna leaf.

Shun Qi Dao Tan Tang, Qi regulating decoction to expell phlegm (proved recipe): Pinellia tuber, tangerine peel, poria, licorice root, fresh ginger, bile treated arisaema tuber, immature bitter orange, aucklandia root, cyperus root.

Si Chong Wan, Four worm pill (proved recipe): Stirfried ground beetle, scorpion, batryticated silkworm, earthworm.

Si Jun Zi Tang, Decoction of four noble drugs (《Formularies of peaceful benevolent dispensary》): Ginseng, white atractylodes rhizome, poria, licorice root.

Si Wu Tang, Decoction of four ingredients (《Formularies of peaceful benevolent dispensary》): Chinese angelica root, chuanxiong rhizome, white peony root, prepared rehmannia root.

Su He Xiang Wan, Storax pill (《Formularies of peaceful benevolent dispensary》): White atractylodes rhizome, cyperus tuber, cinnabar, chebula fruit, sandal wood, eagle wood, musk, benzoin, black rhinoceros horn, cloves, long piper, borneol, dutchmanspipe root, storax oil, frankincense.

Tai Chan Jin Dan, Precious pill for pregnancy (proved recipe): Chinese angelica root, poria, ginseng, white atractylodes rhizome, eucommia bark, swallowwort root, carbonized argyi leaf, ligusticum root, chuanxiong rhizome, red halloysite, dipsacus root, rehmannia root, donkey hide glue bead, cyperus tuber, scutellaria root, eagle wood, licorice root, schisandra fruit, white peony root, myrrh, dodder seed.

Tao Hong Si Wu Tang, Decoction of four ingredients with addition of peach kernel and safflower (《The golden mirror of medicine》): Chinese angelica root, red peony root, rehmannia root, chuanxiong rhizome, peach kernel, safflower.

Tian Ma Gou Teng Yin, Decoction of gastrodia and uncaris (《The new conception of syndromes and treatment of miscellaneous disease》): Gastrodia tuber, uncaria stem with hooks, sea-ear shell, capejasmine fruit, scutellaria root, cyathula root, eucommia bark, motherwort, loranthus, mulberry mistletoe, fleece flower stem, poria with host wood.

Tiao Gan Tang, Liver regulating decoction (proved recipe): Prepared rehmannia root, Chinese yam, Chinese angelica root, white peony root, dogwood fruit, donkey hide glue, bupleurum root, cyperus tuber.

Tiao Ying Yin, Drinks to regulate *ying* (《Standards of diagnosis and treatment of six branches of medicine》): Chinese angelica root, chuanxiong rhizome, red peony root, zedoary, licorice root, asarum, cinnamon bark, chinese pink herb, rhubarb, areca seed, tangerine peel, shell of areca nut, lepidium seed, poria, mulberry bark, corydalis tuber.

Tong Qiao Huo Xue Tang, Decoction for activating blood circulation (《Corrections on the errors of medical works》): Red peony root, chuanxiong rhizome, peach kernel, safflower, fresh ginger, scallion, Chinese date, musk, yellow rice wine.

Tong You Tang, Decoction to pass the pylorus (《A secret book of the orchids chamber》): Honey treated licorice root, safflower, rehmannia root, prepared rehmannia root, cimicifuga rhizome, peach kernel, Chinese angelica root.

Wan Nian Qing injection Rhodea japonica injection fluid (proved recipe): each ml. contains rhodexin 1.3ml.

Wei Ling Tang, Decoction of peptic powder and powder of five drugs with poria (《Required readings for medical professionals》): Atractylodes rhizome, magnolia bark, tangerine peel, licorice root, poria, alismatis rhizome, cinnamon bark, umbellate pore, fresh ginger, Chinese date.

Wu Mei Wan, Bolus of black plum (《Treatise on febrile diseases》): Black plum, asarum herb, Chinese angelica root, coptis root, phellodendron bark, dried ginger, pricklyash peel, cinnamon twig, aconite root, ginseng.

Wu Ren Wan, Pill of five kernels (《Effective formularies tested by physicians for generations》): Peach kernel, bitter apricol kernel, arborvitae seed, pine seed, bush-cherry seed, tangerine peel.

Wu Tou Tang, Sichuan aconite decoction (《Synopsis of prescriptions of the golden chamber》): Sichuan aconite root, ephedra, peony root, astragalus root, licorice root.

Wu Xian Zai Sheng Wan, Resurrection pill of various epileptiform disease (《Yi Shou Tang Fang》): Rhubarb, scutellaria root, eagle wood, bile treated arisaema tuber, phlogopite, alum, prepared Chinese gall.

Wu Zhi An Zhong Yin, Drink of five fluids to comfort the mid-burner (proved recipe): Chives juice, milk, fresh ginger juice, peach juice, lotus root juice.

Xi Huang Wan, Bolus of bezoar and musk (《Life saving book of surgery》): Bezoar, musk, frankincense, myrrh.

Xi Jiao Di Huang Tang, Decoction of rhinoceros horn and rehmannia (《Prescriptions worth a thousand gold for emergencies》): Rhinoceros horn, rehmannia root, white peony root, moutan bark.

Xi Jiao Wan, Rhinoceros horn pill (《Compendium on epidemic febrile disease》): Rehmannia root, honey-suckle flower, forsythia fruit, isatis root, fermented soybean, scrofularia root, rhinoceros horn, grass-leaved sweetflag rhizome, scutellaria root, trichosanthes root, arnebia root, *ren zhong huang* (prepared licorice root).

Xi Lei San, Antimony-like grey powder for buccal ulcer («Supplements to commentaries on synopsis of prescriptions of the golden chamber»): Cow's bezoare, human finger nail, borneol, pearl, ivory powder, natural indigo, *bi qian* (uroetea).

Xi Ling Jie Du Pian, Antiphlogistic pill including rhinoceros and antelope horn (proved recipe): Peppermint, schizonepeta spike, honey suckle flower, forsythia fruit, arctium fruit, lophtharum, prepared soybean, platycoden root, rhinoceros horn, antelope horn, borneol.

Xian Zhu Li Shui, Fresh bamboo juice fluid (proved recipe): Fresh bamboo juice.

Xiang Lian Wan, Pill of aucklandia and coptis («Collections of prescriptions in military board»): Aucklandia root, coptis root.

Xiang Sha Liu Jun Zi Wan, Pill of aucklandia and amomum with six noble ingredients («The golden mirror of medicine»): Ginseng, poria, white atractylodes rhizome, licorice root, tangerine peel, pinellia tuber, aucklandia root, amomum fruit.

Xiang Sha Yang Wei Wan, Stomach pills with cyperus and amomum («Recipe selections and remark of *Ci Xi* empress dowager»): Tangerine peel, cyperus rhizome, ferment leaven, white atracytlodes rhizome, immature bitter orange, pinellia tuber, atractylodes rhizome poria, magnolia bark, platycodon root, coptis root, amomum fruit, aucklandia root, hawthorn fruit, licorice root, stir-fried capejasmine fruit, agastache, chuanxiong rhizome.

Xiao Chai Hu Tang, Minor decoction of bupleurum (《Treatise on febrile diseases》): Bupleurum root, scutellaria root, pinellia tuber, ginseng, licorice root, fresh ginger, Chinese date.

Xiao Huo Luo Dan, The minor bolus for activating the energy flow in channels and collaterals (《Formularies of peaceful benevolent dispensary》): Sichuan aconite root, wild aconite root, earthworm, arisaema tuber, frankincense, myrrh.

Xiao Xian Xiong Tang, Minor decoction for relieving stuffiness in the chest (《Treatise on febrile diseases》): Coptis root, pinellia tuber, trichosanthes fruit.

Xiao Yao Wan, Easy pill (《Formularies of peaceful benevolent dispensary》): Chinese angelica root, white peony root, bupleurum root, poria, white atractylodes root, licorice root, fresh ginger, peppermint.

Xie Bai San, Powder to purge lungs (《Key to therapeutics of children's disease》): Mulberry bark, wolfberry bark, honey-fried licorice root.

Xin Ling Wan, Effective bolus for stimulating the heart (proved recipe): Rhinoceros horn, musk, cow's bezoar, bear gall, toad venom, pearl, borneol, etc.

Xin Xue Ning Pian, Extract tablet of hawthorn and puerarum (proved recipe): Each tablet contains the extract from haw-thorn fruit 0.25g and puerarum root extract 0.15g.

Xing Nao Jing injection, Consciousness restoring injection fluid (proved recipe): Musk, borneol, bezoar, scutellaria root, capejasmint fruit, curcuma root, and others.

Xiong Zhi Shi Gao Tang, Decoction of chuanxiong, dahurian angelica and gypsum (《The golden mirror of medicine》): Chuanxiong rhizome, dahurian angelica root, gypsum, chrysanthemum flower, notopterygium root, ligusticum root.

Xue Fu Zhu Yu Tang, Decoction for removing blood stasis in the chest (《Corrections on the errors of medical works》): Chinese angelica root, rehmannia root, peach kernel, safflower, bitter orange, chuanxiong rhizome, red peony root, bupleurum root, platycodon root, cyathula root, licorice root.

Yang Jiao Fen Wan, Epilepsy pill (proved recipe): Curcuma root, alum, coptis root, rhubarb, magnetite, red tangerine peel, capejasmine fruit, medicated leaven, phellodendron bark, scutellaria root, phlogopite, eagle wood, white mustard seed.

Yang Xin An Shen Wan, Sedative pill of nourishing blood (proved recipe): Eclipta, hair vein agrimony, spatholobus stem, prepared rehmannia root, rehmannia root, fleece flower stem, albizia bark.

Yang Xin Tang, Decoction for nourishing the heart (《Standards of diagnosis and treatment of six branches of medicine》): Astragalus root, poria, poria with hostwood, Chinese angelica root, chuanxiong rhizome, honey fried licorice root, ginseng, cinnamon bark, pinellia (tuber) leaven, biota seed, wild jujuba seed, polygala root, schisandra fruit.

Yang Yin Qing Fei Tang (Wan), Decoction (pill) for nourishing *yin* and clearing the lung heat (《*Chong Lou Yu Yue*》 specialized treatise on branch of larynx): Rehmannia root, zhejiang fritillary bulb, moutan bark, peppermint, white peony root, ophiopogon root, Licorice-root, scrofularia root.

Yi Li Zhi Tong Dan, One pill enough to arrest the pain (proved recipe): Stephania root, musk, frankincense, myrrh, corydalis tuber.

Yi Qi Cong Ming Tang, Qi reinforcing decoction for improving hearing and vision (《*Dong Yuan*'s ten books》): Astragalus, ginseng, pueraria root, white peony root, phellodendron bark, cimicifuga rhizome, honey-fried licorice root, chastetree fruit.

Yi Shen Pai Shi Tang, Decoction to reinforce kidney and expel stones (proved recipe): Rehmannia root, prepared fleece flower root, eucommia bark, moutan bark, pyrrosia leaf, climbing fern spore, talc, grass-leaved sweetflag rhizome.

Yi Wei Tang, Decoction to replenish stomach (《Detailed analysis of epidemic febrile diseases》): Glehnia root, ophiopogon root, rehmannia root, fragrant solomonseal rhizome.

Yi Xin Kou Fu Ye (Pian), Oral fluid or tablet for tonifying the heart (proved recipe): Ginseng, ophiopogon root, schisandra fruit, anemarrhena rhizome and others.

Yin Chen Hao Tang, Oriental wormwood decoction (《Treatise on febrile diseases》): Oriental worm wood, capejasmine fruit, rhubarb.

Yin Chen Wu Ling Wan, Pill of oriental worm-wood and five drugs with poria (proved recipe): Oriental wormwood, poria, atractylodes rhizome, scutellaria root, alismatis rhizome, magnolia bark, white atractylodes rhizome, umbellate pore, hawthorn fruit, licorice root, tangerine peel, fermented leaven, hovenia seed.

Yin Huang injection, Lonicera and scutellaria injection (《Chinese pharmacopia》 1977 edition): Fluid extract of honeysuckle flower and scutellaria root, chlorogenic acid and baicalin mainly.

Yin Qiao Jie Du Wan (Pian), Antiphlogistic pill (tablet) including lonicera and forsythia (proved recipe): Honeysuckle flower, forsythia fruit, platycodon root, peppermint, lophtharum, schizonepeta spike, prepared soybean, arctium fruit, capejasmine fruit, licorice root, reed root water, talcpowder coat.

Yin Qiao San, Powder of lonicera and forsythia (《Treatise on differentiation and treatment of epidemic febrile diseases》): Schizonepeta, peppermint, honeysuckle flower, forsythia fruit, platycodon root, reed root, licorice root, arctium fruit, prepared soybean, lophatherum.

You Gui Wan, The kidney-*yang* reinforcing bolus (《*Jing Yue*'s complete works》): Prepared rehmmania root, dogwood fruit, Chinese yam, Chinese angelica root, wolfberry fruit, antler glue, dodder seed, eucommia bark, cinnamon bark, aconite root.

You Gui Yin, The kidney *yang* reinforcing decoction (《*Jing Yue*'s complete works》): Dogwood fruit, licorice root, cinnamon bark, prepared rehmannia root, Chinese yam, eucommia bark, wolfberry fruit, aconite root.

Yu Gong San, Hydragogue powder (《The confucian school's care of their parents》): Morning gloryseed, common fennel fruit.

Yu Ping Feng San, The jade screen powder (proved recipe): Astragalus root, white atractylodes rhizome, ledebouriella.

Yu Shu Dan, Pleione and Chinese gall powder (《A bit experience from the heart bosom》): Pleione rhizome, Chinese gall, musk, realgar, cinnabar, lathyris seed (removal of oil), Beijing spurge root.

Yuan Hu Zhi Teng Pian, Corydalis tablet for relief of pain (proved recipe): Corydalis tuber.

Yun Nan Bai Yao, White drug powder (proved recipe): White medicinal powder consisting of pulverized notoginseng root and other ingredients.

Zeng Ye Tang, Fluid increasing decoction (《Treatise on differentiation and treatment of epidemic febrile diseases》): Fresh rehmannia root, scrofularia root, ophiopogon root.

Zhen Wu Tang, Decoction of *Zhen Wu* (The god who controls water) (《Treatise on febrile diseases》): Poria, white atractylodes rhizome, white peony root, fresh ginger, prepared aconite root.

Zhi Bai Di Huang Wan (*Tang*), Kidney bolus (decoction) of six drug including rehmannia with addition of anemarrhena and phelladendron (《The golden mirror of medicine》): Rehmannia, dogwood fruit, Chinese yam, moutan bark, poria, alismatis rhizome, amemarrhena rhizome, phellodendron bark.

Zhi Bao Dan, Treasured bolus (《Formularies of peaceful benevolent dispensary》): Benzoin, cinnabar, musk, rhinoceros horn, amber, realgar, hawksbill shell, borneol.

Zhi Gan Cao Tang, Decoction of prepared licorice (《Treatise on febrile disease》): Honey-fried licorice, cinnamon twig, ophiopogon root, ginseng rehmannia root, donkey-hide gelatin, hemp seed, fresh ginger, Chinese date.

Zhi Ke Qing Guo Wan, Pill of Chinese white olive to arrest cough (proved recipe): Coltsfoot flower, sichuan fritillary bulb, aristolochia fruit, gingko seed, pinellia tuber, licorice root, gypsum, bitter apricot seed, lily bulb, scutellaria root, ephedra, mulberry bark, Chinese white olive.

Zhi Mi Fu Ling Wan, Poria bolus from *Zhi Mi* formularies (《Prescriptions worth a thousand gold for emergencies》): Bitter orange, pinellia tuber, poria, mirabilite.

Zhi Xue Hua Yu Tang, Decoction to treat blood stasis

and arrest bleeding (proved recipe): Inula flower, trichosanthes fruit, moutan bark, node of lotus, rhubarb, notoginseng.

Zhi Zi Yan Qin Gao Pian, Tablet of fluid extract of potentilla (proved recipe):Each tablet contains fluid extract of potentilla 0.2g (corresponding to crude drug 1g).

Zhong Man Fen Xiao Wan, Pill to relieve abdominal distension with resolving method (《A secret book kept in orchid chamber》): White atractylodes root, ginseng, honey-fried licorice root, umbellate pore fungus, turmeria, poria, dried ginger, amomum fruit, alismatis rhizome, tangerine peel, anemarrhena rhizome, scutellaria root, coptis root, pinellia tuber, immature bitter orange, magnolia bark.

Zhou Che Wan, Hydragogue pill for relieving ascites (《Jing yue's complete works》): Pharbitis seed, kansui root, genkwa flower, Beijing spurge root, rhubarb, tangerine peel, green tangerine orange peel, aucklandia root, areca seed, calomel.

Zhu Li Da Tan Wan, Phlegm expelling pill including bamboo juice (《A mirror of ancient and modern medicine》): Phlogopite, eagle wood, rhubarb, scutellaria root, bamboo juice, pinellia tuber, red tangerine peel, licorice root, ginger juice, poria, ginseng.

Zhu Sha An Shen Wan, Sedate pill of cinnabar (《A secret book in orchid chamber》): Cinnabar, coptis root, licorice root.

Zi Shen Wan, Kidney nourishing pill (《A secret book

in orchid chamber》): Phellodendron bark, anemarrhena rhizome, cinnamon bark.

Zi Shui Qing Gan Yin, Decoction for nourishing the kidney essence and clearing the liver fire (《The self duty of medicine》): Prepared rehmannia root, dogwood fruit, Chinese yam, wild jujuba seed, moutan bark, alismatis rhizome, poria, Chinese angelica root, white peony root, bupleurum, capejasmine fruit.

Zi Shui Qing Huo Tang, Kidney essence nourishing pill for clearing up the fire (proved recipe): Anemarrhena rhizome, scrofularia root, rehmannia root, asparagus root, phellodendron bark, stir-fried wild jujuba seed, moutan bark, red sage root, mulberry mistletoe.

Zi Xue Dan (San), Purple snowy powder (《Formularies of peaceful benevolent dispensary》): Rhinoceros horn, antelope horn, talc, gypsum, mirabilite, magnetite, dutchmanspipe root, eagle wood, cimicifuga rhizome, cloves, scrofularia root, niter, cinnabar, musk, gold, licorice root.

Zun Sheng Run Chang Wan, Pill to moisten the intestine in Shen's book (《Shen's work on the importance of life preservation》): Chinese angelica root, rehmannia root, peach kernel, hemp seed, bitter orange, bitter apricot kernel, honey to make pill.

Zuo Gui Wan, Kidney tonifying bolus (《*Jing Yue's* complete works》): Prepared rehmmania, dogwood fruit, wolfberry fruit, antler glue, Chinese yam, tortoise plastron glue, dodder seed, cyathula root.

Zuo Gui Yin, Kidney decoction (《*Jing Yue*'s complete works》):Prepared rehmannia, dogwood fruit, Chinese yam, wolfberry fruit, poria, licorice root.

中国针灸中药治疗疑难病症

邵念方 编著

萧琪 左连君 译

萧琪 审校

*

中国山东科学技术出版社出版
(中国济南玉函路 34 号)
中国山东新华印刷厂潍坊厂印刷
(中国潍坊工农路 99 号)
中国国际图书贸易总公司发行
(中国北京车公庄西路 21 号)
中国北京邮政信箱第 399 号 邮政编码 100044
1990 年 3 月第 1 版 1990 年 3 月第 1 次印刷
ISBN 7-5331-0639-3/R·168
03000
14—E—2492P